Exercise Prescription Case Studies
for Special Populations

Exercise Prescription Case Studies
for Special Populations

Revised First Edition

Matthew D. McCabe, Ph.D. and Bradley R. A. Wilson, Ph.D.

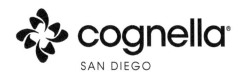

cognella®
SAN DIEGO

Bassim Hamadeh, CEO and Publisher
Carrie Baarns, Manager, Revisions and Author Care
Kaela Martin, Project Editor
Abbey Hastings, Production Editor
Emely Villavicencio, Senior Graphic Designer
Alexa Lucido, Licensing Manager
Natalie Piccotti, Director of Marketing
Kassie Graves, Senior Vice President of Editorial
Jamie Giganti, Director of Academic Publishing

Cover images: Copyright © 2018 iStockphoto LP/FatCamera.
Copyright © 2018 iStockphoto LP/milan2099.
Copyright © 2019 iStockphoto LP/FatCamera.
Copyright © 2019 iStockphoto LP/adamkaz.

Printed in the United States of America.

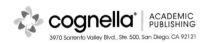

3970 Sorrento Valley Blvd., Ste. 500, San Diego, CA 92121

To Forrest, Anita, Mark, and Andrea McCabe for their continuous love and support.
—MM

To my wife, Frances, for being my partner for life.
—BW

Brief Contents

PREFACE xvii

ACKNOWLEDGMENTS xix

CH 1   Pre-exercise Screening and Evaluation for Special Populations   1

CH 2   Principles of Exercise Testing and Prescription for Special Populations   45

CH 3   Exercise Testing and Prescription for Clients with Diabetes Mellitus   109

CH 4   Exercise Testing and Prescription for Clients with Hypertension   145

CH 5   Exercise Testing and Prescription for Overweight and Obese Clients   177

CH 6   Exercise Testing and Prescription for Clients with Dyslipidemia   201

CH 7   Exercise Testing and Prescription for Clients with Arthritis, Fibromyalgia, and Osteoporosis   227

CH 8   Exercise Testing and Prescription for Clients with Multiple Diseases   257

Detailed Contents

PREFACE   xvii
ACKNOWLEDGMENTS   xix

CH 1   Pre-exercise Screening and Evaluation for Special Populations   1
Introduction   1
Pre-participation Screening   2
Demonstration Case Study 1.1: PAR-Q+   3
Demonstration Case Study 1.2: PAR-Q+   4
Demonstration Case Study 1.3: Exercise Pre-participation Health Screening
    Questionnaire for Exercise Professionals   7
Demonstration Case Study 1.4, 1.5: Exercise Pre-participation Health
    Screening Questionnaire for Exercise Professionals   8
Demonstration Case Study 1.6: ACSM's Pre-participation Health
    Screening Algorithm   11
Demonstration Case Study 1.7: ACSM's Pre-participation Health
    Screening Algorithm   12
Demonstration Case Study 1.8: ACSM's Pre-participation Health
    Screening Algorithm   13
Demonstration Case Study 1.9: ACSM's Pre-participation Health
    Screening Algorithm   14
Pre-participation Evaluation   14
Demonstration Case Study 1.10: Informed Consent   15
Demonstration Case Study 1.11: Cardiovascular Disease Risk Factor Analysis   19
Demonstration Case Study 1.12: Medical History   20
Demonstration Case Study 1.13: Assessment of Pulses   23
Demonstration Case Study 1.14: Assessment of Blood Pressure   25
Demonstration Case Study 1.15: Inspection of Skin and Lower Extremities   26
Demonstration Case Study 1.16: Pulmonary Function Testing   28
Student Case Studies   28
Student Case Study 1.1: PAR-Q+   28
Student Case Study 1.2: PAR-Q+   29
Student Case Study 1.3: PAR-Q+   30
Student Case Study 1.4: Exercise Pre-participation Health Screening
    Questionnaire for Exercise Professionals   30
Student Case Study 1.5: Exercise Pre-participation Health Screening
    Questionnaire for Exercise Professionals   31
Student Case Study 1.6: Exercise Pre-participation Health Screening
    Questionnaire for Exercise Professionals   32

Student Case Study 1.7: ACSM's Pre-participation Health Screening Algorithm 33

Student Case Study 1.8: ACSM's Pre-participation Health Screening Algorithm 34

Student Case Study 1.9: ACSM's Pre-participation Health Screening Algorithm 35

Student Case Study 1.10: Informed Consent 35

Student Case Study 1.11, 1.12: Cardiovascular Disease Risk Factor Analysis 36

Student Case Study 1.13: Cardiovascular Disease Risk Factor Analysis 37

Student Case Study 1.14, 1.15: Cardiovascular Disease Risk Factor Analysis 38

Student Case Study 1.16: Medical History 39

Student Case Study 1.17: Assessment of Pulses 39

Student Case Study 1.18: Blood Pressure Assessment 40

Student Case Study 1.19: Inspection of Skin and Lower Extremities 41

Student Case Study 1.20: Pulmonary Function Testing 41

Student Case Study 1.21: Comprehensive Case Study 42

References 43

CH 2   Principles of Exercise Testing and Prescription for Special Populations   45

Introduction 45

Exercise Testing 46

Exercise Test Selection 48

Demonstration Case Study 2.1: Cardiorespiratory Endurance Test Selection 49

Demonstration Case Study 2.2: Body Composition Test Selection 51

Demonstration Case Study 2.3: Muscle Fitness Test Selection 53

Demonstration Case Study 2.4: Muscle Fitness Test Selection 54

Demonstration Case Study 2.5: Flexibility Test Selection 55

Contraindications for Exercise Testing 55

Demonstration Case Study 2.6, 2.7: Contraindications for Exercise Testing 56

Demonstration Case Study 2.8: Contraindications for Exercise Testing 57

Test Termination Criteria 57

Demonstration Case Study 2.9, 2.10: Exercise Testing Termination Criteria 59

Demonstration Case Study 2.11: Exercise Testing Termination Criteria 60

Exercise Test Interpretation 60

Demonstration Case Study 2.12: Cardiorespiratory Fitness
    Test Interpretation: YMCA Cycle Test 62

Demonstration Case Study 2.13: Cardiorespiratory Fitness Test
    Interpretation: Astrand-Rhyming Cycle Test 64

Demonstration Case Study 2.14: Cardiorespiratory Fitness Test
    Interpretation: Submaximal Treadmill Test 64

Demonstration Case Study 2.15: Cardiorespiratory Fitness Test
    Interpretation: Maximal Treadmill Protocol 65

Demonstration Case Study 2.16: Muscular Strength Testing: Chest Press 67

Demonstration Case Study 2.17: Skinfold Assessment: Seven-Sites 70

Demonstration Case Study 2.18: Skinfold Assessment: Three-Sites 70

Demonstration Case Study 2.19: Girth Measurements 71

Demonstration Case Study 2.20: Flexibility Test Interpretation: Sit-and-Reach 72

Exercise Prescription 72

Demonstration Case Study 2.21: Cardiorespiratory Exercise Prescription 75

Demonstration Case Study 2.22: Muscular Fitness Exercisc Prescription 79

Student Case Study 2.1: Exercise Test Selection 80

Student Case Study 2.2: Exercise Test Selection 81

Student Case Study 2.3: Exercise Test Selection 82

Student Case Study 2.4: Exercise Test Selection: Critical Thinking 83

Student Case Study 2.5: Contraindications for Exercise Testing 84

Student Case Study 2.6: Contraindications for Exercise Testing 85

Student Case Study 2.7: Contraindications for Exercise Testing: On Your Own 86

Student Case Study 2.8: Exercise Test Termination 86

Student Case Study 2.9: Exercise Test Termination 87

Student Case Study 2.10: Exercise Test Termination: On Your Own 88

Student Case Study 2.11: Exercise Test Interpretation: YMCA Cycle Test 88

Student Case Study 2.12: Exercise Test Interpretation: YMCA Cycle Test 89

Student Case Study 2.13, 2.14: Exercise Test Interpretation: Astrand-Rhyming
Cycle Test 91

Student Case Study 2.15: Exercise Test Interpretation: Submaximal
Treadmill Test 92

Student Case Study 2.16: Exercise Test Interpretation: Submaximal
Treadmill Test 93

Student Case Study 2.17: Exercise Test Interpretation: Maximal Treadmill Test 94

Student Case Study 2.18: Muscular Strength 95

Student Case Study 2.19: Muscular Strength 96

Student Case Study 2.20: Body Composition Test Interpretation: Skinfolds 97

Student Case Study 2.21: Body Composition Test Interpretation: Skinfolds 98

Student Case Study 2.22: Exercise Prescription: Cardiorespiratory Endurance 98

Student Case Study 2.23: Exercise Prescription: Cardiorespiratory Endurance 99

Student Case Study 2.24: Exercise Prescription: Muscular Strength 100

Student Case Study 2.25: Exercise Prescription: Muscular Endurance 100

Student Case Study 2.26: Exercise Testing and Prescription: Comprehensive
Case Study 101

References 106

CH 3 **Exercise Testing and Prescription for Clients with Diabetes Mellitus** **109**

Introduction 109

Glucometabolic Responses to Exercise 110

Type I Diabetes Mellitus 111

Type II Diabetes Mellitus 111

Demonstration Case Study 3.1: Differentiating Diabetes Mellitus 112

Exercise Testing for Clients with Diabetes 113

Demonstration Case Study 3.2: Exercise Testing and Diabetes Mellitus 114

Demonstration Case Study 3.3, 3.4: Exercise Testing and Diabetes Mellitus 115

Exercise Prescription for the Client with Diabetes 116

Demonstration Case Study 3.5: Cardiorespiratory Exercise Prescription and
Diabetes Mellitus 118

Demonstration Case Study 3.6: Cardiorespiratory Exercise Prescription and
Diabetes Mellitus 120

Demonstration Case Study 3.7: Muscular Fitness Exercise Prescription and
Diabetes Mellitus 122

Demonstration Case Study 3.8, 3.9: Safety Considerations for Clients
with Diabetes 125

Demonstration Case Study 3.10: Safety Considerations for Clients
with Diabetes 126

Student Case Study 3.1: Exercise Test Selection for Clients with Diabetes 126

Student Case Study 3.2: Exercise Test Selection for Clients with Diabetes 127

Student Case Study 3.3: Exercise Test Selection for Clients with Diabetes 128

Student Case Study 3.4: Exercise Test Interpretation: YMCA Cycle Test 129

Student Case Study 3.5: Exercise Test Interpretation: Astrand-Rhyming
Cycle Test 130

Student Case Study 3.6: Exercise Test Interpretation: Submaximal
Treadmill Test 131

Student Case Study 3.7: Muscular Strength Testing for Clients with Diabetes 132

Student Case Study 3.8: Body Composition Test Interpretation: Skinfolds 133

Student Case Study 3.9: Exercise Prescription for Clients with Diabetes:
Cardiorespiratory Endurance 134

Student Case Study 3.10: Exercise Prescription for Clients with Diabetes:
Cardiorespiratory Endurance 135

Student Case Study 3.11: Exercise Prescription for Clients with Diabetes:
Muscular Fitness 136

Student Case Study 3.12: Exercise Prescription for Clients with Diabetes:
Muscular Fitness 136

Student Case Study 3.13: Exercise Testing and Prescription:
Comprehensive Case Study 137

Student Case Study 3.14: Safety Considerations for Clients with Diabetes 142

References 143

CH 4   Exercise Testing and Prescription for Clients with Hypertension   145

Introduction 145

Acute and Chronic Blood Pressure Responses to Exercise 147

Demonstration Case Study 4.1: Exercise Responses 148

Demonstration Case Study 4.2, 4.3: Exercise Responses 149

Exercise Testing for Clients with Hypertension 149

Demonstration Case Study 4.4: Exercise Testing and Hypertension 150

Demonstration Case Study 4.5: Exercise Testing and Hypertension 151

Demonstration Case Study 4.6, 4.7: Exercise Testing and Hypertension 152

Exercise Prescription for Clients with Hypertension   153

Demonstration Case Study 4.8: Cardiorespiratory Exercise Prescription and
    Hypertension   154

Demonstration Case Study 4.9: Cardiorespiratory Exercise Prescription and
    Hypertension   156

Demonstration Case Study 4.10: Muscular Fitness Exercise Prescription and
    Hypertension   157

Student Case Study 4.1: Exercise Test Selection for Clients with Hypertension   159

Student Case Study 4.2: Exercise Test Selection for Clients with Hypertension   160

Student Case Study 4.3: Exercise Test Selection for Clients with Hypertension   161

Student Case Study 4.4: Exercise Test Interpretation: YMCA Cycle Test   162

Student Case Study 4.5: Exercise Test Interpretation: Astrand-Rhyming
    Cycle Test   164

Student Case Study 4.6: Exercise Test Interpretation: Submaximal
    Treadmill Test   164

Student Case Study 4.7: Muscular Strength Testing for Clients
    with Hypertension   165

Student Case Study 4.8: Body Composition Test Interpretation: Skinfolds   166

Student Case Study 4.9: Exercise Prescription for Clients with Hypertension:
    Cardiorespiratory Endurance   167

Student Case Study 4.10: Exercise Prescription for Clients with Hypertension:
    Cardiorespiratory Endurance   168

Student Case Study 4.11: Exercise Prescription for Clients with Hypertension:
    Muscular Fitness   169

Student Case Study 4.12: Exercise Testing and Prescription: Comprehensive
    Case Study   170

References   175

CH 5   Exercise Testing and Prescription for Overweight and Obese Clients   177

Introduction   177

The Role of Exercise on Energy Expenditure and Energy Deficit   178

Demonstration Case Study 5.1: Exercise and Energy Expenditure   179

Exercise Testing for Overweight or Obese Clients   180

Demonstration Case Study 5.2, 5.3: Exercise Testing for Overweight
    or Obese Clients   180

Exercise Prescription for Overweight and Obese Clients   181

Demonstration Case Study 5.4: Cardiorespiratory Exercise Prescription for
    Overweight or Obese Clients   183

Demonstration Case Study 5.5: Cardiorespiratory Exercise Prescription for
    Overweight or Obese Clients   184

Student Case Study 5.1: Exercise Test Selection for Overweight
    or Obese Clients   185

Student Case Study 5.2: Exercise Test Selection for Overweight
or Obese Clients   186

Student Case Study 5.3: Exercise Test Selection for Overweight
or Obese Clients   187

Student Case Study 5.4: Exercise Test Interpretation: YMCA Cycle Test   188

Student Case Study 5.5: Exercise Test Interpretation: Submaximal
Treadmill Test   189

Student Case Study 5.6: Muscular Strength Testing for Overweight
or Obese Clients   190

Student Case Study 5.7: Exercise Prescription for Overweight
or Obese Clients: Cardiorespiratory Endurance   191

Student Case Study 5.8: Exercise Prescription for Overweight
or Obese Clients: Cardiorespiratory Endurance   192

Student Case Study 5.9: Exercise Prescription for Overweight
and Obese Clients: Muscular Fitness   193

Student Case Study 5.10: Exercise Testing and Prescription:
Comprehensive Case Study   194

References   199

CH 6   Exercise Testing and Prescription for Clients with Dyslipidemia   201

Introduction   201

Lipids' Role in the Body   202

Demonstration Case Study 6.1: Role of Lipids in the Body   203

Demonstration Case Study 6.2: Role of Lipids in the Body   204

Basic Lipid Metabolism and the Influence of Diet and Exercise   205

Demonstration Case Study 6.3: Role of Diet and Exercise on Lipids   206

Exercise Testing for Clients with Dyslipidemia   207

Demonstration Case Study 6.4, 6.5: Exercise Testing for Clients
with Dyslipidemia   208

Exercise Prescription for Clients with Dyslipidemia   209

Demonstration Case Study 6.6: Cardiorespiratory Exercise Prescription for
Clients with Dyslipidemia   210

Student Case Study 6.1: Exercise Test Selection for Clients with Dyslipidemia   212

Student Case Study 6.2: Exercise Test Selection for Clients with Dyslipidemia   213

Student Case Study 6.3: Exercise Test Interpretation: YMCA Cycle Test   214

Student Case Study 6.4: Exercise Test Interpretation: Submaximal
Treadmill Test   215

Student Case Study 6.5: Muscular Strength Testing for Clients
with Dyslipidemia   216

Student Case Study 6.6: Exercise Prescription for Clients with Dyslipidemia:
Cardiorespiratory Endurance   217

Student Case Study 6.7: Exercise Prescription for Clients with Dyslipidemia:
Cardiorespiratory Endurance   218

Student Case Study 6.8: Exercise Prescription for Clients with Dyslipidemia:
    Muscular Fitness   219
Student Case Study 6.9: Exercise Testing and Prescription:
    Comprehensive Case Study   220
References   225

CH 7   **Exercise Testing and Prescription for Clients with Arthritis, Fibromyalgia, and Osteoporosis**   **227**
Introduction   227
Arthritis   228
Exercise Testing for Clients with Arthritis   229
Demonstration Case Study 7.1: Exercise Test Selection for Clients
    with Arthritis   229
Exercise Prescription for Clients with Arthritis   230
Demonstration Case Study 7.2: Exercise Prescription for Clients
    with Arthritis   231
Fibromyalgia   232
Exercise Testing for Clients with Fibromyalgia   233
Demonstration Case Study 7.3: Exercise Test Selection for Clients with
    Fibromyalgia   233
Exercise Prescription for Clients with Fibromyalgia   235
Demonstration Case Study 7.4: Exercise Prescription for Clients with
    Fibromyalgia   235
Osteoporosis   237
Exercise Testing for Clients with Osteoporosis   237
Demonstration Case Study 7.5: Exercise Testing for Clients
    with Osteoporosis   238
Exercise Prescription for Clients with Osteoporosis   238
Demonstration Case Study 7.6: Exercise Prescription for Clients with
    Osteoporosis   239
Student Case Study 7.1: Exercise Testing and Prescription for Clients with
    Arthritis: Comprehensive Case Study   241
Student Case Study 7.2: Exercise Testing and Prescription for Clients with
    Fibromyalgia: Comprehensive Case Study   246
Student Case Study 7.3: Exercise Testing and Prescription for Clients with
    Osteoporosis: Comprehensive Case Study   250
References   253

CH 8   **Exercise Testing and Prescription for Clients with Multiple Diseases**   **257**
Introduction   257
Exercise Testing and Prescription for Clients with Multiple Diseases   258
Demonstration Case Study 8.1: Exercise Testing and Prescription
    for Clients with Multiple Diseases   258

Student Case Study 8.1: Exercise Testing and Prescription for Clients with
    Multiple Diseases   261
Student Case Study 8.2: Exercise Testing and Prescription for Clients with
    Multiple Diseases   263
Student Case Study 8.3: Exercise Testing and Prescription for Clients with
    Multiple Diseases   265
References   267

Preface

WITHOUT QUESTION, REGULAR exercise participation provokes a series of physiological adaptations, which leads to an overall reduction in chronic disease risk. For this reason, among many others, regular exercise participation is highly recommended by healthcare professionals for virtually all individuals. With such a recommendation, exercise science students and current exercise professionals will have a myriad of opportunities to write exercise prescriptions.

As presented in our previous publication, *Exercise Prescription Case Studies for Healthy Populations*, exercise prescription is a lengthy process. Exercise prescription involves pre-exercise screening and evaluation, exercise testing, exercise test interpretation, and the application of the FITT-VP principle. This process was established, over many years of rigid research and professional application, to promote the safety and efficacy of an exercise program. As detailed as this process is, more detail is required when prescribing exercise for individuals with controlled chronic diseases.

Regular exercise participation is not only beneficial for minimizing chronic disease risk; it can actually help manage many diseases as a compliment, not supplement or replacement, to traditional medical care. Regular exercise participation can help manage many chronic diseases, including diabetes, hypertension, dyslipidemia, obesity, metabolic syndrome, peripheral vascular disease, arthritis, osteoporosis, asthma, and cancer. Therefore, it is highly likely that an exercise student or current exercise professional will encounter individuals with one of the previously stated conditions. Thus an in-depth understanding of the principles of exercise testing and prescription, general knowledge of various diseases and exercise physiology, and special considerations are required to safely prescribe exercise for clients with chronic diseases.

We wrote this book to provide students with the opportunity to apply the knowledge they have learned in the classroom to situations they are likely to encounter when writing exercise prescriptions in professional settings. The purpose of this book is not to teach students all of the concepts involved with developing exercise prescriptions for special populations but rather to review and synthesize information learned in the classroom into practical applications. In addition, completing the case studies in this book will help prepare students for the American College of Sports Medicine (ACSM) Certified Exercise Physiologist® exam.

The case studies presented will closely follow the guidelines established by the ACSM. These are clearly outlined in *ACSM's Guidelines for Exercise Testing and Prescription, 11th edition.* Since this book states very specific information about conducting exercise tests, interpreting the results, and writing exercise prescriptions, we believe that all exercise science students and exercise physiologists should have the most recent edition as part of their libraries and regularly use it as a reference. While the guidelines in the book are very detailed and concise, they do not provide all of the background explanations required for good student understanding. Therefore, other resources are required to provide that information. Our book is an effort to fill in some of those gaps.

The focus of this book is on exercise testing and prescription for clients with chronic diseases. Special populations presented in this book include clients with diabetes, hypertension, dyslipidemia, obesity, metabolic syndrome, arthritis, osteoporosis, fibromyalgia, other unique conditions. This book presents case studies that involve the continuum of information from screenings to writing the exercise prescriptions for clients with chronic diseases.

Further, the first two chapters focus on pre-exercise screening, evaluation, and principles of exercise testing and prescription. Information presented in these chapters build into proceeding chapters until procedures for pre-exercise screening, evaluation, exercise testing, and prescription are tied to serving clients with various diseases. Lastly, overviews of various diseases and special considerations will be presented. This will help students break the process into pieces and then put them all together. We hope that students will find the case studies interesting and enjoyable. In the end, students should have better skills for developing exercise programs, scoring well on certification exams, and meeting the specific needs of their clients.

Acknowledgments

THE AUTHORS WOULD like to offer their gratitude to all of the exercise professionals who have contributed to the knowledge needed for the writing of exercise prescriptions over the years. Without them, there would be no reason to write this book. Special credit goes to the past and current leaders of the American College of Sports Medicine for establishing and updating the guidelines used for safe exercise testing and prescription.

We would also like to recognize Cognella Academic Publishing for helping us to make this book a reality. We extend our sincere appreciation to Jennifer Codner and Michelle Piehl for their exceptional guidance and continual support.

Pre-exercise Screening and Evaluation for Special Populations

INTRODUCTION

EXERCISE, UNDOUBTINGLY, PROMOTES many positive adaptations to physiology and metabolism at both the cellular and systems levels. In sum, these adaptations improve normal function, physical performance, and fitness; delay pathologies; and, as it pertains to the text, help manage chronic diseases. In 2021, it is accepted that any form of exercise will result in improvements to some aspect of human physiology. It is for this reason that exercise professionals claim that any form of exercise is better than not engaging in exercise at all. Moreover, it is accepted that the benefits of regular exercise outweigh the risks. These benefits include decreases in the risks for cardiovascular diseases, metabolic diseases, and certain cancers.

Despite the benefits of regular exercise participation more often than not outweighing the risks, there are still risks that must be considered. In general, the primary risk associated with exercise is musculoskeletal injury. The risk for musculoskeletal injury can largely be mitigated by the exercise professional. Methods such as emphasizing technique over intensity, direct supervision, and exercise selections based on an individual's needs, goals, and health/fitness status can be implemented to reduce a client's/patient's risk of musculoskeletal injury.

However, there are certain exercise-induced adverse health events that are often beyond the capacity of an exercise professional to control through proper exercise prescription and supervision. Consider clients with known underlying cardiovascular disease pathology. Such pathology can result in fatal dysrhythmias, acute coronary syndrome, and fatal complications from hypertrophic cardiomyopathy in response to an acute bout of exercise. When examining the numbers, underlying cardiovascular disease pathologies account for approximately six exercise-induced cardiac events per 10,000 during exercise testing.[1] While the risk for severe adverse cardiac events during exercise is extraordinarily low, exercise professionals seek to further lower the risk and promote safety during exercise.

The risks associated with exercise increase when a client has a known chronic disease. To lower the already low risk of exercise-induced adverse health events or complications, even when controlled diseases are present, exercise professionals must conduct pre-exercise screenings and evaluations. Together, this can be considered a comprehensive exercise evaluation.

There are several goals of comprehensive exercise evaluations. First, comprehensive exercise evaluations seek to identify individuals who need medical clearance before initiating an exercise program or continuing with a current exercise program and screen for clinically significant disease. This aspect of the comprehensive exercise evaluation is called pre-participation screening. Second, comprehensive exercise evaluations seek to gather additional information—beyond pre-participation screening—that can be used for exercise prescription to determine indications and contraindications for exercise and exercise testing and to determine the need for medical clearance or more testing. This aspect of the comprehensive exercise evaluation is called the pre-exercise evaluation.

The purpose of this chapter is to teach students how to apply their knowledge of special populations to determine if clients can exercise safely. On completion of the case studies, students will be able to achieve the following:

1. Evaluate a client's symptoms of cardiovascular, metabolic, and renal diseases
2. Identify a client's known medical conditions
3. Assess a client's current physical activity status
4. Determine if a client needs to consult a physician prior to beginning a moderate or vigorous physical activity program
5. Determine the number of cardiovascular risk factors a client has
6. Evaluate physical examination data
7. Interpret basic laboratory tests

PRE-PARTICIPATION SCREENING

The first set of case studies presented in this chapter involves using the Physical Activity Readiness Questionnaire for Everyone (PAR-Q+), the Physical Activity Readiness Medical Evaluation (ePARmed-X+; if needed), the Exercise Pre-participation Health Screening Questionnaire for Exercise Professionals, and the American College of Sports Medicine's (ACSM) Pre-participation Screening Algorithm. Before tackling these case studies, it is helpful to be familiarized to the process and each prescreening tool. An excellent starting point is to administer a self-guided questionnaire to gather generalized information about a client.

The first self-guided questionnaire is the PAR-Q+.[2] The PAR-Q+ is a prescreening tool that is used by exercise professionals and administered to clients to determine whether exercise is safe for them. The PAR-Q+ consists of several questions covering four pages. The first page of the PAR-Q+ consists of seven initial questions. These initial questions are intended to make exercise professionals or exercise participants aware of known cardiac conditions, hypertension, signs or symptoms suggestive of cardiorespiratory ailments, other known chronic diseases, prescribed medications, musculoskeletal abnormalities, or physician-ordered supervision of physical activity. These seven questions "guide" exercise professionals or exercise participants toward the next steps of exercise participation or screening. Should a client answer "no" to all of the first seven questions of the PAR-Q+, then exercise professionals or participants can feel confident that exercise is safe and proceed to pre-exercise evaluations and exercise testing. However, should the client answer "yes" to any of the first seven questions, then the client should answer the follow-up questions on pages 2 and 3. The questions presented on pages 2 and 3 of the PAR-Q+ further probe clients for more information about existing medical conditions that can be used to determine whether exercise is safe. With these follow-up questions, should a client answer "yes" to any question, the client would need to complete a more in-depth questionnaire called the ePARmed-X+.

The ePARmed-X+[3] is a follow-up questionnaire to the PAR-Q+. The ePARmed-X+ enables exercise professionals and participants to further probe for additional medical information. Once complete, the client is either cleared for participation in regular exercise or referred to a physician for medical clearance. The ePARmed-X+, unlike the PAR-Q+, is specifically completed online at www.eparmedx.com. It is highly likely, that clients with known chronic diseases will need to complete the ePARmed-X+ when self-guided prescreening techniques are employed. From an exercise leadership standpoint, exercise professionals should assist clients in the completion of the ePARmed-X+ as the questions are more technical than the PAR-Q+.

When serving special populations, exercise professionals will make one of two recommendations to a client following the completion of the PAR-Q+ and/or ePARmed-X+. These recommendations are similar to the recommendations that are made to apparently healthy populations. The first recommendation is for the client to consult a physician prior to becoming more physically active. In this scenario, the client answered "yes" to one of the first seven questions of the PAR-Q+, answered "yes" to at least one follow-up PAR-Q+ question, and provided answers to the online ePARmed-X+ that suggest exercise may not be safe for the client. Therefore, to ensure the safety of the client, exercise professionals would refer the client for medical clearance. The second recommendation is that exercise is safe, and the client can become more physically active. The level of exercise that is safe will depend on the person's previous activity level. Sedentary people should begin with low- to moderate-intensity exercise. Those who have been exercising at moderate levels can progress to vigorous exercise. Lastly, should a client be 45 years of age or older, an exercise professional should make a reasonable judgment as to the beginning exercise intensity. If the client is regularly exercising and has no major symptoms, perhaps progression to vigorous-intensity exercise is appropriate. Otherwise, a previously sedentary client should begin at low- to moderate-intensity exercise levels.

Demonstration Case Study 1.1

PAR-Q+

Bart is a 58-year-old male who has decided to begin an exercise program, as he believes it will help him manage his high blood pressure. Bart goes to a local health-fitness facility where he meets with the director of wellness, Bridget. Bridget tells Bart that it is the facility's policy to have all members interested in a supervised fitness program complete a PAR-Q+ and, if necessary, the ePARmed-X+.

So Bart and Bridget sit down to complete the PAR-Q+. On the first page of the PAR-Q+, Bart gives the following answers: (1) "no" to having a heart condition, (1a) "yes" to having high blood pressure, (2) "no" to experiencing chest pain or shortness of breath, (3) "no" to dizziness or balance issues, (4) "no" to other chronic diseases, (5) "yes" to medications (he is taking Lisinopril), (6) "no" to musculoskeletal issues, and (7) "no" to being ordered by a physician to perform only medically supervised exercise.

As a result of these responses to the first seven questions of the PAR-Q+, Bridget correctly asserts that Bart needs to answer questions on pages 2 and 3 of the PAR-Q+. On the second page, Bart answers "no" to all questions with the exception of question 4b. Here Bart answers "yes" as his blood pressure is greater than 160/90 mmHg at rest when he is not taking his Lisinopril. On page 3, Bart answers "no" to all questions. Bridget then correctly instructs Bart to complete the ePARmed-X+ because he answered "yes" to at least one question on pages 2 and 3 of the PAR-Q+.

Bridget helps Bart take the ePARmed-X+ online. Bart answers "no" to the first two questions. The third question asks if Bart has high blood pressure, and Bart answers "yes." The next question asks if a physician is managing Bart's blood pressure, and Bart answers "yes." The fifth question asks if Bart's blood pressure is less than 160/90 mmHg, between 160/90 and 200/110 mmHg, or above 200/110 mmHg. Bart selects less than 160/90 mmHg as he is currently taking Lisinopril to lower his blood pressure. The ePARmed-X+ then indicates that Bart is ready to become more physically active.

However, Bridget's questioning and information gathering are not complete. She has to determine whether Bart should exercise at moderate or vigorous intensity. Therefore, she asks Bart about his current exercise habits. Bart claims to exercise only on occasion, about one or two days per week. Bridget sees that Bart is over the age of 45. She then asks about signs and symptoms of major diseases. Bart reassures Bridget that he has never experienced such signs or symptoms. Therefore, given Bart's inconsistency in participating in regular exercise and being over the age of 45, Bridget suggests that Bart should start an exercise program performing low to moderate-intensity exercises.

Demonstration Case Study 1.2

PAR-Q+

Joy is a 64-year-old female who has battled osteoporosis and arthritis for nearly ten years. She recently read an article in a women's health magazine that suggested regular exercise can help slow the progression of osteoporosis and even manage some of the limitations and pain associated with arthritis. Thus Joy makes an appointment with an exercise physiologist at the local hospital's women's health exercise facility. The exercise physiologist assures Joy that the information she obtained from her women's health magazine is largely true. This excites Joy, and she insists on getting started with exercise. The exercise physiologist, Angelina, tells Joy that before she receives an exercise prescription and is granted access to the facilities' exercise equipment, she has to complete the PAR-Q+.

Angelina sits down with Joy to assist her through the PAR-Q+. On the first page of the PAR-Q+, Joy provides the following answers: (1) "no" to having a heart condition; (1a) "no" to having high blood pressure; (2) "no" to experiencing chest pain or shortness of breath with activities of daily living or physical activity; (3) "no" to having dizziness or balance issues; (4) "yes" to having a chronic medical condition other than heart disease or high blood pressure, as she has osteoporosis; (5) "yes" to medications, as she takes Boniva for her osteoporosis and Aleve for her arthritis; (6) "yes" to having musculoskeletal issues, as she has osteoporosis and arthritis; and (7) "no" to having been ordered to perform only medically supervised exercise. After reading Joy's responses, Angelina correctly claims that Joy needs to complete the follow-up questions on pages 2 and 3 of the PAR-Q+.

Angelina continues to assist Joy, this time through the follow-up PAR-Q+. Right away, Joy answers "yes" to the first question on page 2, specifically 1b. For this question, Joy claimed that she had pain associated with joint problems, mainly pain from her arthritis. Angelina encouraged Joy to answer the remaining questions for which Joy responded "no" to all of them. Angelina rightfully suggests that Joy complete the ePARmed-X+ because she has answered "yes" to one of the follow-up questions.

Angelina then allows Joy to use her computer to answer questions from the ePARmed-X+. The first question provided to Joy asks if she is pregnant or may be pregnant. Joy answers "no." The second question, however, asks if Joy has multiple chronic diseases. Joy currently has osteoporosis and arthritis, therefore she answers "yes." The survey immediately ends and suggests that Joy seek physician consultation or consultation from a university-trained exercise professional. Luckily, Angelina is a university-trained exercise professional. Despite this training, Angelina accepts her limitations and insists that Joy seek medical clearance from a physician. Angelina assures Joy that she is referring her to a physician first because she wants to make absolutely sure that she maximizes Joy's safety throughout an exercise program. Therefore, Joy agrees to see a physician, and Angelina signs the ePARmed-X+ physician referral form. Joy was medically cleared three days later.

After Joy's medical clearance, Angelina gathered information about Joy's exercise history. Joy told Angelina that she has never exercised a day in her life. Given Joy's sedentary lifestyle coupled with her advancing age, Angelina correctly suggests that Joy begin her exercise program with low to moderately intense exercises.

PRE-PARTICIPATION SCREENING (*CONTINUED*)

As previously stated, the first set of case studies presented in this chapter involves using the PAR-Q+, ePARmed-X+, Exercise Pre-participation Health Screening Questionnaire for Exercise Professionals, and ACSM's Pre-participation Screening Algorithm. So far, the self-guided pre-participation screening tools have been discussed and their applications presented in demonstration case studies. Now, the focus of pre-participation screening can be placed on the administration of professionally guided pre-participation screening tools. Professionally guided pre-participation screening tools are more technical and can help exercise professionals gather more pertinent medical information from their clients. It should be noted that the administration of self-guided or professionally guided pre-participation screening tools would be acceptable when working with clients who have chronic diseases. However, because of the fact that professionally guided pre-participation screening tools are more technical and require greater interaction between exercise professionals and exercise participants, professionally guided pre-participation screening tools are often preferred over self-guided tools, especially when serving clients with chronic diseases. Before completing case studies using professionally guided pre-participation screening tools, it is beneficial to be familiarized with the processes. To do this, the Exercise Pre-participation Health Screening Questionnaire for Exercise Professionals and the ACSM's Pre-participation Screening Algorithm will be discussed individually.

The Exercise Pre-participation Health Screening Questionnaire for Exercise Professionals[4] is a simplified checklist for exercise professionals to use when prescreening clients. This checklist is divided into three steps: (1) symptoms, (2) current physical activity, and (3) current or past medical conditions. By using this checklist, exercise professionals can quickly make recommendations for their clients. These recommendations include (1) to begin an exercise program, (2) continue a current exercise program, (3) continue a current exercise program at only low to moderate exercise intensity, or (4) seek medical clearance from a licensed physician.

To begin, exercise professionals will ask their clients a series of questions intended to identify whether the client has experienced a major sign or symptom suggestive of cardiometabolic or renal diseases. These signs and symptoms include chest discomfort with exertion (angina), unreasonable breathlessness (dyspnea), dizziness, fainting, or blackout (syncope or near syncope); ankle swelling (pitting ankle edema); forceful or rapid heartbeats (palpitations); lower leg cramps with exertion (claudication); and known heart murmurs. Following these questions, the simplicity of the Exercise Pre-participation Health Screening Questionnaire for Exercise Professionals starts to kick in. Should clients claim that they have experienced one of the aforementioned signs or symptoms, the recommendation will always be for the client to seek medical clearance from a licensed physician.

If a client does not claim to have experienced a major sign or symptom suggestive of cardiometabolic or renal diseases in the first step of the Exercise Pre-participation Health Screening Questionnaire for Exercise Professionals, then the exercise professional can proceed to the second and third steps. The second step probes the client about his or her current physical activity level. Here being regularly physically active is defined as exercising at least three days per week, 30 minutes per day, at a moderate intensity, and having done so for at least the previous three months. This is a simple "yes" or "no" question. Regardless of the client's answer, the exercise professional will proceed to step 3.

In step 3 of the Exercise Pre-participation Health Screening Questionnaire for Exercise Professionals, the exercise professional asks clients whether they have or have had one of the following medical conditions: (1) myocardial infarction (heart attack); (2) heart surgery, cardiac catheterization, or coronary angioplasty; (3) pacemaker or defibrillator placement; (4) heart failure; (5) heart transplantation; (6) congenital heart disease; (7) diabetes (type I or type II); or (8) renal disease. Once step 3 is complete, recommendations can be made. The following recommendations are made based on select scenarios: (1) begin exercise if no medical conditions are selected in step 3; (2) begin or continue exercise at low to moderate intensity only if medical conditions are selected in step three, and "yes" was answered in step 2 (medical clearance required for vigorous-intensity exercise); (3) medical clearance is needed if the client answers "no" in step 2 and has one of the medical conditions listed in step 3; or (4) if "yes" is answered in step 2 and no medical conditions identified in step 3, no medical clearance is required, and the client can begin exercising.

Demonstration Case Study 1.3

Exercise Pre-participation Health Screening Questionnaire for Exercise Professionals

Hugh is a 55-year-old male who has noticed significant weight gain over the previous three years. He is concerned that his recent, yet gradual, weight gain will be detrimental for his overall health as he approaches his retirement years. Therefore, he visits a weight-loss clinic at his local hospital. There, he meets the lead exercise physiologist, Ryan. Ryan tells Hugh that because he is obese, the first step to becoming physically active is to gather some necessary medical and past exercise history. Thus Ryan decides to administer the Exercise Pre-participation Health Screening Questionnaire. Ryan begins asking Hugh questions about symptoms. Hugh tells Ryan that he has never felt chest pain with exertion, unusual breathlessness, or dizziness; has never fainted or blacked out; has never noticed any forceful or rapid heartbeats; and has never had any lower leg cramps. Ryan decides to be thorough in his screening of Hugh and chooses to view Hugh's ankles himself. Ryan determines that Hugh does not have any ankle swelling.

Since Hugh has apparently never experienced a major sign or symptom suggestive of cardiometabolic or renal diseases, Ryan moves on to step 2 of the Exercise Pre-participation Health Screening Questionnaire. Here Hugh tells Ryan that his only exercise is performing his job duties as a contractor. Ryan correctly tells Hugh that though being a contractor is physical work, it does not count as regular exercise. Ryan then moves on to step 3. Here Ryan asks Hugh a series of questions regarding his past medical history. Ryan determines that Hugh has been fighting type I diabetes mellitus since he was seven years old. Other than type I diabetes mellitus, Hugh has never had a cardiovascular disease or procedure, and his renal health is good.

Ryan then reads over the results of the Exercise Pre-participation Health Screening Questionnaire to make an immediate recommendation regarding Hugh's pursuit of regular exercise. Ryan points out two key findings: (1) Hugh does not exercise regularly, and (2) Hugh has type I diabetes mellitus. Therefore, Ryan strongly recommended that Hugh receive medical clearance from a licensed physician.

Demonstration Case Study 1.4

Exercise Pre-participation Health Screening Questionnaire for Exercise Professionals

Elsa is a 42-year-old female who recently had her cholesterol and blood glucose checked as a part of her company's employee wellness program. When Elsa received her results, the form indicated that she has high low-density lipoprotein cholesterol (LDL-c) levels suggesting dyslipidemia. She then visited her physician, who prescribed Elsa Atorvastatin to lower her LDL-c. Her physician also suggested that Elsa should begin exercise to help control her blood lipid levels. Elsa decided to follow through on her physician's recommendation and promptly scheduled a visit with the local health-fitness facility's lead exercise physiologist, Rebecca.

Upon meeting Elsa, Rebecca states that Elsa needs to answer a series of questions prior to exercise testing and exercise participation. Rebecca relies on the Exercise Pre-participation Health Screening Questionnaire to prescreen Elsa. Rebecca begins asking Elsa questions about signs and symptoms. Elsa tells Rebecca that she has never experienced chest pain with activity, uncomfortable shortness of breath, dizziness, fainting, or blackouts. In addition, Elsa claims she has never noticed unusual or rapid heartbeats and has never had any lower leg cramps. Rebecca decides to examine Elsa's ankles for edema. Rebecca notes some swelling in one of Elsa's ankles. The swelling is associated with redness of the skin. Rebecca probes Elsa further and finds out that Elsa has some pain in that ankle and lower leg. Rebecca cannot rule out venous insufficiency or deep vein thrombosis on her own. Therefore, the only recommendation that Rebecca can offer is for Elsa to seek medical clearance prior to exercise from a licensed physician.

Demonstration Case Study 1.5

Exercise Pre-participation Health Screening Questionnaire for Exercise Professionals

Deacon is a 67-year-old male who has noticed an increase in his blood pressure as he regularly checks it at home. Deacon recently heard a public service announcement on the radio that claimed exercise is an excellent way to help manage blood pressure. Therefore, Deacon decided to visit a personal trainer at the local YMCA.

His personal trainer, Leslie, tells Deacon that she needs to ask him some questions about his symptoms, physical activity, and past medical history. Leslie tells Deacon this is necessary because of his blood pressure and his age. Leslie uses the Exercise Pre-participation Health Screening Questionnaire for Exercise Professionals to gather this information. For step 1, Deacon tells Leslie that he never experienced chest pain, breathlessness, dizziness, or fainting; forceful or rapid heartbeats; or lower leg cramps.

Leslie examines Deacon's ankles and finds no swelling. Therefore, Leslie proceeds to steps 2 and 3.

Leslie asks Deacon about his exercise history. Deacon tells Leslie that he walks two days per week for 60 minutes each time he walks. Leslie tells Deacon this is a great start, but it doesn't count as regular exercise. Therefore, Leslie checks "no" for current activity. Leslie then moves on to step 3, which involves asking Deacon about his past medical history. Deacon tells Leslie that he has never been diagnosed with any disease and has never surgery.

Leslie then reads over the results of the Exercise Pre-participation Health Screening Questionnaire for Exercise Professionals to make an immediate recommendation regarding Deacon's pursuit of regular exercise. The only key finding Leslie discovers is that Deacon does not engage in regular exercise. Therefore, Leslie recommends that Deacon proceed to exercise testing and regular exercise starting at a moderate-intensity. Moderate intensity is recommended because Deacon is not classified as a regular exerciser because he does not exercise three times per week.

PRE-PARTICIPATION SCREENING (*CONTINUED*)

The final method of pre-participation screening, and a professionally guided prescreening tool, is the ACSM's Pre-participation Health Screening Algorithm. The ACSM's Pre-participation Health Screening Algorithm[5] is a relatively new prescreening tool and is a more intensive prescreening method for identifying individuals at risk for cardiovascular complications during exercise. Therefore, it is highly recommended that exercise professionals use the ACSM's Pre-participation Health Screening Algorithm when serving all clients but especially so for clients with chronic diseases.

The ACSM's Pre-participation Screening Algorithm is based on a client's current exercise participation, known cardiovascular, metabolic, and renal diseases, and signs or symptoms suggestive of cardiovascular, metabolic, and renal diseases. The following recommendations are made following the application of this screening algorithm: (1) medical clearance is not required, and the client can exercise or continue exercise at a low or moderate-intensity level and progress to vigorous exercise; (2) medical clearance is only needed for vigorous-intensity exercise; (3) medical clearance is required before exercise; or (4) discontinue exercise pending medical clearance. To make these recommendations using the algorithm, four steps need to be followed. These steps are (1) determining whether a client is a regular exerciser; (2) identifying previous signs and symptoms suggestive of cardiometabolic or renal diseases; (3) identifying known cardiovascular, metabolic, or renal diseases; and (4) determining the exercise intensity to be performed during an exercise program.

The first step in using the ACSM's Pre-participation Health Screening Algorithm is to identify whether a client is a regular exerciser. Knowing whether a client is a regular exerciser dictates the recommendations that are made following questions regarding symptoms and past medical history. Regular exercise, for the purposes of pre-participation health screening, is defined as performing at least moderate-intensity exercise for at least 30 minutes per day, three days per week, for the previous three months. Once a client's current exercise status is identified, exercise professionals move to questioning a client's experience with signs or symptoms suggestive of cardiovascular, metabolic, or renal diseases.

The major signs or symptoms suggestive of cardiovascular, metabolic, or renal diseases are as follows: (1) angina, (2) dyspnea, (3) dizziness or syncope, (4) orthopnea or paroxysmal nocturnal dyspnea, (5) ankle edema (particularly pitting edema), (6) palpitations, (7) intermittent claudication, (8) heart murmur, and (9) unusual fatigue or shortness of breath. These signs and symptoms are caused by a number of factors. One of the main factors is a reduction in blood flow caused by atherosclerosis. A reduction in blood flow to the myocardium can result in angina and/or palpitations, while a reduction in blood flow to the muscles of the lower leg can result in claudication. Another factor is left ventricular dysfunction or impairment, which leads to the inability of the heart to sufficiently pump enough oxygenated blood. Several symptoms can result because of left ventricular dysfunction or impairment, including dyspnea, orthopnea, paroxysmal nocturnal dyspnea, ankle edema, or unusual fatigue or shortness of breath. In addition, damage to the heart or venous valves can result in the presence of ankle edema or heart murmurs.

Exercise professionals must be able to recognize the major signs and symptoms suggestive of cardiometabolic and renal diseases. Beyond recognition, exercise professionals also have to be able to explain these signs and symptoms to their clients when administering prescreening tools. To begin, angina can be described as "heavy, constricting, and crushing" substernal chest pain that radiates to the back, neck, arms, or jaw. This type of angina is typical angina and is most common in men. Atypical angina can be described as feelings of nausea and fatigue. This type of angina is most common in women. Next, dyspnea is described as excessive shortness of breath during usual activities. Orthopnea differs from dyspnea in that shortness of breath occurs in the recumbent position and is relieved with a change of position. Paroxysmal nocturnal dyspnea is shortness of breath that occurs during sleep and is relieved with a change of position. Syncope is a loss of consciousness because of reductions in blood flow to the brain. Intermittent claudication occurs in a similar manner to angina and is described as lower leg pain occurring during walking/running that resolves with rest. Heart palpitations are described as a forceful and/rapid heartbeat. Ankle edema is swelling of the ankles that occur because of either inefficient heart pump action or insufficient venous return. A heart murmur can be found by listening to a client's heart sounds. Here, extra heart sounds may indicate valvular complications or coronary artery disease. Lastly, a catch-all symptom is feelings of unusual fatigue or shortness of breath with regular activity. Unusual fatigue or shortness of breath could be indicative of left ventricular dysfunction.

The third step in using the ACSM's Pre-participation Health Screening Algorithm is to determine whether a client has a known cardiovascular, metabolic, or renal disease. There are several examples of each type of disease. To keep things simple, a cardiovascular disease is any disease that affects the heart or vasculature. Common examples of cardiovascular disease include coronary artery disease, valvular heart disease, myocardial infarction, cardiac arrhythmias, peripheral vascular disease, dissections and aneurysms, pulmonary embolism, and deep vein thrombosis. A metabolic disease can be characterized as a disease that interferes with the normal chemical reactions occurring in the body. This could include a wide array of specific diseases. However, the most common metabolic disease is diabetes mellitus (type I and type II). Other common metabolic diseases include hypo/hyperthyroidism, mitochondrial disorders, and various muscle wasting disorders. Lastly, renal diseases are characterized as a set of diseases that alter kidney function. A common kidney disease is renal failure, which may or may not be accompanied by renal replacement therapy (dialysis or transplant).

The final step in using the ACSM's Pre-participation Health Screening Algorithm is determining the desired exercise intensity to be performed by the client. This step comes down to whether a client wants to exercise at a low to moderate intensity or vigorous intensity. Moderate-intensity exercise can be defined as exercise performed at 40–60 percent of heart rate/maximal oxygen uptake reserve or at a perceived exertion of 12–13 or more on the 6–20 Borg scale.[6,7] Vigorous exercise intensity can be defined as exercise performed above 60 percent of heart rate/maximal oxygen uptake reserve or a perceived exertion of 14–17 on the 6–20 Borg scale. Identifying the level of desired exercise intensity is ultimately critical in making recommendations regarding exercise participation or referral for medical clearance.

Once the previous steps have been completed, exercise professionals then make recommendations regarding exercise participation or medical clearance. The first recommendation that can be made is that the client does not need medical clearance and can exercise or continue exercise at low or moderate intensity and progress to vigorous exercise. This recommendation can only be made when a client does not have a known cardiovascular, metabolic, or renal disease or major sign or symptom suggestive thereof. The second recommendation that can be made is that medical clearance is only needed for vigorous-intensity exercise. This recommendation is made when a client is a regular exerciser; has a known cardiovascular, metabolic, or renal disease; is asymptomatic; and has *not* been medically cleared to perform vigorous-intensity exercise within the previous 12 months. The third recommendation that can be made is that medical clearance is required prior to participating in *any* exercise program. This recommendation is made when a client is a nonexerciser and has either a known cardiovascular, metabolic, or renal disease or has experienced signs or symptoms suggestive thereof. The last recommendation that can be made is that a current exerciser needs to discontinue exercise and receive medical clearance. This recommendation is made when a current exerciser has experienced any sign or symptom suggestive of cardiovascular, metabolic, or renal diseases.

Demonstration Case Study 1.6

ACSM's Pre-participation Health Screening Algorithm

Chloe is a 48-year-old female who has a family history of type II diabetes mellitus. Therefore, she regularly checks her fasting blood glucose. Recently, she noticed her blood glucose levels have increased. Her fasting blood glucose is regularly 115 mg/dL.

In light of this, she decides to become more physically active, as she was recently made aware of the fact that exercise can help prevent type II diabetes.

Chloe visits a women's fitness club and meets with Brittany, the lead personal trainer. Brittany tells Chloe that before she can exercise at the facility, she needs to go through a prescreening process. Given Chloe's family history of type II diabetes, Brittany decides the most appropriate prescreening tool is the ACSM's Pre-participation Health Screening Algorithm. Initially, Brittany probes Chloe regarding her exercise behavior. Chloe tells Brittany that she exercises on a recumbent cycle ergometer at an intensity equal to approximately 33 percent of her heart rate reserve. Chloe indicates she has done this three days per week, for the last three months, for 30 minutes each exercise session. Brittany notes that while this is a good habit, it is not intense enough to qualify as being a regular exerciser. Next, Brittany asks Chloe about her current symptoms. Chloe claims that she occasionally feels winded when she exercises but that it resolves once she gets more "into" the exercise. Other than this, Chloe reports experiencing no major sign or symptom suggestive of cardiovascular, metabolic, or renal diseases. Brittany ponders her symptom of shortness of breath and easily links this to the rapid phase of oxygen consumption in response to an acute bout of exercise. Therefore, Brittany does not identify any major signs or symptoms. Next, Brittany asks Chloe about her past medical history. Chloe indicates that she has asthma, but has never been diagnosed with a cardiovascular, metabolic, or renal disease. Lastly, Brittany determines an initial exercise intensity for Chloe. Given that Chloe only exercises at a low intensity, moderate intensity is likely an appropriate starting point.

Taking all of the gathered information into account, Brittany makes her recommendation regarding exercise participation and medical clearance. Brittany tells Chloe that since she has never experienced a major sign or symptom suggestive of cardiometabolic or renal diseases nor has she ever been diagnosed with a cardiovascular, metabolic, or renal disease, she may begin an exercise program following exercise testing without the need for medical clearance. Brittany then progresses to the pre-exercise evaluation.

Demonstration Case Study 1.7

ACSM's Pre-participation Health Screening Algorithm

Titus is a 51-year-old male who has a family history of cardiovascular disease. Given this family history, Titus is concerned he may develop cardiovascular disease if he does not change his lifestyle. Currently, Titus has hypertension, dyslipidemia, trouble managing his blood glucose, and is classified as obese. Therefore, he has made the decision to visit a personal trainer at the local health-fitness facility.

Justin, the personal trainer, meets with Titus before conducting exercise tests and writing an exercise prescription. Justin tells Titus that since he has hypertension, dyslipidemia, high blood glucose, and is classified as obese, it is best to do a prescreening using the ACSM's Pre-participation Health Screening Algorithm. Justin starts by inquiring about Titus's current physical activity level. Titus tells Justin that he exercises on the elliptical three days per week, 30 minutes per session, at an intensity equal to 75 percent of his maximum heart rate. Justin determines that the intensity of Justin's exercise is approximately 65 percent of his heart rate reserve. Justin then correctly asserts this is good enough for Titus to be considered a regular exerciser. Next, Justin tries to identify signs and symptoms suggestive of cardiovascular, metabolic, or renal diseases. Titus tells Justin that he has never suffered any sign or symptom. From here, Justin asks Titus about his past medical history, particularly his blood glucose issues. Justin gets Titus to admit he was diagnosed with type II diabetes last year. Justin asks Titus whether he had been medically cleared to exercise within the past year. Titus says that he has not sought medical clearance.

With all of the information gathered, Justin then makes his recommendation regarding exercise participation and medical clearance. Justin makes the recommendation that Titus can exercise at a moderate intensity without medical clearance, but he needs medical clearance before progressing to vigorous-intensity exercise. Justin makes this recommendation because Titus is a regular exerciser, has never experienced a major sign or symptom suggestive of cardiometabolic or renal diseases, and has not been medically cleared to exercise within the past 12 months.

Demonstration Case Study 1.8

ACSM's Pre-participation Health Screening Algorithm

Frida is a 40-year-old female aerobics instructor. She has always been very physically active. She works out five days per week, 60 minutes per day, at a vigorous intensity. She really enjoys circuit training and boot camp. Therefore, she has made the decision to enroll in a CrossFit gym in hopes of one day competing in CrossFit competitions.

Prior to beginning classes at the gym, Frida meets with the lead instructor, Mollie. Mollie tells Frida that since the exercises to be performed in classes are of vigorous intensity that she needs to conduct a thorough prescreening process to enhance safety. Frida agrees that this is appropriate. Mollie then proceeds to administer the ACSM's Pre-participation Health Screening Algorithm. She first determines that Frida is clearly a regular exerciser. Mollie then asks about symptoms. Frida then provides the following response, "I have never experienced any chest pain, shortness of breath, unusual fatigue or shortness of breath, heart palpitations, leg cramps, nor have I been diagnosed with a heart murmur. However, I have noticed some pain and swelling of my right ankle and calf." This response raises Mollie's suspicion, and she insists on examining Frida's right ankle. Mollie notes that the ankle is indeed swollen, as is the lower calf, and the whole area is red and painful. Following this observation, Mollie abruptly ends the screening. Mollie makes an immediate recommendation that Frida see a physician for medical clearance. Frida was unhappy and demanded an explanation. Mollie tells Frida that she is not a physician, but she is concerned that the right ankle swelling may be due to a vascular condition and that she insists on being cautious. Mollie tells Frida that it is most appropriate to stop exercising immediately and visit a physician.

Demonstration Case Study 1.9

Juan is a 55-year-old male who has a family history of coronary artery disease and myocardial infarction. In fact, Juan suffered a minor myocardial infarction two years ago and had angioplasty with a coronary artery stent placed in his circumflex coronary artery. Juan completed cardiac rehabilitation one year ago but has not exercised since. Juan realizes that exercise is important for preventing a future myocardial infarction and, therefore, he decides to visit the local hospital's health and wellness fitness facility.

Juan meets with Brett, the facility's clinical exercise physiologist to discuss an exercise program. Given Juan's history with heart disease, Brett wants to conduct an intensive prescreening and chooses to administer the ACSM's Pre-participation Health Screening Algorithm. First, Brett asks about Juan's current physical activity level. Juan tells Brett that he has not exercised since completing phase II cardiovascular rehabilitation. Brett then asks about signs and symptoms and past medical history, just to be thorough. Juan tells Brett that he hasn't experienced a sign or symptom since he experienced angina during his myocardial infarction. Then Juan tells Brett that his only medical history is the myocardial infarction.

Brett takes all of the information into consideration and makes a recommendation regarding exercise participation and medical clearance. Brett tells Juan that since he is not a regular exerciser and has a known cardiovascular disease, he needs medical clearance prior to exercise testing, exercise prescription, and exercise training. Brett then offers to help Juan make an appointment with one of the hospital's cardiologists.

PRE-PARTICIPATION EVALUATION

When serving clients with chronic diseases, it is prudent for exercise professionals to obtain as much information about the clients as possible. It is highly likely that such detailed information will not be obtained during pre-exercise screening. Therefore, exercise professionals should seek further information about their clients through a series of evaluations. Pre-participation evaluations serve as a bridge between pre-screening and exercise testing.[8] Further, pre-participation evaluations can help exercise professionals elucidate any contraindications for exercise testing and participation and further determine whether medical clearance should be recommended prior to beginning exercise testing or participation. The components of a thorough pre-participation evaluation covered in this text include informed consent, cardiovascular risk factor analysis, medical history, physical examination, and pulmonary function testing.

Pre-participation evaluations should always begin with obtaining informed consent from the client. Even if the client is a minor, informed consent must be obtained, and the minor's guardian(s) need to sign the form. Obtaining informed consent is of legal and ethical importance. By obtaining informed consent from clients, exercise professionals can ensure that the client fully knows and understands the purposes and the risks that are associated with exercise testing and exercise participation. It must be noted that even if an exercise professional obtains informed consent from the client, it in no way absolves the exercise professional from negligence. Therefore, proper prescreening and evaluation, exercise testing, exercise prescription, and supervision must be at the forefront of an exercise professional's mind.

It is important for exercise professionals to make sure that their clients completely understand the information presented in an informed consent document. For this reason, informed consent documents should be written at a middle school reading level, and the exercise professional should verbally explain everything in the document. At a minimum, informed consent documents should include statements that indicate several items. First, informed consent documents need to outline the purposes of the exercise program and any procedures. Second, the informed consent document should state that the client has been given an opportunity to ask questions about every aspect of the exercise program. Next, informed consent documents should clearly outline all conceivable benefits and risks of the exercise program. When working with special populations, the risks of an exercise program are greater than with apparently healthy adults, and these risks need to be highlighted in the informed consent document. Once benefits and risks are presented, the informed consent document needs to include a statement assuring client confidentiality, especially when medical information is collected. After statements of confidentiality, the informed consent document should indicate emergency procedures and the treatment protocols should injuries or illnesses occur during the exercise program. Lastly, informed consent documents always have to make it clear that the client is free to withdraw from the exercise program at any time. For questions concerning informed consent, exercise professionals should not hesitate in seeking legal consultation.

Demonstration Case Study 1.10

Informed Consent

Christina and Anna are experienced clinical exercise physiologists. They each have worked in cardiovascular and pulmonary rehabilitation for ten years. Now they have decided that, together, they are going to start an exercise clinic for serving individuals at risk for or having been diagnosed with chronic diseases. Christina and Anna are going to name the clinic "Exercise for Health." After obtaining the appropriate financing, purchasing a facility and equipment, and developing a market strategy, Christina and Anna focus on some legal matters. The first legal matter that Christina and Anna address is writing an informed consent document. Since Christina and Anna will be serving clients with chronic diseases or at risk thereof, they want to be thorough. Christina and Anna meet with an attorney, and it was recommended that their document include verbiage that indicates that their clients have the opportunity to ask questions, all possible benefits and risks, protection of client confidentiality, emergency and treatment procedures, and that the client is free to withdraw from an exercise program at any time. Therefore, Christina and Anna developed the following informed consent document (see Figure 1.1).

Figure 1.1 This is an example of how to construct an informed consent document for clients entering a fitness program

Exercise for Health

Document of Informed Consent

- Purpose and Explanation of Exercise for Health's Exercise Program:

  o Exercise for Health's exercise programs are designed to help reduce clients' risks for developing many chronic diseases or to help clients better manage current chronic medical conditions. All exercise programs begin with questions about exercise, symptoms of medical conditions, and medical history. Then clients will be given a recommendation about seeking a doctor's clearance to exercise. Once it is deemed safe for a client to exercise, they will complete a fitness test. The fitness test will be on a treadmill or cycle. The test will last about ten minutes, and an exercise professional will take the client's heart rate and blood pressure before, during, and after the test. The client has the ability to stop the test at any time. An exercise professional will stop the test if the client experiences health complications. After an exercise test, an exercise professional will write an exercise plan. All clients will be supervised during exercise training.

- Risks and Benefits:

  o During or after fitness testing or exercise, there is a slight risk for high or low blood pressure, dizziness, muscle cramps, drops or increases in blood sugar, muscle or joint injury, heart attack, or stroke. The benefits of participation include improved fitness, improved blood pressure, improved blood sugar, weight loss, decreased disease risk, improved alertness, and improved ability to do regular activities.

- Statement of Confidentiality:

  o All demographic, fitness, and medical information will be securely kept at the facility. Medical information may only be shared with medical professionals in the event of an emergency given the client's consent.

- In the Event of Emergency:

  o Should a client have a medical emergency, emergency aid will be provided on-site. Emergency medical services will be contacted if needed and transport decisions will be made by emergency medical services, clients, and families. Automated External Defibrillators (AEDs) and oxygen supplementation are available on-site. Exercise professionals routinely check blood pressure, heart rate, blood sugar, electrocardiogram (ECG), and oxygen saturation.

(Continued)

Figure 1.1 This is an example of how to construct an informed consent document for clients entering a fitness program (Continued)

- Questions:
  - All clients may ask, and are encouraged to ask, questions about any aspect of the exercise program, confidentiality, or emergency procedures.

- Freedom of Consent and Withdraw:
  - By signing this document, the client acknowledges voluntary participation. All clients may withdraw from any aspect of the exercise program at any time.

Signature of Client or Guardian: _____

Date: _____

Signature of Exercise Professional: _____

Date: _____

PRE-PARTICIPATION EVALUATION (*CONTINUED*)

Another component of a thorough pre-participation evaluation is a cardiovascular disease risk factor analysis. The cardiovascular disease risk factor analysis is very useful for exercise professionals and clients alike. This is particularly true when serving clients with chronic diseases, as these clients oftentimes have an elevated risk for cardiovascular disease or a repeat cardiovascular disease event, such as a myocardial infarction. Consider clients with hypertension. Individuals with hypertension have a life expectancy of approximately five years less than individuals without hypertension and can expect fewer years free from cardiovascular disease.[9] Similar data hold true for many of the other cardiovascular disease risk factors, which highlights the importance of cardiovascular disease risk factor analysis when working with special populations.

The cardiovascular disease risk factor analysis[10] keeps the client and exercise professional aware of present risk factors, which helps capture a controllable aspect of a client's overall health. A well-designed exercise program for clients with chronic diseases should always address controllable risk factors for cardiovascular disease. Therefore, identifying cardiovascular disease risk factors, especially controllable risk factors, can aid in establishing exercise program goals and serve as a tracking method to determine the effectiveness of an exercise program.

Cardiovascular disease risk factor analysis begins with a recognition of each cardiovascular disease risk factor and each of their criterion. There are eight major risk factors that have been linked to the development of atherosclerotic cardiovascular disease. Two of these risk factors are not controllable. These noncontrollable risk factors are age and family history. For a client to have age as a risk factor, a male client has to be 45 years old or older and a female client has to be 55 years old or older. For a client to have the family history risk factor, a client has to have a first-degree biological relative (mother, father, brother, or sister) who had a myocardial infarction, coronary revascularization, or sudden death. Further, the previous events have age cutoffs for male and female relatives, before 55 for male relatives and before 65 for females.

Of the eight cardiovascular disease risk factors, six are controllable and, therefore, can be reduced/improved in response to an exercise program. The first of these controllable risk factors is arguably the most controllable: cigarette smoking and exposure to secondhand smoke. A client would have the cigarette smoking risk factor if he or she has smoked or been regularly exposed to secondhand smoke within the previous six months. The second controllable risk factor is physical inactivity. Physical inactivity is defined as not exercising at least 75–150 minutes of moderate—vigorous intensity exercise per week or 500–1,000 MET-min/week.

MET-min/week = (exercising $\dot{V}O_2$ in ml/kg/min/3.5) x minutes of exercise per week

Moderate-intensity exercise is defined as exercise performed at an equivalent of 40–60 percent of heart rate or oxygen uptake reserve or at a perceived exertion of 12–13 on the 6–20 Borg scale.[11,12] The next controllable risk factor is hypertension. Here the cutoff is systolic blood pressure is equal to or greater than 130 mg/dL and/or a diastolic blood pressure equal or greater than 80 mg/dL or treatment of hypertension with antihypertensive medication(s). The fourth controllable risk factor is dyslipidemia. The criteria for dyslipidemia are LDL-c equal to or greater than 130 mg/dL, or high-density lipoprotein cholesterol (HDL-c) lower than 40 mg/dL, for men, an LDL-c lower than 50 mg/dL for women, or total serum cholesterol greater than or equal to 200 mg/dL, non HDL-c equal to or greater than 160 mg/dL, or the client is being treated with an antilipemic medication.

Obesity is another controllable risk factor. There are many methods to determine whether a client meets the criteria for the obesity risk factor. The first method involves calculating a client's body mass index (BMI). The BMI is equal to the client's weight in kilograms divided by the person's height in meters squared. If the BMI is equal to or greater than 30 kg/m² the person is classified as obese. It should be noted that BMI is merely a height to weight ratio and does not take into account a client's muscle mass. Nevertheless, epidemiological data still suggest that a BMI equal or greater than 30/kgm² increases the likelihood of developing cardiovascular disease. Sometimes, exercise professionals choose to assess the obesity risk factor by performing a waist circumference measurement. The reason for this is that abdominal adiposity is highly associated with the development of cardiovascular disease. A male client is given the obesity risk factor if his waist circumference is greater than 40 inches. A female client is given the obesity risk factor if her waist circumference is greater than 35 inches.

Given the strong relationship between diabetes mellitus and cardiovascular disease,[13] diabetes is an important controllable risk factor. It should be noted that not all cases of diabetes are controllable. For instance, type I diabetes is an autoimmune disease that results in the inability of the pancreas to produce and secrete insulin. However, blood glucose levels are largely controllable and regular exercise has a potent influence on glucose metabolism. A fasting plasma glucose concentration greater than or equal to 100 mg/dL would warrent diabetes as a risk factor for cardiovascular disease. Another assessment that can be used to identify the diabetes risk factor is the oral glucose tolerance test. Here, if the two-hour plasma glucose following ingestion is greater than or equal to 140 mg/dL, then the client would be given the diabetes risk factor. Also, exercise professionals can assess a client's glycolated hemoglobin value (HbA1c). With this test, an HbA1c value greater than or equal to 5.7 percent, not 6.5 percent would warrant the diabetes risk factor. As with the hypertension and dyslipidemia risk factors, if a client is being medicated to control diabetes, then the diabetes risk factor is given.

The aforementioned risk factors are considered positive risk factors because of their association with the development of cardiovascular disease. During a cardiovascular disease risk factor analysis, whenever an exercise professional cannot obtain data regarding certain risk factors, that risk factor should be considered a positive risk factor until proven otherwise. Also, there is one negative risk factor. This risk factor is a high HDL-c level. Higher levels of HDL-c have been shown to be cardioprotective. Therefore, when a client has an HDL-c level greater than 60 mg/dL, a negative risk factor is given, and this, by all intents and purposes, removes a positive risk factor.

Demonstration Case Study 1.11

Cardiovascular Disease Risk Factor Analysis

Mikhail is the newly hired lead exercise physiologist working for his hospital's preventive health-fitness clinic. His first client is Gene. Gene was referred to the program by his primary care physician to help aid his recovery from cancer treatment. Following pre-participation screening and informed consent, Mikhail conducts a cardiovascular risk factor analysis on Gene because Mikhail recognizes that exercise programs for special populations should aim to improve these risk factors. Mikhail has all the resources he needs to conduct the analysis, and he obtains the following information about Gene:

1. Age = 60 years old
2. Family History = mother had a myocardial infarction at age 66, father had open heart surgery at the age of 58, brother had cancer at 65, and his sister was diagnosed with type II diabetes at the age of 52
3. Height = 70 inches
4. Weight and Waist Circumference = 220 pounds, 40 inches
5. Smoking History = never smoked, wife smokes a pack per day in the house
6. Physical Activity = no exercise in the last six months, he was too fatigued and ill from chemotherapy

7. Blood Pressure = 130/78 mmHg, no medications
8. Lipid Profile = LDL-c = 135 mg/dL, HDL-c = 30 mg/dL, total cholesterol = 203 mg/dL, no medications
9. Blood Glucose = HbA1c = 6.6 percent, no medications

After reviewing these data, Mikhail identifies six positive risk factors. These risk factors are age (60 years old), obesity (BMI = 32.6 kg/m^2), cigarette smoking (wife smokes in the house), physical inactivity (no exercise within the last six months), dyslipidemia (LDL-c = 135 mg/dL, HDL-c = 30 mg/dL, and total cholesterol = 203 mg/dL), hypertension (systolic blood pressure = 130 mmHg) and diabetes (HbA1c = 6.6 percent). Mikhail did not identify any negative risk factors.

PRE-PARTICIPATION EVALUATION (*CONTINUED*)

The third aspect of the pre-participation evaluation is obtaining a client's medical history. If an exercise professional does not have enough resources to perform a cardio-vascular risk factor analysis, it is useful to attempt to obtain a client's medical history. A medical history is extraordinarily valuable for exercise professionals working with special populations. The information gathered from a client's medical history helps exercise professionals identify indications/contraindications for exercise testing and exercise participation, the needs that should be addressed in an exercise program, and medical conditions or medicine requiring special considerations to be administered as a part of an exercise program.

Obtaining a client's medical history can be tricky, especially if exercise professionals are not directly employed by a healthcare facility or rendering a medical service, such as cardiopulmonary rehabilitation. Therefore, it is likely that most exercise professionals will have to have their clients complete a medical history questionnaire. Regardless of the method used to obtain a client's medical history, exercise professionals must always keep the information strictly confidential and in accordance with the Health Insurance Portability and Accountability Act (HIPAA). Ideally, an exercise professional should obtain the following information as a part of a client's medical history: (1) medical diagnoses; (2) physical examination findings; (3) laboratory values; (4) history of symptoms; (5) surgical procedures; (6) illnesses; (7) medications; (8) drug allergies; (9) tobacco, alcohol, and drug use; 10) exercise history; 11) work history; and 12) family history.

Demonstration Case Study 1.12

Medical History

Christina and Anna have successfully opened their exercise clinic for serving individuals at risk for or having been diagnosed with chronic diseases, Exercise for Health. To design safe and effective exercise programs for their clients, Christina and Anna decide that it is necessary and of utmost value to obtain information about their clients' medical histories. Since Christina and Anna's facility is not a part of a hospital, and they do not provide medically billable services, they have to obtain their clients' medical histories by administering a medical history questionnaire. Christina and Anna want to make sure they obtain the most information as possible but not overwhelm their clients with paperwork. They designed the following brief medical history questionnaire (see Figure 1.2).

Figure 1.2 This is an example of a medical history questionnaire designed to gather information necessary for an adequate pre-participation health screening

Exercise for Health

Medical History Questionnaire

Has a doctor ever told you that you have chronic medical conditions?

_____ yes _____ no

If so, list all conditions:

_____

_____

Do you currently take any medications?

_____ yes _____ no

If so, list all medications and any drug allergies:

_____

_____

Have you had surgery before?

_____ yes _____ no

If so, list all surgeries and when they were performed:

_____

_____

(Continued)

Figure 1.2 This is an example of a medical history questionnaire designed to gather information necessary for an adequate pre-participation health screening (Continued)

Have you had any recent illnesses?

_____ yes _____ no

If so, list all recent illnesses:

_____

_____

Have you ever exercised?

_____ yes _____ no

If so, list your favorite exercises:

_____

_____

What is your occupation? _____

Has a doctor expressed any concerns about you exercising?

_____ yes _____ no

If so, what were the concerns?

_____

_____

PRE-PARTICIPATION EVALUATION (*CONTINUED*)

When exercise professionals work with clients who have chronic diseases, an abbreviated physical examination should be conducted. The reasons for conducting this examination are to uncover physical findings that may have recently developed, identify physical conditions that can be worsened during exercise or by completing certain exercises, identify physical conditions that need to be monitored during exercise, and identify physical conditions that would warrant having a client seek medical clearance prior to exercise testing or participation. It is important to note that exercise professionals are not physicians and thus cannot make diagnoses. Therefore, physical examinations conducted by exercise professionals are intended to gather more information pertinent for designing a safe exercise program and identify physical findings that need medical attention. The components of a physical examination that can be competently performed by an exercise professional are pulses, blood pressure, inspection of the skin and extremities, and pulmonary function testing.

One of the first assessments conducted as a part of a physical examination is a basic assessment of cardiac function. Here, exercise or healthcare professionals will assess a client's resting apical pulse and radial pulse. The reason both are assessed is to determine if there is a deficit (more apical than radial). A deficit between apical and radial pulse indicates abnormal cardiac function, whereby ventricular contractions do not result in optimal blood flow to the periphery. This could indicate one of three abnormal cardiac conditions: (1) atrial fibrillation (several weak atrial contractions leading to limited ventricular filling), (2) ventricular ectopy (several premature ventricular beats), and (3) pacemaker rhythms. If a difference between the apical and radial pulse is noted, assess the client one more time to ensure accuracy, and if present again, a referral for medical clearance should be made to investigate the possibility of the client having an abnormal cardiac dysrhythmia capable of compromising the normal hemodynamic response to exercise.

To assess apical pulse, exercise professionals should have the client in a seated position with both feet flat on the floor and spine rested comfortably against a seat back. Then an exercise professional places the diaphragm of the stethoscope at the fifth intercostal space, midclavicular line, on the left side of the body. This should be the location of the apex of the heart, which is the point of maximal impulse. Here exercise professionals will listen for the heart sounds S1 and S2. These sounds are "lub dub." Each "lub dub" combination represents one heartbeat. The heartbeats are counted for a full 60 seconds.

After the apical pulse has been recorded, a client's radial pulse is assessed. To assess radial pulse, exercise professionals palpate the flexor tendons below the base of the client's thumb. Then with the middle and fourth fingers, the exercise professional will palpate laterally until the radial pulse is felt. Each pulse is counted for a full 60 seconds. At this point, the exercise professional will note whether the pulses occurred at a consistent rate, the rate was between 60 and 100 beats per minute, or if there was a deficit in the apical pulse rate. Should a client's heart rate be irregular without known atrial fibrillation, well outside the normal heart rate range, or there is significant deficit between apical and radial pulse, the client should seek medical consultation prior to exercise.

Demonstration Case Study 1.13

Assessment of Pulses

Jennifer is an exercise physiologist working for an employee wellness program at a Fortune 500 company. She meets with Dave, a software developer who has sought an exercise program to better control his high blood pressure and cholesterol. Jennifer administers the ACSM's Pre-participation Health Screening Algorithm and finds that Dave does not need medical clearance to participate in exercise testing and an exercise program. Jennifer, realizing that she is working with a client who has comorbidities, decides to perform an abbreviated physical examination. The first exam that Jennifer conducts is an apical and radial pulse. She notes an apical pulse of 70 beats per minute and a radial pulse of 60 beats per minute. Jennifer then double-checks Dave's medical history and does not find atrial fibrillation as a known medical condition. Therefore, Jennifer does another apical and radial pulse assessment to make sure she did not make a mistake. The second attempt shows a similar deficit. Thus Jennifer recommends that Dave seek medical consultation to investigate the apical-radial pulse deficit.

PRE-PARTICIPATION EVALUATION (*CONTINUED*)

Another assessment of cardiovascular function that can be conducted as a part of an abbreviated physical examination is the assessment of blood pressure. Blood pressure refers to the pressure exerted against the blood vessel walls by circulating blood. There are two types of blood pressure: (1) systolic blood pressure and (2) diastolic blood pressure. Systolic blood pressure reflects the pressure exerted against the artery walls during ventricular systole. Diastolic blood pressure, on the other hand, reflects the pressure exerted against artery walls during ventricular diastole. Assessing a client's blood pressure is always a good idea, especially when working with special populations. Consider this, when an individual is hypertensive for long periods of time, the blood vessels harden to prevent bursting because of excess pressure. Hardened blood vessels are not as distensible, and, therefore, pressure is greater in more rigid blood vessels. This explains why long-term hypertension fuels continued hypertension. Moreover, should an individual have an existing unknown aneurysm, prolonged hypertension may result in a catastrophic cardiovascular event.

The assessment of blood pressure really begins at least the day before the assessment is performed. The exercise professional must communicate with the client to ensure the client avoids eating, tobacco use, and caffeine consumption at least 60 minutes prior to assessment and avoid exercising for at least three hours before assessment. Upon arrival, the exercise professional should instruct their client to remove bulky sleeves and sit with his or her feet flat on the floor for five minutes before assessment. Then the exercise professional will circle the blood pressure cuff over the brachial artery, correctly aligning the arrow on the cuff over it. It should be noted that the exercise professional should ensure that the cuff size is correct. Once the blood pressure cuff is in place, the exercise professional will place the earpieces of a stethoscope in his or her ears with the binaurals facing forward. Then the diaphragm of the stethoscope is firmly placed on the antecubital fossa as the client supinates at the wrist. Next, the exercise professional raises the client's arm to heart level while fulling supporting the client's arm. The exercise professional will then inflate the blood pressure cuff to 20 mmHg above the last Korotkoff sound and then slowly release the air at a rate of 2–3 mmHg per second. The exercise professional will listen for two consecutive Korotkoff sounds. If two consecutive Korotkoff sounds are heard, then the position of the needle on the sphygmomanometer at the time of the first sound is noted as the systolic blood pressure. At this point, the exercise professional will keep deflating the cuff until the Korotkoff sounds dissipate. The position of the needle on the sphygmomanometer at the time when the sounds are no longer heard is noted as the diastolic blood pressure. It is possible that the Korotkoff sounds will be heard until zero. In this case, record the point when the sounds become muffled over zero (i.e., 120/80/0). The exercise professional should repeat this procedure for both arms and record the highest of the two blood pressures, and for subsequent measures, use the arms with the highest blood pressure.

Similar to apical and radial pulse assessment, should significantly abnormal blood pressure be recorded, an exercise professional should recommend that the client seek medical consultation. The problem with making a recommendation regarding blood pressure is that there isn't a set cutoff or specific criterion for a referral to medical care. More often than not, the decision to recommend that a client seek medical consultation is based on that client's symptoms. Therefore, if high or low blood pressure is recorded, an exercise professional should match these recordings with a client's current symptoms, and if symptoms are consistent with high or low blood pressure, then make a recommendation for medical consultation. In addition, if resting blood pressure values are extreme, medical consultation should be recommended. As it pertains to exercise testing, if the resting systolic blood pressure is greater than 200 mmHg and/or the resting diastolic blood pressure is greater than 110 mmHg, then an exercise test should not be conducted without physician approval or supervision.[14] At the very least, when abnormally high or low blood pressure is recorded, these values need to be monitored during exercise testing and throughout an exercise program.

Demonstration Case Study 1.14

Assessment of Blood Pressure

Francine is a personal trainer at a local fitness center. She sees Caroline, a client who is seeking an exercise program to help her manage her weight. Francine is very thorough and determines, initially, that Caroline does not need a medical exam after administering the ACSM's Pre-participation Health Screening Algorithm. However, given that Caroline is obese, Francine wants to conduct some physical examination assessments, one of them being blood pressure. Francine records a Caroline's blood pressure as 190/96 mmHg. This is very high, so Francine probes Caroline about her symptoms. As it turns out, Caroline has frequent headaches. Francine notes that headaches are a symptom associated with high blood pressure. So since Francine records a high blood pressure and matches symptoms associated with high blood pressure, she recommends that Caroline see her primary care physician for medical consultation prior to beginning an exercise program.

PRE-PARTICIPATION EVALUATION (*CONTINUED*)

A third physical examination assessment that an exercise professional can conduct when serving clients with chronic diseases is an inspection of the skin and extremities. Here exercise professionals should specifically examine first the feet, ankles, and lower legs. The rationale for this is to make sure a client does not have ankle edema that can be associated with poor venous return because of vascular or cardiac abnormalities. Such conditions include heart failure, venous insufficiency, or deep vein thrombosis.

If a client has heart failure, the heart cannot contract sufficiently enough to generate the pressure necessary to facilitate optimal venous return. Therefore, fluid can accumulate in the feet, ankles, and lower legs. A key characteristic of such fluid accumulation is bilateral pitting edema. This means that if an exercise professional pushes on the area of edema, a "pit" will be briefly left. Next, if a client has venous insufficiency, some of the "one-way" valves in the veins of the lower legs are damaged. This will impair the ability of blood to return to the heart through the venous network and fluid will accumulate in the lower leg. Here, a client would have unilateral pitting edema. Third, if a client has a deep vein thrombosis, a blood clot has developed in one or more of the veins of the lower legs. Deep vein thrombosis not only results in edema but also the skin will be red and warm. It is important to note that whenever these physical findings are recorded, the client should be required to have medical clearance prior to exercise testing and exercise training.

Next, exercise professionals should examine their clients' skin. This is especially important when serving clients with dyslipidemia or diabetes mellitus. A specific concern with clients who have dyslipidemia is that their cholesterol and lipid levels are not being controlled either because of a lack of treatment or adherence to treatment. When cholesterol levels get too high, fatty deposits called xanthomas appear. Although the presence of xanthomas would not necessarily require medical clearance prior to exercise, the findings need to be communicated with the client, and possibly the client's physician, and monitored throughout the exercise program. A major concern with clients who have diabetes mellitus is the presence of sores or blisters. These clients are slow wound healers, and all efforts must be made to avoid making any blister or wound worse and developing new ones.

Demonstration Case Study 1.15

Inspection of Skin and Lower Extremities

Andrew is a business analyst working for a major bank. He spends most of his day sitting at a desk and often finds himself too tired to exercise when he gets off work. Andrew saw a nurse practitioner at a health clinic, and the nurse practitioner determined that Andrew has dyslipidemia and diabetes. He was medically cleared at that time to exercise. One week later, Andrew decided to start exercising, and he visited Sharon, an exercise physiologist at his company's employee wellness facility. Sharon administered a brief prescreening since Andrew was already cleared to exercise. However, since Andrew has dyslipidemia and diabetes, Sharon wants to examine his skin for sores, blisters, and xanthomas. After inspecting Andrew's skin, Sharon notes not finding the aforementioned, but she finds some swelling and redness around Andrew's right ankle and lower leg. She asks Andrew if he has lower leg pain and Andrew replied, "Yes, I have noticed a lot of pain in my right lower leg, but I have assumed the pain was from not moving enough." Sharon tells Andrew that he needs to have a medical exam to rule out something more serious.

PRE-PARTICIPATION EVALUATION (*CONTINUED*)

The final physical examine assessment discussed in this text is the pulmonary function test. A pulmonary function test is an assessment that is used for a variety of reasons. These reasons include screening for the presence or severity of obstructive or restrictive lung disease, determining the progress of therapy, documenting the progression of pulmonary disease, presurgery evaluation, and patient education. Exercise professionals conduct these tests when a client is a smoker and is 45 years and older or when a client presents with dyspnea, wheezing, chronic cough, or excessive mucus production.[15]

Pulmonary abnormalities can be grouped into two main categories: (1) obstructive defects or (2) restrictive defects. This grouping is based on spirometry measures of the flow and volume of air moved in and out of the lungs in one breath. Generally, if flow is reduced, then the defect is obstructive, and if the volume is diminished, then the defect is restrictive. Before discussing the pulmonary function test in more detail, exercise professionals need to be aware that in diagnostic settings, a pulmonary function test is conducted after the administration of a bronchodilator medicine. Therefore, in an exercise setting, no bronchodilators are used, and findings are not an indication of obstructive or restrictive diseases. Exercise professionals merely make recommendations for follow-up testing.

The common measurements of a pulmonary function test are forced vital capacity, one-second forced expiratory volume, one-second forced expiratory volume to forced vital capacity ratio, and peak expiratory flow. The forced vital capacity is the amount of air that can be voluntarily expired from the lungs. In men, the average forced vital capacity is approximately 5 liters, and in women, it is approximately 4 liters. If these values are diminished, the client may have a restrictive lung disorder, such as pneumonia, pleural effusion, or cancer. The one-second forced expiratory volume is the amount of air a client can expire in one second. The peak expiratory flow is the peak velocity of expiration. In obstructive pulmonary disorders, such as chronic obstructive pulmonary disease, both the peak expiratory flow and the one-second forced expiratory volume to forced vital capacity ratio are diminished. If the one-second forced expiratory volume to forced vital capacity ratio is less than 80%, then a referral should be made for follow-up testing.

The pulmonary function test is oftentimes an effort-based test. This is because the pulmonary function test requires a client to inhale as deeply as possible and then immediately and forcefully expel the most amount of air as possible, as fast as possible.

To conduct a pulmonary function test, exercise professionals will place a nose clip over the client's nose so that no air can escape through the nostrils. Then the client will place his or her teeth and lips around a pneumotach so that all air goes into the mouthpiece. It is important for an exercise professional to instruct the client to inhale as much air as possible and then blow it all out as fast as possible, exhaling for at least six seconds. Encouragement can be useful; therefore, the exercise professional should cheer the client on as they exhale the air, "Blow, blow, blow, squeeze all the air out, go, go, go." The best of three trials is recorded.

Demonstration Case Study 1.16

Pulmonary Function Testing

Derek is an exercise physiologist working for a preventive wellness fitness center. He regularly serves clients with chronic diseases. His most recent client was Robert. Robert is 46 years old and is obese, has hypertension, is sedentary, and a 15-year smoker. After prescreening, Derek decided to perform an abbreviated physical examination. All previous assessment findings did not warrant a recommendation for medical consultation. Given Robert is a smoker, Derek decides a pulmonary function test is appropriate. After three trials, the following data were the highest recorded:

> Forced Vital Capacity = 4.8 liters
>
> One-Second Forced Expiratory Volume = 3.99 liters

Derek determines that 4.8 liters for forced vital capacity is near normal for males. Thus Derek moves on to calculate the one-second forced expiratory volume to forced vital capacity ratio. This ratio was 83%. Therefore, Derek does not note any abnormalities and doesn't make a recommendation for medical consultation. However, Derek does recommend smoking cessation classes.

STUDENT CASE STUDIES

Student Case Study 1.1

PAR-Q+

Jerry is a 72-year-old, avid baseball fan who spent the last 45 years writing a highly successful baseball column for a major newspaper. During the baseball season, Jerry was very much physically inactive but did try to exercise in spurts during the off-season. Despite never regularly and consistently exercising, Jerry is in relatively good health with the exception of having high blood pressure. Otherwise, Jerry does not have any other medical conditions. Now that Jerry has more free time, he wants to exercise regularly to better manage his blood pressure and ward off the development of cardiovascular disease. He comes to the fitness facility and asks about membership options. Per facility policy all new members are required to complete the PAR-Q+ as a part of a prescreening process. Jerry's blood pressure is 170/92 mmHg at rest without taking his medication, Catopril. His primary care physician is managing his blood pressure, and during his last doctor's visit, his resting blood pressure was 162/90 mmHg. Jerry has never experienced chest pain, dizziness, syncope, or dyspnea nor does he have any orthopedic issues, mental issues, or spinal issues. Jerry was never told by his physician that he needs medically supervised exercise. He completes all pages of the PAR-Q+. What would Jerry's next steps be based on these results?

1. Does he need to complete pages 2 and 3 of the PAR-Q+ and why?
2. Does he need to complete the ePARmed-X+ and why?
3. Can he begin the exercise program without consultation with a physician or advanced trained exercise professional? Why?
4. Should Jerry perform moderate or vigorous exercise? Why?

Student Case Study 1.2

PAR-Q+

Samantha is a 60-year-old, recently retired school teacher. Samantha is a fan of the outdoors. She frequently hikes through the mountains, participates in amateur swimming events at the lake, and occasionally rides her bike through the metropolitan park trails. She loves to exercise. Samantha exercises five days a week, 60 minutes per day, at moderate to vigorous intensities. Samantha has had this exercise routine for 15 years. Recently, Samantha has expressed interest in preparing for a marathon. She has come to a strength and conditioning facility to participate in an expert-supervised training program. Per facility policy, all members must complete an annual PAR-Q+. Samantha notes the following regarding her health and exercise history: (1) type I diabetes for 50 years; (2) no other medical conditions; (3) no orthopedic or spinal conditions; (4) never experienced chest pain, dizziness, or dyspnea; (5) takes Lantus for her diabetes; (6) no physician orders for a medically supervised exercise program; (7) she has never had issues controlling her blood glucose nor had any signs or symptoms of hypo or hyperglycemia; (8) she desires vigorous exercise intensity; (9) she does not have signs of vascular or kidney disease and has never showed signs or symptoms of neuropathy or retinopathy; and (10) she is not pregnant nor will become pregnant. Samantha completes all pages of the PAR-Q+. What should be Samantha's next steps based on these results?

1. Does she need to complete pages 2 and 3 of the PAR-Q+ and why?
2. Does she need to complete the ePARmed-X+ and why?

3. Can she begin the exercise program without consultation with a physician or advanced trained exercise professional? Why?
4. Should Samantha perform moderate or vigorous exercise? Why?

Student Case Study 1.3

PAR-Q+

Camila is a 41-year-old, mother of three. Camila recently gave birth to her third child and is having trouble losing her pregnancy weight. Therefore, she has decided to seek out a supervised fitness program for weight loss at a health-fitness facility. Per facility policy, all new members must complete a PAR-Q+. Camila is told the purpose of the PAR-Q+ and then the survey is administered. Camila notes the following regarding her health and exercise history: (1) asthma; (2) no other medical conditions; (3) no orthopedic or spinal conditions; (4) never experienced chest pain, dizziness, or dyspnea; (5) takes albuterol for her asthma; (6) no physician orders for a medically supervised exercise program; (7) she has never had issues controlling her asthma or experienced any cardiovascular or respiratory symptoms; (8) she never needed a rescue inhaler; (9) she has never had a physician say her oxygen levels are too low or that she has pulmonary hypertension; (10) she is not pregnant nor will she become pregnant; and (11) she used to do yoga before her last pregnancy but hasn't exercised in 12 months. Camila completes all pages of the PAR-Q+. What should Samantha's next steps be based on these results?

1. Does she need to complete pages 2 and 3 of the PAR-Q+ and why?
2. Does she need to complete the ePARmed-X+ and why?
3. Can she begin the exercise program without consultation with a physician or advanced trained exercise professional? Why?
4. Should Camila perform moderate or vigorous exercise? Why?

Student Case Study 1.4

Exercise Pre-participation Health Screening Questionnaire for Exercise Professionals

Mark is a 50-year-old male who is obese and has recently been diagnosed with osteo-arthritis. Mark has always been concerned with his weight, and now with his arthritis, he is more concerned about his weight. Mark fears that he will only continue to gain weight, thus making him even more susceptible to cardiovascular disease. However, with his arthritis, he isn't sure as to what kind of exercises he can safely perform. Therefore, he visits his local hospital's weight-loss exercise clinic for help. He meets with the lead exercise physiologist. He tells Mark that he needs to conduct a prescreening survey to make sure it is safe for him to exercise. The Exercise Pre-participation Health Screening Questionnaire for Exercise Professionals is administered. Mark says that he has never felt chest pain with exertion, unusual breathlessness, or dizziness; has never fainted or blacked out; has never noticed any forceful or rapid heartbeats; and has never had any lower leg cramps. The exercise physiologist decides to be thorough in the screening of Mark and chooses to examine Marks's ankles. Mark does not have any ankle swelling.

He moves on to step 2 of the questionnaire. Here Mark tells that he does not exercise, as he is afraid of hurting himself. Then he moves on to step 3 of the questionnaire. Here, it is determined that Mark does not have any existing cardiovascular, metabolic, or renal diseases. Also, Mark has never had a cardiovascular surgery

1. Does Mark have any major signs or symptoms suggestive of cardiovascular, metabolic, or renal diseases? If so, which ones? If not, explain why not.
2. Is Mark physically active? Why or why not?
3. Based on the results of the Exercise Pre-participation Health Screening Questionnaire for Exercise Professionals, does Mark need medical clearance from a licensed physician before beginning or continuing an exercise program? Why or why not?
4. Based on the results of the Exercise Pre-participation Health Screening Questionnaire for Exercise Professionals, can Mark exercise at low to moderate exercise intensity? Why or why not?
5. Based on the results of the Exercise Pre-participation Health Screening Questionnaire for Exercise Professionals, can Mark exercise at vigorous exercise intensity? Why or why not?

Student Case Study 1.5

Exercise Pre-participation Health Screening Questionnaire for Exercise Professionals

Bethany is a 61-year-old female who recently visited her physician for an annual physical. After the physical, Bethany's physician recommended lab work to check her lipids and glycosylated hemoglobin. A follow-up physician visit was scheduled to go over the lab results. The lab results revealed high LDL-c levels and total cholesterol suggesting dyslipidemia. Also, the lab results showed high glycosylated hemoglobin. Because of the high lipid and glucose levels, Bethany's physician recommended regular exercise and an appointment with an endocrinologist. The endocrinologist conducted a two-hour oral glucose tolerance test and diagnosed Bethany with type II diabetes mellitus.

Bethany follows through with her physician's recommendation to begin an exercise program. She meets with the lead exercise physiologist at a health-fitness facility. Upon meeting with Bethany, she answers a series of questions prior to exercise testing and exercise participation. The Exercise Pre-participation Health Screening Questionnaire for Exercise Professionals is administered to prescreen Bethany. Bethany is asked questions about signs and symptoms. Bethany says that she has never experienced chest pain with activity, uncomfortable shortness of breath, dizziness, fainting, blackouts, or lower leg cramps. Bethany does claim to have experienced irregular heartbeats. Bethany's ankles are examined for edema. There is swelling in Bethany's left ankle and no swelling in the right ankle. The swelling appears to be nonpitting, and there is no warmth or redness. Bethany then mentions that she sprained her ankle three days ago walking to her car.

The exercise physiologist continues questioning Bethany. Bethany tells that she stays active by gardening and stretching every day when she wakes up. She moves on to step 3 of the questionnaire. Here it is determined that Bethany has type II diabetes mellitus but no other cardiometabolic or renal diseases. It is also found that Bethany had an aortic valve replacement when she was a child because of a birth defect.

1. Does Bethany have any major signs or symptoms suggestive of cardiovascular, metabolic, or renal diseases? If so, which ones? If not, explain why not.
2. Is Bethany physically active? Why or why not?
3. Based on the results of the Exercise Pre-participation Health Screening Questionnaire for Exercise Professionals, does Bethany need medical clearance from a licensed physician before beginning or continuing an exercise program? Why or why not?
4. Based on the results of the Exercise Pre-participation Health Screening Questionnaire for Exercise Professionals, can Bethany exercise at low to moderate exercise intensity? Why or why not?
5. Based on the results of the Exercise Pre-participation Health Screening Questionnaire for Exercise Professionals, can Bethany exercise at vigorous exercise intensity? Why or why not?

Student Case Study 1.6

Exercise Pre-participation Health Screening Questionnaire for Exercise Professionals

Samuel is a 44-year-old male who has battled asthma since he was a child. He has noticed his symptoms worsen with everyday activity, and he feels it is necessary to begin an exercise program to hopefully limit shortness of breath with daily activities. Therefore, Samuel decides to visit the wellness facility at his company's corporate headquarters.

He meets with the company's health and fitness specialist. She tells Samuel that he needs to answer some questions about his symptoms, physical activity, and past medical history. She uses the Exercise Pre-participation Health Screening Questionnaire for Exercise Professionals to gather this information. For step 1, Samuel says that he never experienced chest pain, dizziness, or fainting; forceful or rapid heartbeats; or lower leg cramps. He does say that he experiences shortness of breath during normal activities, such as walking up stairs, standing from a seated position, and when walking longer than three minutes. Samuel's ankles show no swelling.

Next, she asks Samuel about his exercise history, and he says that he gets too short of breath, therefore, he doesn't exercise. They move on to step 3 of the questionnaire, which involves asking Samuel about his past medical history. Samuel says that he has never been diagnosed with any disease, except asthma, and has never had surgery.

1. Does Samuel have any major signs or symptoms suggestive of cardiovascular, metabolic, or renal diseases? If so, which ones? If not, explain why not.
2. Is Samuel physically active? Why or why not?
3. Based on the results of the Exercise Pre-participation Health Screening Questionnaire for Exercise Professionals, does Samuel need medical clearance from a licensed physician before beginning or continuing an exercise program? Why or why not?
4. Based on the results of the Exercise Pre-participation Health Screening Questionnaire for Exercise Professionals, can Samuel exercise at low to moderate exercise intensity? Why or why not?
5. Based on the results of the Exercise Pre-participation Health Screening Questionnaire for Exercise Professionals, can Samuel exercise at vigorous exercise intensity? Why or why not?

Student Case Study 1.7

ACSM's Pre-participation Health Screening Algorithm

Alana is 44-year-old female who is burdened by lower leg cramps. These cramps limit Alana's ability to walk longer distances and are hampering her capacity to fully enjoy life. She recently heard that exercise could help with her condition and thus decides to visit the hospital's vascular rehabilitation clinic. There she meets with the head clinical exercise physiologist. He tells Alana that since the facility is a hospital-based exercise program, all new participants need to go through a thorough prescreening process to maximize exercise safety. The prescreening tool used is the ACSM's Pre-participation Health Screening Algorithm.

He begins the screening by asking Alana about her exercise behavior. Alana says that since it hurts too bad to walk longer distances, the only exercise she does is with resistance bands. Alana says that she uses light resistance bands to exercise three days per week and that each training session lasts 25 minutes. Alana has done this exercise routine for the last two years. Since this is a hospital-based program, the exercise physiologist has access to Alana's health records, and he notices the following: (1) asthma diagnosis in 2002, (2) meningitis diagnosis in 2003, (3) fibromyalgia diagnosis in 2008, (4) arthroscopic knee surgery in 2013, and (5) peripheral vascular disease diagnosis in 2017. He then asks Alana about her signs and symptoms that could be associated with cardiovascular, metabolic, or renal diseases. Alana claims that she has never experienced chest pain, shortness of breath, dizziness, fainting, or blackout with exertion. Alana also says that she has never felt short of breath while lying down or sleeping, never felt rapid and forceful heartbeats, and no unusual shortness of breath. Alana notes that she has lower leg pain and cramps while walking and that the pain and cramping goes away with rest.

1. Should she get medical clearance before beginning? Why?
2. Should she perform moderate or vigorous exercise? Why?
3. Should she get medical clearance before progressing to higher intensities? Why?

Student Case Study 1.8

ACSM's Pre-participation Health Screening Algorithm

Barry is 59-year-old male, recently retired college baseball coach. Barry was incredibly active during his coaching years and has no intentions of slowing down. Barry's main concern about exercise is that he had a small "brain bleed" when coaching at the age of 45. He visits an exercise facility to begin a supervised exercise program.

Being concerned with Barry's past "brain bleed," the exercise physiologist decides to be thorough and administers the ACSM's Pre-participation Health Screening Algorithm as a prescreening tool. Barry is an excellent client and brings his full medical history. In Barry's medical history the exercise physiologist finds the following: (1) knee ligament repair (anterior cruciate ligament) surgery in 2000, (2) herniated L5 vertebra disc in 2002, (3) pneumonia in 2003, and (4) subarachnoid hemorrhage because of cerebrovascular aneurysm in 2004. Barry is then asked about signs and symptoms suggestive of cardiovascular, metabolic, or renal diseases. Barry provides the following information: (1) no chest pain with exertion, (2) no shortness of breath with exertion or when laying down or sleeping, (3) no rapid and forceful heartbeats, (4) no lower leg cramps, (5) no ankle swelling, (6) no known murmurs, (7) dizziness in 2004 with the "brain bleed," and (8) no unusual fatigue or shortness of breath. Then, Barry is asked about his exercise habits, and Barry says that he exercises every day of the week. Three days per week, Barry runs five miles at a heart rate equal to 60 percent of his heart rate reserve, two days per week Barry lifts weights, and two days per week Barry golfs and never rides in the cart. To be thorough, the exercise physiologist asks Barry when the last time he was cleared to exercise by his doctor. Barry says he was last evaluated and cleared by his doctor 13 months ago.

1. Should he get medical clearance before beginning? Why?
2. Should he perform moderate or vigorous exercise? Why?
3. Should he get medical clearance before progressing to higher intensities? Why?

Kylie is 29-year-old female, school teacher. Kylie has noticed some weight gain and is terrified about becoming obese and developing cardiovascular disease like her mother and father. In light of this recent weight gain, Kylie decides to visit a women's health and exercise clinic. There she meets with the facilities lead wellness coordinator. She briefly interviews Kylie and finds out she wants to be held accountable for exercising regularly and that she feels it's best to follow a rigid exercise protocol.

She tells Kylie that she wants to conduct a prescreening using the ACSM's Pre-participation Health Screening Algorithm. She starts by asking Kylie about her current exercise habits. Kylie claims to exercise three days per week by walking on the treadmill, 30 minutes each session, for the last two years. She further probes Kylie about her exercise. She asks her about her heart rate during exercise, and she claims to exercise at a heart rate of 150 beats per minute. She determines this is equivalent to 55 percent of Kylie's heart rate reserve.

Moving on with the screening, she asks Kylie about her past medical history. She finds out that Kylie was diagnosed with hypothyroidism in 2016, dysmenorrhea in 2014, and an eating disorder in 2013. Other than these conditions, Kylie has not been diagnosed with any medical condition. She then asks Kylie when was the last time she was cleared to exercise by a physician. Kylie states she was last cleared eight months ago. She lastly asks about Kylie's symptoms, and she provides the following information: (1) no chest pain with exertion, (2) no shortness of breath with exertion or when laying down or sleeping, (3) no rapid and forceful heartbeats, (4) no lower leg cramps, (5) no ankle swelling, (6) no known murmurs, (7) no dizziness or syncope, and (8) no unusual fatigue or shortness of breath.

1. Should she get medical clearance before beginning? Why?
2. Should she perform moderate or vigorous exercise? Why?
3. Should she get medical clearance before progressing to higher intensities? Why?

Two friends decide to open up an exercise facility to serve clients who are obese. They will offer abbreviated physical examinations, exercise testing, exercise prescriptions, exercise and diet education, and supervised exercise programing. Once the facility and equipment are procured, they need to write a document of informed consent. Write all necessary information for a client at the facility to provide voluntary consent to participate in the services. Be sure the writing is thorough yet easily comprehendible by prospective clients. The writing should include information about (1) explanation and purpose of services, (2) procedures of offered services, (3) benefits and risks, (4) how you will ensure confidentiality, (5) emergency procedures, (6) opportunities for clients to ask questions, and (7) freedom of voluntary consent and withdraw.

Student Case Study 1.11

Cardiovascular Disease Risk Factor Analysis

An exercise physiologist is serving a client with type II diabetes. The client completed diabetes rehabilitation one year ago and wants to exercise under the supervision of an advanced trained exercise professional. Following prescreening, it was determined that the client needed physician's approval to complete exercise testing and an exercise program. The approval was granted one week ago. The exercise physiologist wants to be thorough in gathering information from the client and track her cardiovascular disease risk factors. The following information about the client is found: (1) female, age 53, smoked one pack per day for 15 years, quit five months ago; (2) drinks alcohol on Friday and Saturday nights; (3) height = 63 inches, weight = 175 pounds; (4) blood pressure = 142/78 mmHg; (5) total cholesterol = 210 mg/dL; (6) fasting blood glucose = 128 mg/dL; (7) HDL-c = 41 mg/dL; (8) LDL-c = 132 mg/dL; (9) 160 minutes of exercise per week at moderate intensity for the last four months, and (10) father had a heart attack at age 65.

1. What are the positive risk factors for cardiovascular disease?
2. Why is each risk factor in question 1 qualified as a positive risk factor?
3. What is the negative risk factors for cardiovascular disease?
4. Why is each risk factor in question 3 qualified as a negative risk factor?
5. Which risk factors does the client not have?
6. Why is each risk factor in question 5 not qualified as a risk factor?
7. How many risk factors does the client have?
8. What lifestyle changes would you recommend? Why?

Student Case Study 1.12

Cardiovascular Disease Risk Factor Analysis

A weight-loss consultant serves a client who has battled overweightness and obesity for many years. The client has tried fad diets and novel exercise programs in the past and now wants to exercise under the supervision of a clinical exercise professional. Following prescreening, it was determined that the client did not need a physician's approval to complete exercise testing and an exercise program. The exercise physiologist decides that since the client is considered to be a part of a special population, she should track and monitor his cardiovascular disease risk factors. She obtains the following information about the client: (1) male, age 45; (2) quit smoking 7 months ago; (3) height = 75 inches, weight = 230 pounds; (4) blood pressure = 128/88 mmHg; (5) LDL-c = 100 mg/dL, HDL-c = 62 mg/dL; (6) fasting blood glucose = 104 mg/dL; (7) exercises four days per week, moderate aerobic exercise intensity, last two months; and (8) mother had a heart attack at age 64 and father died of suddenly following cardiac symptoms at the age of 75.

1. What are the positive risk factors for cardiovascular disease?
2. Why is each risk factor in question 1 qualified as a positive risk factor?
3. What is the negative risk factors for cardiovascular disease?
4. Why is each risk factor in question 3 qualified as a negative risk factor?
5. Which risk factors does the client not have?
6. Why is each risk factor in question 5 not qualified as a risk factor?
7. How many risk factors does the client have?
8. What lifestyle changes would you recommend? Why?

Student Case Study 1.13

Cardiovascular Disease Risk Factor Analysis

A clinical exercise physiologist is serving a client who has a history of metabolic syndrome. The client has put forth minimal effort in controlling this condition but now wants to put forth the effort and thus seeks to exercise under the supervision of an exercise professional. Following prescreening, it was determined that the client did not need a physician's approval to complete exercise testing and an exercise program. The exercise professional decides that since the client has a history of metabolic syndrome, she wants to track and monitor her cardiovascular disease risk factors. She obtains the following information about the client: (1) female, age 55; (2) quit smoking five months ago; (3) height = 66 inches, weight = 140 pounds; (4) blood pressure = 132/84; (5) no lipid values available; (6) fasting blood glucose = 89 mg/dL; (7) 75 minutes of exercise per week at a vigorous intensity for the previous five months; and (8) mother had a coronary artery bypass graft at age 64.

1. What are the positive risk factors for cardiovascular disease?
2. Why is each risk factor in question 1 qualified as a positive risk factor?
3. What is the negative risk factors for cardiovascular disease?
4. Why is each risk factor in question 3 qualified as a negative risk factor?
5. Which risk factors does the client not have?
6. Why is each risk factor in question 5 not qualified as a risk factor?
7. How many risk factors does the client have?
8. What lifestyle changes would you recommend? Why?

Cardiovascular Disease Risk Factor Analysis

A clinical exercise physiologist is serving a client who recently defeated breast cancer. The client has been physically limited during her cancer treatment but is now ready to begin an exercise program to help build back up her physical health. Following prescreening, it was determined that the client did not need a physician's approval to complete exercise testing and an exercise program. The exercise physiologist decides that since the client had cancer, she wants to assess her cardiovascular disease risk factors. She obtains the following information about the client: (1) female, age 54; (2) nonsmoker; (3) height = 71 inches, weight = 205 pounds; (4) waist circumference = 36 inches; (5) blood pressure = 118/82 mmHg; (6) takes enalapril; (7) LDL-c = 110 mg/dL, HDL-c = 44 mg/dL, total cholesterol = 197 mmHg; (8) fasting blood glucose = 127 mg/dL; (9) nonexerciser; and (10) mother was diagnosed with chronic obstructive pulmonary disease at the age of 60, father passed away of a stroke at the age of 66.

1. What are the positive risk factors for cardiovascular disease?
2. Why is each risk factor in question 1 qualified as a positive risk factor?
3. What is the negative risk factors for cardiovascular disease?
4. Why is each risk factor in question 3 qualified as a negative risk factor?
5. Which risk factors does the client not have?
6. Why is each risk factor in question 5 not qualified as a risk factor?
7. How many risk factors does the client have?
8. What lifestyle changes would you recommend? Why?

Cardiovascular Disease Risk Factor Analysis

A clinical exercise physiologist is serving a client who recently completed vascular rehabilitation. The client saw improvements in her claudication threshold and now wants to continue with an exercise program at a facility. Following prescreening, it was determined that the client did not need a physician's approval to complete exercise testing and an exercise program. The exercise physiologist decides that since the client has a history of vascular disease, she wants to track and monitor the client's cardiovascular disease risk factors. She obtains the following information about the client: (1) female, age 65; (2) smokes two packs of cigarettes per day; (3) height = 64 inches, waist circumference = 34 inches; (4) blood pressure = 104/68 mmHg; (5) LDL-c = 129 mg/dL, HDL-c = 62 mg/dL; (6) takes the medication atorvastatin; (7) fasting blood glucose = 120 mg/dL; (8) exercises on the treadmill 5 days per week, 30 minutes per session, at a perceived exertion of 15, for the last 7 months; and (9) mother had lung cancer at age 61, father died of a heart attack at age 81.

1. What are the positive risk factors for cardiovascular disease?
2. Why is each risk factor in question 1 qualified as a positive risk factor?
3. What are the negative risk factors for cardiovascular disease?
4. Why is the risk factor in question 3 qualified as a negative risk factor?
5. Which risk factors does the client not have?
6. Why is each risk factor in question 5 not qualified as a risk factor?
7. How many risk factors does the client have?
8. What lifestyle changes would you recommend? Why?

Student Case Study 1.16

Medical History

An exercise physiologist just recently successfully opened a weight-loss exercise facility intended to serve clients who are either overweight or obese. The mission of the facility is clear: to help reduce the risk for chronic disease among those with trouble controlling their body weight. In fulfilling this mission, it is necessary to obtain information about clients' medical histories. Since the facility is not a part of a hospital and does not provide medically billable services, the facility has to obtain the clients' medical histories by administering a medical history questionnaire. Write a medical history questionnaire that is most appropriate for the facility. Be sure the writing is comprehendible for the clients and is intended to obtain the following information: (1) medical diagnoses; (2) physical examination findings; (3) laboratory values; (4) history of symptoms; (5) surgical procedures; (6) illnesses; (7) medications; (8) drug allergies; (9) tobacco, alcohol, and drug use; (10) exercise history; (11) work history; and (12) family history.

Student Case Study 1.17

Assessment of Pulses

An exercise physiologist is working for a risk reduction fitness clinic. She meets with Simon, a passenger jet pilot who is seeking an exercise program to help lower his blood glucose and cholesterol. She administers the ACSM's Pre-participation Health Screening Algorithm and finds that Simon does not need medical clearance to participate in exercise testing and an exercise program. Since she is serving a client with a higher risk for cardiovascular, metabolic, and renal disease. She decides to perform an abbreviated physical examination. The first exam that she conducts is an assessment of apical and radial pulse. She records an apical pulse of 100 beats per minute and a radial pulse of 85 beats per minute. She checks Simon's medical history, and she does not find any cardiac medical conditions. Therefore, she does another apical and radial pulse assessment to make sure she did not make a mistake. The second attempt shows similar results.

1. Describe how to assess Simon's apical pulse. Be sure to include the specific anatomical location of where the stethoscope should be placed, why the stethoscope should be placed there, and what specific sounds are to be heard.
2. What sounds would be indicative of one full heart beat?
3. Describe how to assess Simon's radial pulse. Be sure to include the anatomical location of where to place the fingers. Which fingers should be used to feel for a radial pulse? Why?
4. What is the normal heart rate range?
5. Does Simon's heart rate fall within this range?
6. Does an apical-radial pulse deficit exist? If so, how so? If not, why not? What could an apical-radial pulse deficit indicate?
7. What recommendation should be made regarding Simon's immediate participation in exercise testing and programming? Why was this recommendation made?

Student Case Study 1.18

Blood Pressure Assessment

A personal trainer is working for a corporate wellness program aimed at reducing the company's employees' risk for developing chronic diseases. The personal trainer meets with Jamie, a client who is seeking an exercise program to help her manage her type I diabetes. The personal trainer determines, initially, that Jamie does not need a medical exam after administering the Pre-participation Exercise Health Screening Questionnaire for Exercise Professionals. He decides to conduct some physical examination assessments, one of them being blood pressure. He records Jamie's blood pressure at 184/92 mmHg. This is a notably high blood pressure, so he asks Jamie about her symptoms and history with hypertension. Jamie notes being treated for hypertension with medication, but she forgot to take her medication that morning. Jamie also mentions not feeling any symptoms associated with high blood pressure.

1. Describe the complete process for assessing a client's blood pressure.
2. How long before a blood pressure assessment should a client avoid consuming food and caffeinated beverages? How about using tobacco? How about exercise?
3. What specifically should be listened for when trying to record systolic blood pressure?
4. What specifically should be listened for when trying to record diastolic blood pressure?
5. Should Jamie seek medical consultation prior to exercise testing and participation in regular exercise? Why or why not?

Student Case Study 1.19

Clayton is an accountant working for a large manufacturer. He spends most of his day sitting at a desk. Clayton is very much physically inactive, and his diabetes, cholesterol, and blood pressure have all gotten worse. In light of these changes in Clayton's health, his physician medically cleared him to begin exercising two weeks ago. Now, Clayton reports to a fitness facility. The lead exercise specialist wants to conduct some physical examination assessments. One of the appropriate assessments is an inspection of the skin and lower extremities.

1. Why would it be appropriate to assess Clayton's skin? Are there specific health conditions that Clayton has that would warrant this inspection?
2. What specifically should one be looking for on Clayton's skin? If these things are present, what may have caused their appearance?
3. Why would it be appropriate to assess Clayton's lower extremities? Are there specific health conditions that Clayton has that would warrant this inspection?
4. What specifically should one be looking for on Clayton's lower extremities? What would cause those abnormal findings?
5. What findings would need to be monitored during exercise training? Why?
6. What findings would warrant a recommendation for medical consultation? Why?

Student Case Study 1.20

Pulmonary Function Testing

An exercise physiologist is working for an employee health clinic. A client, Gary, is 50 years old, has hypertension, dyslipidemia, is obese, and a 30-pack per year cigarette smoker. After prescreening, it is determined that Gary needs medical clearance to exercise as he is physically inactive and had a myocardial infarction seven years ago. After physician clearance, an abbreviated physical examination is performed. All previous assessment findings did not warrant a recommendation for medical consultation. Given that Gary is a smoker, the exercise physiologist decides to conduct a pulmonary function test. After three trials, the following data were the highest recorded:

Forced Vital Capacity = 4.4 liters

One-Second Forced Expiratory Volume = 3.52 liters

1. Was Gary's force vital capacity within normal limits? If not, why? If Gary's forced vital capacity was not normal, would it be indicative of a restrictive or obstructive pulmonary disorder?

2. What was Gary's one-second forced expiratory volume to forced vital capacity ratio?
3. Should Gary follow up with a physician regarding any of his findings? Why or why not?

Student Case Study 1.21

Comprehensive Case Study

An exercise professional is working at Stay in Motion, a health-fitness facility that provides fitness programming for clients of special populations. The exercise professional meets with Sandra, a new client interested in enrolling in a fitness program. After conducting a prescreening and evaluation of Sandra, the following health, exercise, and medical information was found:

Demographics: (1) female, (2) 55 years old, (3) environmental exposure to cigarette smoke, and (4) walks 3 days per week, 25 minutes per day, 45 percent of heart rate reserve, previous 3 months.

Family History: (1) grandmother had a fatal stroke at age 66, (2) grandfather had a fatal myocardial infarction at age 62, (3) grandmother died of natural causes at age 85, (4) grandfather died of cancer at age 71, (5) father died of kidney failure at age 67, (7) mother had triple coronary artery bypass surgery at age 54, and (8) younger sister had a fatal asthma attack at age 45.

Biometrics: (1) resting heart rate = 75 beats per minute; (2) apical pulse = 82 beats per minute; (3) radial pulse = 77 beats per minute; (4) resting blood pressure = 142/76 mmHg; (5) LDL-c = 129 mg/dL, HDL-c = 41 mg/dL, total cholesterol = 199 mg/dL; (6) glycosylated hemoglobin = 5.6 percent; and (7) height = 68 inches, weight = 185 pounds, waist circumference = 41 inches

Medical Diagnoses: (1) type I diabetes mellitus, (2) polymyositis, (3) polycystic kidney disease, (4) asthma, (5) rheumatoid arthritis, (6) fibromyalgia, and (7) last medical examination and clearance was 14 months ago

Medications: (1) lovastatin, (2) metoprolol, (3) NovoLog, (4) Prednisone, (5) formoterol, and (6) quinapril

Symptoms: (1) signs and symptoms associated with type I diabetes, (2) inconsistent management of blood glucose, (3) chest pain with exertion, (4) paroxysmal forceful heartbeats, and (5) right ankle pain, redness, and edema.

Physical Examination Findings: (1) apical pulse = 82 beats per minute, (2) radial pulse = 77 beats per minute, (3) resting seated blood pressure = 142/86 mmHg, (4) standing blood pressure = 144/76 mmHg, (5) supine blood pressure = 142/78 mmHg, (6) xanthomas above the eyes, (7) unhealed blisters on the inferior surfaces of the feet, (8) right ankle edema, (9) right lower leg edema and redness, (10) forced vital capacity = 4.5 liters, and (11) one-second forced expiratory volume = 4.05 liters

1. By using the PAR-Q+ and ePARmed-X+, if necessary, make a recommendation for Sandra regarding the need for medical clearance prior to exercise testing and participation. Why was this recommendation made?
2. By using the Exercise Pre-participation Health Screening Questionnaire for Exercise Professionals, make a recommendation for Sandra regarding the need for medical clearance prior to exercise testing and participation. Why was this recommendation made?
3. By using the ACSM's Pre-participation Health Screening Algorithm, make a recommendation for Sandra regarding the need for medical clearance prior to exercise testing and participation. Why was this recommendation made?
4. Was the recommendation regarding medical clearance different among any of the prescreening tools in questions 1 through 3? If differences are noted, what would be the professional implication for prescreening clients with chronic diseases?
5. What are the positive risk factors that Sandra has for cardiovascular disease? Why is each considered a risk factor?
6. What, if any, physical examination findings would be concerning to Sandra's exercise trainer? Why?
7. Why was an inspection of the skin and lower extremity performed on Sandra?
8. Why was a pulmonary function test conducted on Sandra?
9. Should Sandra consult with a physician regarding her pulmonary function?
10. Taking in all of the presented information, can Sandra proceed to exercise testing, prescription, and participation without having sought medical clearance? Why or why not?

REFERENCES

1. American College of Sports Medicine, *ACSM's Guidelines for Exercise Testing and Prescription*, 11th ed. (Philadelphia: Wolters Kluwer Health, 2022).
2. S. S. Bredin, N. Gledhill, V. K. Jamnik, and D. E. Warburton, "PAR-Q+ and ePARmed-X+: New Risk Stratification and Physical Activity Clearance Strategies for Physicians and Patients Alike," *Canadian Family Physician* 59, no. 3 (2013): 273–77.
3. ibid.
4. M. Magal and D. Riebe, "New Preparticipation Health Screening Recommendations: What Exercise Professionals Need to Know," *ACSM Health Fitness Journal* 20, no. 3 (2022): 22–27.
5. American College of Sports Medicine, *ACSM's Guidelines*, 2022.
6. ibid.
7. G. A. Borg, *Borg's Perceived Exertion and Pain Scales* (Champaign, IL: Human Kinetics, 1998).
8. American College of Sports Medicine, *ACSM's Guidelines*, 2022.

9. A. S. Go, D. Mozzaffarian, R. L. Veronique, et al. "Heart Disease and Stroke Statistics—2014 Update: A Report from the American Heart Association," *Circulation* 129, no. 3 (2014): e28–e92.

10. American College of Sports Medicine, *ACSM's Guidelines*, 2022.

11. ibid.

12. Borg, *Borg's Perceived*, 1998.

13. C. S. Fox, S. H. Golden, C. Anderson, et al. "Update on Cardiovascular Disease in Adults with Type 2 Diabetes Mellitus in Light of Recent Evidence: A Scientific Statement from the American Heart Association and the American Diabetes Association," *Circulation*, 132 (2015): 691–718.

14. American College of Sports Medicine, *ACSM's Guidelines*, 2022

15. ibid.

CHAPTER 2

Principles of Exercise Testing and Prescription for Special Populations

INTRODUCTION

I N THE FIRST chapter, the focus was on reducing the risk of exercise-induced negative health events when serving clients with chronic diseases. This was accomplished by introducing the purposes and procedures for various pre-exercise screening and evaluation methods. This chapter will introduce and discuss the next three steps in developing exercise programs for special populations: exercise testing, exercise test interpretation, and exercise prescription. Specifically, this chapter will discuss how common exercise tests are selected and conducted, how they can be modified for special populations, and how these tests are interpreted. As with other chapters, relevant case studies will be provided.

Like serving apparently healthy clients, to write safe and effective exercise prescriptions, exercise professionals need to understand the fitness levels and limitations of their clients. This is accomplished by conducting a series of exercise tests. Ideally, exercise tests should evaluate each component of health-related physical fitness.[1] These components are cardiorespiratory endurance, body composition, muscular strength, muscular endurance, and flexibility.[2] When serving special populations, the procedures for conducting exercise tests are fairly like conducting exercise tests on apparently healthy populations. However, it is important for exercise professionals to understand that clients with certain medical conditions and diseases will need to have exercise test procedures modified to accommodate specific needs. In general, when conducting exercise tests on clients with chronic diseases, exercise professionals need to pay very close attention to their client's physiological responses to exercise, any abnormal signs or symptoms, pretest medication status, and individual contraindications for testing. Each of these will be discussed as they pertain to specific special populations in later chapters.

Following exercise testing and interpretation, exercise professionals begin to develop an exercise prescription for their clients. Exercise prescriptions are put together with all possible available information. The information gathered for the development of an exercise prescription is obtained not only from exercise test results, but they are put together with knowledge of a client's exercise goals, medical history, cardiovascular disease risk factors, and exercise history. Together this information provides an exercise professional with enough data to construct and individualize an exercise prescription. An important truth about an exercise prescription is that the more an exercise prescription is individualized, the more desirable the result will be. This is an incredibly important truth for exercise professionals to keep in mind when prescribing exercise to clients with chronic diseases. After all, a primary goal of a client with a chronic disease is to better control, manage, or attenuate that disease.

As with writing exercise prescriptions for apparently healthy clients, exercise prescriptions for special populations are written according to the FITT-VP principle.[3] Here, the frequency, intensity, time, type, volume, and progression are individualized to meet a client's needs and goals. When serving clients with chronic diseases, the FITT-VP principle frequently needs to be modified. Modification of the FITT-VP principle for individual special populations will be presented in later chapters. This chapter will focus on the application of the FITT-VP principle for writing an initial exercise prescription for improving cardiorespiratory endurance, muscle fitness, and flexibility.

The purpose of this chapter is to teach students how to apply their knowledge of exercise testing and prescription for special populations. On completion of the case studies, students will be able to achieve the following:

1. Determine appropriate exercise tests for assessing cardiorespiratory endurance, body composition, muscle fitness, and flexibility
2. Identify the contraindications for exercise testing
3. Identify the criteria for stopping an exercise test
4. Interpret cardiorespiratory, body composition, muscle fitness, and flexibility tests
5. Use exercise test data to design an exercise prescription for improving cardiorespiratory endurance, muscle fitness, and flexibility in accordance with the FITT-VP principle
6. Use metabolic equations to set exercise intensity for cardiorespiratory endurance
7. Use maximal strength estimates to prescribe exercise intensity for muscle fitness

EXERCISE TESTING

Exercise testing primarily serves as a method to obtain baseline data for designing an exercise prescription and to obtain data that can be tracked and monitored over the course of an exercise program. This enables exercise professionals to constantly make changes and alterations to initial exercise prescriptions to bring about the desired physiological outcomes in their clients. Oftentimes, when serving clients from special populations, the desired physiological outcome is paramount in managing a given disease or comorbidity. Moreover, when clients see improvements in their exercise tests, it helps to increase exercise adherence.

Ideally, exercise professionals will select exercise tests that evaluate each component of health-related physical fitness. At the very least, when exercise professionals serve clients with chronic diseases, cardiorespiratory endurance must be assessed. The rationale for this is a powerful indirect correlation between cardiorespiratory endurance and the development of cardiometabolic diseases and comorbidities.[4] When selecting exercise tests, it is important for exercise professionals to consider safety, validity, reliability, availability of equipment, and specificity.

Safety begins with pre-exercise screening and evaluation, as discussed in Chapter 1. Clients with orthopedic limitations, who are deconditioned or have chronic or acute diseases or illnesses need to be tested in a manner that limits the likelihood of exercise-induced health complications. Examples of ensuring safety include knowing the contraindications for testing, test termination criteria, and monitoring appropriate physiological variables during a test.[5]

To ensure validity, exercise tests must evaluate the specific component of health-related physical fitness being targeted for improvement during exercise training. Simply, an exercise test must test what it is supposed to test. For instance, if an established goal of an exercise program is improving cardiorespiratory endurance, then the test must elicit a progressive cardiovascular and respiratory response. This means an appropriate test would be one that results in the gradual increase in cardiac output, blood pressure, and minute ventilation. Thus a test like the push-up test would not be a valid test for evaluating cardiorespiratory endurance. Instead, a test such as the Bruce treadmill test would be most appropriate.

When conducting exercise tests, exercise professionals should ensure that the exercise test results are repeatable. This is the characteristic of reliability. Reliability is highest when exercise professionals adhere to strict testing procedures. For instance, when conducting a maximal strength test, the procedures for adding resistance and rest and recovery time from one trial to the next must be the same from one test to the next. Otherwise, factors like fatigue may blunt the test result from one client to the next or from one data collection point to the next. Such errors in testing lead to the development of poor exercise prescriptions and the failure of clients to achieve their goals. From a practical standpoint, when working with special populations, the failure of a client to achieve his or her exercise goals can have a negative influence on a client's overall health.

The availability of equipment is always a concern when conducting exercise tests. Oftentimes, the most accurate test is the most expensive test. Therefore, exercise professionals should conduct the most accurate tests with the equipment and budgetary resources they have available. A classic example of this is the assessment of body composition. Tests like hydrostatic weighing, air displacement plethysmography, and duel-energy X-ray absorptiometry are more accurate assessments of body composition than a simple bioelectrical impedance test. However, these assessments are highly expensive and require advanced training for professionals. Thus a less expensive test would be enough, so long as the exercise professional adheres to testing procedures.

Lastly, specificity must be considered. Specificity, in an exercise testing context, refers to selecting exercise tests that evaluate aspects of physical fitness that align with a client's exercise goals. The reasons for this are that a client's goals need to be tracked throughout an exercise program, and a client's exercise prescription is based, in part, on these goals. An example of specificity would be testing waist circumference for clients who are obese with the goal of reducing central adiposity.

EXERCISE TEST SELECTION

Exercise test selection begins with an analysis of a client's needs, goals, and physical limitations with issues of safety, validity, reliability, and specificity kept in mind. When working with special populations, exercise professionals will have to determine aspects of the client's physiology needs to be addressed to better control or manage a given medical condition. Then exercise professionals must consider what a client wants to accomplish through regular exercise. By accounting for a client's goals, adherence to an exercise program will be improved. An equally important consideration to be made when working with special populations is a client's physical limitations. The rationale for knowing a client's physical limitations is that certain tests cannot be physically performed by the client or estimates regarding physical fitness from certain tests may be skewed. With this knowledge, exercise professionals will be able to select exercise tests based on the principle of specificity.

Cardiorespiratory Endurance Testing

Given the importance of cardiorespiratory endurance for overall health, selecting an appropriate cardiorespiratory fitness test will likely be the first exercise testing decision made by an exercise professional. Cardiorespiratory endurance tests evaluate the capacity of the heart, lungs, and vasculature to deliver oxygenated blood to working muscles. The maximal capacity of the heart, lungs, and vasculature to deliver oxygenated blood to working muscles is referred to as $\dot{V}O_{2max}$. Therefore, cardiorespiratory endurance tests evaluate either estimated $\dot{V}O_{2max}$ via submaximal effort protocols or by assessing expiratory gasses during maximal effort protocols.

The best method for determining $\dot{V}O_{2max}$ is to conduct a maximal effort cardiorespiratory endurance test while collecting expired gases using a metabolic cart. However, this test is expensive, and it often poses unnecessary health risks for special populations. Consider an obese client who is sedentary. In this case, a maximum effort test may not be physically feasible or safe. Also, clients with orthopedic conditions may not have the capability to perform a maximal effort test. In general, although maximal effort cardiorespiratory endurance tests are the most accurate, they should be avoided when serving special populations unless the test is absolutely necessary, and the facility is equipped with the appropriate instruments and exercise or medical personnel.

Most often, submaximal cardiorespiratory endurance tests are preferred when serving clients with chronic diseases. Here the use of mathematical formulas estimate $\dot{V}O_{2max}$

based on the client's heart rate response during the test. Typically, $\dot{V}O_{2max}$ is estimated by submaximal workloads or heart rates and projecting them to an estimated maximum workload or heart rate. Such estimates can be made because there is an assumed direct linear relationship between the workload of exercise and heart rate.

There are several cardiorespiratory endurance tests. These tests include maximal- and submaximal-graded exercise tests, single-stage submaximal tests, and field tests. Further, cardiorespiratory fitness tests can be conducted using treadmills, cycles, arm cycles, and even a simple step. Equations exist to estimate $\dot{V}O_{2max}$ for tests performed using each of these modalities. The specific modality chosen depends on several factors, including a client's needs, goals, physical limitations, and availability of equipment and staff members. Consider testing obese clients. Here it may be uncomfortable for the client to complete a cycle test or exercise on a cycle; thus, a treadmill test may be preferred. Also, physical limitations, such as certain orthopedic conditions, may necessitate the selection of non-weight-bearing cardiorespiratory endurance tests.

Demonstration Case Study 2.1

Cardiorespiratory Endurance Test Selection

Carlos is an exercise physiologist working at a health and wellness facility. His newest client is Amanda. Amanda is 45 years old, has never exercised before, is obese, and has dyslipidemia. Carlos determined that Amanda did not need medical clearance prior to exercise and there were no major findings from the physical examinations. Amanda is seeking a supervised fitness program to help her lose weight and manage her blood lipids. Carlos's facility has one other exercise physiologist, four treadmills, five cycle ergometers, and two stair steppers. The facility has no metabolic carts and only one automated external defibrillator.

To choose a cardiorespiratory endurance test, Carlos takes into account Amanda's needs, goals, physical limitations, and availability of equipment and staff. From the start, Carlos rules out a maximal effort test while collecting expiratory gasses, as there is no metabolic cart at the facility. However, this does not rule out a maximal effort test altogether. Next, Carlos considers Amanda's needs. Given that Amanda is obese and has dyslipidemia, she has a need to lose weight and increase her metabolic rate. In this respect, Amanda's goals line up with her needs, and Carlos realizes that cardiorespiratory exercises will be necessary to meet Amanda's needs and goals. This alone doesn't clear up whether Carlos chooses to conduct a maximal or submaximal test. Carlos then considers Amanda's physical limitations. With Amanda's obesity and physical inactivity, Carlos feels she will likely be limited in her physical capacity to perform a maximal effort test and rules that test out. Carlos then homes in on a testing modality. Since Amanda is obese, Carlos feels a cycle test would be uncomfortable. Thus Carlos chooses a more natural test for Amanda and chooses to have her complete a submaximal treadmill test.

Body Composition Testing

Given that poor body composition is associated with poorer health outcomes, it makes sense to track and monitor body composition measures when serving clients with chronic diseases. Numerous methods have been developed for assessing body composition. Some of the more common methods of assessing body composition rely on a two-compartment model. A two-compartment model suggests that body weight is equal to the sum of fat mass and fat-free mass. Body composition assessments using the two-compartment model incorporate the principles of hydrostatic weighing, which is the gold standard of body composition assessment. Such assessments include air displacement plethysmography, skinfold assessment, and bioelectrical impedance.

Hydrostatic weighing is based on the assumption of the two-compartment model. In this model, fat-free mass is assumed to have a density of 1.10 kg/L, and fat mass is assumed to have a density of 0.90 kg/L. Therefore, the density of the human body will be between 0.90 and 1.10 kg/L, as no individual is either 100 percent fat or fat-free mass. The density of the human body depends on the relative amounts of fat and fat-free mass. Hydrostatic weighing is one of the most accurate methods of determining body density. Once body density is known (or estimated, such as in skinfolds), it can be converted into a body fat percentage by using the Siri equation.[6]

A major issue with hydrostatic weighing is the availability of equipment. Often, health facilities are not equipped with underwater weighing equipment. Also, should the equipment be available, hydrostatic weighing is not always the best testing option. Hydrostatic weighing requires clients to expel air from their lungs while being submerged underwater. This poses an uncomfortable stimulus onto clients for which the test results are not of utmost importance for exercise prescription. Exercise prescription and the tracking of body composition data can be based on estimates from other non-intensive tests. So, unless research is being conducted or a client pays for and specifies a desire for hydrostatic weighing, the test should be avoided.

A popular method for assessing body composition in "higher-end" facilities is air displacement plethysmography. Air displacement plethysmography is very similar to hydrostatic weighing. Here, instead of displacing water volume, the subject will displace air volume. Clients are weighed, their lung volumes and gastric gas volumes are estimated, and then they are placed in a Bod Pod™. This test may be an issue for clients who are claustrophobic. Another issue with air displacement plethysmography is that the test may overestimate body fat in large, muscular clients. Otherwise, should a facility have access to air displacement plethysmography and a client is comfortable with the assessment, it is a viable and accurate method for evaluating body composition.

An inexpensive method for assessing body composition is the skinfold assessment. The skinfold assessment was derived from performing hydrostatic weighing and skinfolds on a large sample of subjects. From here, predictive equations were established to estimate body density from skinfold thickness. Commonly used equations have been developed for seven- and three-site skinfold procedures. An average of three trials at each site is recorded. These averages are then summed and entered into site- and sex-related predictive equations for estimating body density.[7] Skinfold measurement assumes that the fat immediately under the skin is proportional to the amount of total body fat. In this assumption, it is assumed that approximately a third of total body fat is subcutaneous. In subjects with a large amount of visceral adiposity, skinfold assessment becomes less valid and reliable. Thus with such individuals, other body composition assessments are ideal.

Another inexpensive method for assessing body composition is bioelectrical impedance. Bioelectrical impedance assessment to estimate body composition is based on the following principle: a small, alternating current flowing between two electrodes passes more rapidly through hydrated fat-free body tissues compared to fat mass. Impedance to the electrical current flow relates to the amount of body water, which in turn relates to the amount of fat and fat-free mass. Bioelectrical impedance analysis requires measurement under standardized conditions, particularly hydration status and recent physical activity. Dehydration and recent sweat loss from physical activity will result in a higher body fat estimate. So long as hydration is controlled, bioelectrical impedance is a reliable assessment of body composition for any special population.

Lastly, girth measurements are an excellent method for assessing body composition among obese or overweight individuals (where a large portion of body fat is visceral) where the goal of an exercise program is weight loss. It is also useful for corporate wellness programs and clinical settings where skinfold assessment may be difficult to conduct in a timely and comfortable manner. Girth measurements should be taken at the waist and the hips where a waist-to-hip ratio can be obtained.

Demonstration Case Study 2.2

Body Composition Test Selection

McKenna is an exercise physiologist working at an executive health facility that serves specifically clients with chronic disease. Her newest client is Joseph. Joseph is 51 years old, has only exercised in brief and inconsistent spurts, is obese, has a larger amount of visceral fat, and has medically controlled hypertension. McKenna determined that Joseph did not need medical clearance prior to exercise, and there were no major findings from the physical examinations.

Joseph is seeking a supervised exercise program to help him lose weight. McKenna's facility has an indoor swimming pool with underwater weighing equipment, a Bod Pod, skinfold calipers, bioelectrical impedance, and anthropomorphic measuring tape. With all of the equipment available for testing body composition, McKenna asks Joseph a couple of questions. First, she asks about his feelings of being submerged in water. Joseph tells McKenna that he gets very nervous when his face gets wet, as he nearly drowned as a child. McKenna then asks Joseph if he is claustrophobic. Joseph says that he is not, as he spent years as a coal miner.

McKenna now has the information she needs to make a test selection decision. She determines that body composition assessment is necessary, as Joseph is obese and he wants to lose weight, particularly body fat. McKenna then rules out skinfold assessment, as Joseph has a great amount of visceral fat, which can interfere with the accuracy of the test. She then rules out underwater weighing because Joseph is afraid of being underwater. She decides between air displacement plethysmography, bioelectrical impedance, and girth measurements. McKenna decides that to be the most accurate, she will select air displacement plethysmography. She also feels that if Joseph sees improvement in his waist circumference, he is more likely to stick with the exercise. Therefore, McKenna selects two body composition assessments: air displacement plethysmography and waist and hip circumference.

Muscle Fitness Testing

Like cardiorespiratory fitness tests, muscle fitness tests are very useful for exercise professionals. Knowing a client's muscular fitness helps an exercise professional with exercise prescription design and client education. Mistakenly, many people associate muscular fitness with athletic performance only. However, muscular fitness has many benefits for overall health and can help special populations better control and manage their medical conditions. Therefore, it is very much appropriate for exercise professionals to conduct muscle fitness tests on clients with chronic diseases, especially if the exercise program will involve resistance training exercises.

Within the umbrella term "muscle fitness" are three distinct components. These components include muscular strength, endurance, and power. Muscular power is certainly beneficial for overall health. However, it is most important for athletic performance. Also, without some level of muscular strength or endurance, muscular power will not be optimal. Moreover, having clients with chronic diseases, who are likely not regular weight lifters, perform muscular power tests may pose an unnecessary risk. Therefore, when conducting muscle fitness tests on clients with chronic diseases, muscular power is often not tested.

Muscular endurance is defined as the ability of muscle to perform over time without fatigue. This means that the test selected will involve the completion of the most repetitions as possible, and the resistance will not be as high. Muscular strength, on the other hand, is defined as the ability of skeletal muscle to exert force. Accordingly, muscular strength tests involve the client completing fewer repetitions and overcoming higher resistances.

Determining muscular strength in special populations can be challenging. The primary assessment for muscular strength is the one-repetition maximum (1RM) test. A problem with 1RM tests is that with each trial of the test, the client becomes more fatigued and safety can become an issue. Also, forcefully straining to overcome a resistance may result in not only musculoskeletal injury, but it can also cause undue spikes in blood pressure, myocardial demand, or injuries associated with certain chronic diseases. Therefore, maximal strength is more appropriately assessed in special populations by estimating maximal strength from a five-repetition maximum (5RM) strength test. Such a test reduces the strain required to overcome resistances and thus limits the risk for adverse health events. Another alternative option to the 1RM test is to use a dynamometer. However, a downfall with dynamometer testing is that muscle strength is not assessed throughout a full range of motion.

A general issue with muscle fitness testing is that there are many joints in the human body, and the muscles responsible for moving the joints will have different levels of strength. Exercise professionals need to determine specific muscle groups to test. Comprehensive muscle fitness testing will assess the strength or endurance of the major muscle groups. These groups include the muscles of the chest, lumbo-pelvic hip complex, shoulders, knee extensors, and knee flexors. However, the muscle groups chosen for testing should be in line with the client's goals and needs.

For muscular endurance, the muscle group to test must be identified as well. The most commonly used muscular endurance tests are push-ups, sit-ups, isometric planks, body squats, and bench/chest press. The ACSM recently announced that the sit-up test is not recommended as the test may cause low back injuries.[8] It should be noted that there are several different push-up protocols, so it is important to follow the specific testing guidelines for the normative data that will be used.

As with all exercise testing, muscle fitness test selection requires that exercise professionals pay attention to their clients' needs, goals, and physical limitations. For example, should a client have the need to improve muscular endurance, muscular endurance tests should be selected. Moreover, exercise tests need to be as specific as possible to the exercises to be completed. For instance, if the exercise prescription will involve the upper and lower body, then muscle fitness tests that evaluate the strength or endurance of the major muscle groups of the upper and lower body should be selected. In addition, muscle fitness tests must be valid, reliable, and safe.

Demonstration Case Study 2.3

Muscle Fitness Test Selection

Emily is an exercise physiologist working for a phase III cardiovascular rehabilitation program that focuses on helping patients control their comorbidities associated with heart disease. Emily prides herself on individualizing her exercise prescriptions to meet her patients' needs. Her most recent patient is Hubert. Hubert is 48 years old, has exercised regularly since having his heart attack, has a healthy body weight, has type II diabetes mellitus without neuropathy, and has medically controlled dyslipidemia and hypertension. Hubert was medically cleared to exercise, and Emily did not observe any major findings during her physical examinations of Hubert.

Hubert established the following exercise goals: (1) improve his muscular strength so that he can continue his contractor work and (2) manage his hypertension, blood glucose, and blood lipids through exercise. Emily determines that a series of muscular strength tests are required. Emily also realizes that being a contractor requires the upper body, lower body, and core strength. Therefore, Emily wants to design an exercise prescription that targets these areas. Thus for muscle fitness testing, Emily decides to assess Hubert's lumbo-pelvic hip strength via a leg press test, chest and anterior shoulder muscle strength via an incline chest press test, and core strength via a seated crunch test. Emily wants to maximize safety and thus selects the 5 repetition maximum (RM) method for assessing muscular strength.

Demonstration Case Study 2.4

Muscle Fitness Test Selection

Nate is an exercise physiologist working for a phase III cardiovascular rehabilitation program that focuses on helping patients control their comorbidities associated with heart disease. He, like his coworker Emily, prides himself on individualizing his exercise prescriptions to meet his patients' needs. His most recent patient is Rita. Rita is 73 years old, has exercised regularly since having an aortic valve replacement, is slightly overweight, and has osteoporosis. Rita was medically cleared to exercise, and Nate did not observe any major findings during her physical examinations.

Rita has the following exercise goals: (1) improve her muscular endurance so that she can continue and complete progressively more intense weight-bearing exercises and (2) maintain muscle fitness to better manage her osteoporosis. Nate determines that a series of muscular endurance tests are required. Nate recognizes that progressively intense weight-bearing exercises will require adequate muscular endurance of the lower body and core. Therefore, Nate wants to design an exercise prescription that targets these areas. Thus for muscle fitness testing, Nate decides to assess Rita's lumbo-pelvic hip muscular endurance via a maximal repetition body squat test and core endurance via an isometric prone plank test.

Flexibility Testing

Flexibility refers to the ability to move a joint through its complete and full range of motion. Flexibility is an important component of health-related physical fitness. Optimal flexibility is needed for carrying out activities of daily living. Flexibility has a carryover influence on many aspects of health. For instance, improvements in flexibility may have a role in injury prevention. Thus it can be useful to assess flexibility when serving clients with chronic diseases.

A challenge for flexibility assessment is that flexibility is very joint specific. For instance, the range of motion available at the shoulder joint is greater than the range of motion available at the knee joint. Therefore, unlike cardiorespiratory fitness, there is no one single flexibility assessment that can evaluate total body flexibility. Instead, a series of flexibility tests need to be conducted for each major joint. This type of assessment can be quite time-consuming. Therefore, the sit-and-reach assessment is usually the only flexibility assessment conducted during a comprehensive fitness evaluation. More in-depth flexibility assessments are conducted on clients with needs and/or goals of improving range of motion at specific joints. An example would be a breast cancer survivor seeking to improve the range of motion of the glenohumeral joint following a mastectomy. Here an exercise professional may choose to select a flexibility assessment specific to the shoulder.

Glenn is an exercise physiologist working for a total body wellness facility. Here, Glenn primarily serves clients with limited mobility. One of his clients is Clyde. Clyde is a cancer survivor and spent a lot of time lying down during his treatment. Because of being sedentary in this manner, Clyde has lost significant mobility and has some issues with his gait. Glenn contributes some of Clyde's mobility limitations to a loss of hamstring flexibility. Therefore, following prescreening and evaluation, Glenn decides to have Glenn perform a sit-and-reach test. Glenn feels that this is a very specific test and can also serve to motivate Clyde during the exercise program.

CONTRAINDICATIONS FOR EXERCISE TESTING

Ensuring client safety is of the utmost importance when conducting exercise tests on clients with chronic diseases. Prior to exercise tests, particularly cardiorespiratory endurance and strenuous muscle fitness tests, exercise professionals need to know the contraindications for testing. When exercise professionals collect client data during pre-exercise screening and evaluation, they must identify any signs, symptoms, or medical conditions that can be worsened and present an immediate threat to a client's health during an exercise test.

Some signs, symptoms, or medical conditions may be considered relative or absolute contraindications for exercise testing. When relative contraindications are present, the benefits of conducting an exercise test may outweigh the risks. When absolute contraindications are present, the benefits of conducting an exercise test never outweigh the risks. Therefore, when relative contraindications are present, an exercise professional may be able to conduct an exercise test, whereas an exercise test is never conducted when absolute contraindications are present. A general rule of thumb for exercise professionals is to only conduct an exercise test when relative contraindications are present if it is ordered directly by a physician.

Conditions such as unstable angina, uncontrolled arrhythmias, aortic aneurysm or dissection, or decompensated heart failure may be immediately exacerbated by exercise and pose life-threatening events. When a client presents with any of these types of conditions, the client would have an absolute contraindication to exercise testing and thus an exercise test should never be conducted. On the other hand, conditions such as advanced atrioventricular blocks, left main coronary artery stenosis, or tachyarrhythmias may be worsened by exercise, but the benefits of the exercise test may outweigh the risks. Therefore, under these circumstances, only physicians should determine whether the benefits of the exercise test outweigh the risks. The ACSM publishes a full list of relative and absolute contraindications for exercise testing.[9] It should also be noted that while this list only contains a handful of contraindications, whenever an exercise professional is uncomfortable with conducting an exercise test on a client with chronic diseases, it is always reasonable to err on the side of caution and not conduct an exercise test without medical clearance and/or physician supervision.

Demonstration Case Study 2.6

Contraindications for Exercise Testing

Mae is an exercise specialist working for a weight-loss clinic. She is charged with designing and supervising exercise programs for high-risk clients with multiple comorbidities and the need to lose weight. Mae's newest client is Brandon. Brandon has a BMI of 37 kg/m^2, hypertension, dyslipidemia, and osteoarthritis. Brandon's medical history reveals that he had surgery to repair a dissecting aortic aneurysm. He has not experienced signs or symptoms of this condition since his surgery and was medically cleared to exercise two months prior. During a pre-exercise abbreviated physical examination, Mae reported the following data: (1) apical pulse = 110 beats per minute; (2) radial pulse = 110 beats per minute; (3) resting blood pressure = 180/112 mmHg; (3) no acanthosis nigricans, open wounds, or xanthomas; and (4) forced one-second expiratory volume to forced vital capacity ratio = 90 percent. The facility where Mae works has nurses and exercise specialists on staff.

Mae is first drawn to the fact that Brandon had surgery to repair a dissecting aortic aneurysm. Mae correctly asserts that since the dissecting aneurysm was corrected by surgery and is not an acute condition, then it is not a contraindication for exercise testing. Mae then determines that Brandon has one contraindication for exercise testing: high resting diastolic blood pressure (diastolic blood pressure greater than 110 mmHg). Mae understands that this is a relative contraindication for testing and that testing Brandon may provide benefits that outweigh the risks. However, Mae does not have a physician on-site to order or supervise an exercise test. Therefore, Mae refers Brandon to a physician for his high blood pressure and delays exercise testing.

Demonstration Case Study 2.7

Contraindications for Exercise Testing

Jimmy is an exercise physiologist at an employee wellness gym for a large hospital. Jimmy's newest client is Cameron. Cameron is 62 years old and has the following cardiovascular disease risk factors: (1) age; (2) positive family history, as his father died of a myocardial infarction at the age of 54; (3) obesity with a waist circumference of 43 inches; (4) dyslipidemia with LDL-c blood concentration of 136 mg/dL; (5) hypertension because of medication; and (6) physical inactivity. Cameron's medical history reveals that he had a myocardial infarction four years ago and skin cancer one year ago. Cameron was last medically cleared to exercise a year and a half ago.

At the time of the pre-exercise evaluation, Cameron told Jimmy that he has been having frequent chest pains that sometimes go away with rest, and sometimes the chest pain persists. During a pre-exercise abbreviated physical examination, Jimmy reported the following data: (1) apical pulse = 84 beats per minute, (2) radial pulse = 84 beats per minute, (3) resting blood pressure = 160/108 mmHg, (3) xanthomas under the eyes, and (4) forced one-second expiratory volume to forced vital capacity ratio = 81 percent. The facility where Jimmy works has immediate access to physicians.

Jimmy easily observed that Cameron was not in optimal health and that exercise testing may be tricky. Jimmy immediately recalls Cameron's comments regarding his chest pain. Not only does chest pain require medical clearance to participate in exercise testing and an exercise program but also the chest pain Cameron described aligns with the description of unstable angina. Jimmy immediately refers Cameron to a physician, as unstable angina is extraordinarily dangerous and the risk for another myocardial infarction is very high, as the myocardial ischemia cannot be predictively relieved.

Demonstration Case Study 2.8

Contraindications for Exercise Testing

Bethany is a clinical exercise physiologist working for a regional hospital's exercise and disease management clinic. She is responsible for all patient intakes, which includes the responsibility of conducting pre-exercise testing. The most recent patient is Thomas. Thomas presents to the clinic with a recent diagnosis of type II diabetes mellitus. Thomas has never experienced cardiac signs or symptoms but was treated for a type I second-degree atrioventricular block three years prior. During a pre-exercise physical examination, Bethany recorded the following data: (1) apical pulse = 66 beats per minute, (2) radial pulse = 60 beats per minute, (3) resting blood pressure = 130/68 mmHg, (3) no open wounds or nerve-related pain, and (4) forced one-second expiratory volume to forced vital capacity ratio = 85 percent. Given Bethany works for a hospital, she also has access to an ECG to monitor patients before, during, and after exercise testing.

In addition to Thomas's type II diabetes, Bethany's attention was drawn to his type I second-degree atrioventricular block. With Thomas's deficit between apical and radial pulse, Bethany suspects Thomas's atrioventricular block may be back. Bethany connects Thomas to the ECG, and, indeed, the ECG reveals a type I second-degree atrioventricular block. Bethany immediately calls her clinic's supervising physician for assistance. The physician decides that since Thomas is asymptomatic, there is more benefit than risk in conducting an exercise test. Therefore, Bethany conducts the exercise test.

TEST TERMINATION CRITERIA

Exercise tests can be terminated at a predetermined end point as is the case with submaximal effort tests or with volitional fatigue, which is the case with maximal effort tests. However, since a major theme in exercise prescription for clients with chronic diseases is that exercise professionals must always ensure safety, this section of the text will highlight the need for exercise professionals to remain observant during the completion of exercise tests. Ensuring safety begins with pre-exercise screening and evaluation and continues through to exercise participation. Despite thorough attempts to identify known or underlying health conditions in pre-exercise screening and evaluation, it is possible that asymptomatic clients make it all the way to exercise testing without being referred to a physician for medical clearance. It is for this reason that exercise professionals must be attentive and observant to a client's physiological responses to acute exercise.

Upon initial movement and each subsequent increase in the work rate of exercise, several predictable physiological events occur to meet the rise in metabolic and oxygen demand. The circulatory system will increase in heart rate, stroke volume, and systolic blood pressure. In addition, arterioles within the vascular network will dilate toward the direction of working muscles. The result with the circulatory system is an increase in cardiac output and the delivery of nutrient- and oxygen-rich blood to actively contracting skeletal muscles. The respiratory system also goes through acute changes by increasing respiratory rate and minute ventilation.

The acute physiological changes will occur over two- to three-minute increments with the initial movement of an increase in exercise intensity. This denotes the rapid phase of the oxygen response to acute exercise. Following the initial two to three minutes of exercise, an individual will reach steady state. Failure of these changes to occur will manifest in a client or patient's volitional fatigue or present significant cardiorespiratory signs or symptoms, which may be accompanied by electrocardiographic changes.

The cardiorespiratory signs and symptoms that clients or patients may experience can be divided into absolute or relative indications for terminating an exercise test.[10] Like absolute and relative contraindications for conducting an exercise test, the ACSM publishes a full list of absolute and relative indications for terminating a symptom-limited maximal exercise test.[11] Also, like with contraindications for exercise testing, absolute test termination criteria when present suggest that if the test were to continue, the client's or patient's immediate health would be in danger. Examples of absolute indications for terminating an exercise test include ST-segment elevation, a ten-point or more decrease of systolic blood pressure with an increase in exercise intensity, the presence of any major cardiac sign or symptom, equipment issues, or a client's or patient's desire to stop. Thus whenever absolute indications are present, then exercise professionals must terminate the test immediately. Relative indications for terminating an exercise test, when present, could suggest imminent health concerns. However, the benefit of continuing a test whenever relative indications are present may be greater than the risk of continuing the test. As a rule, exercise professionals should defer to the judgment of a licensed physician whenever relative indications for terminating an exercise test occur.

Demonstration Case Study 2.9

Exercise Testing Termination Criteria

Davis is an exercise physiologist at an occupational health center. As a part of his responsibilities, Davis conducts cardiorespiratory fitness tests on the city's fire and police personnel. His first several tests of the day were completed with no complications. Davis, awaiting the end of the workday, had to conduct one more test on Antonio, a firefighter. Antonio started the test without complications. His heart rate, blood pressure, and minute ventilation increased with each increase in exercise intensity. Further, no abnormal electrocardiographic changes occurred. In stage three of the exercise test, Antonio developed chest discomfort but did not communicate this to Davis, nor did Davis inquire about Antonio's perceptions of the exercise. Given the unremarkable events of the first two stages and throughout the day, Davis chose to ignore the ECG in stage three. Had Davis looked, he would have observed a 3-millimeter, ST-segment depression in the inferior leads. Although this is a relative indication for terminating the test, Davis could've informed the physician nearby.

Davis continued with the exercise test to stage four. In stage four, Antonio started feeling more chest pain and experienced shortness of breath. Davis still did not inquire about Antonio's perceptions. Finally, Davis was alerted to the ECG as an alarm sounded. Davis then noted a two-millimeter, ST-segment elevation in the inferior leads, Antonio was having an active myocardial infarction. At that time, Davis terminated the test and alerted the health center's STEMI (ST elevation myocardial infarction) alert system. Antonio's myocardial infarction was treated, and he was released from the hospital four days later. Davis was placed on administrative leave and became a case study highlighting the importance of continued observation throughout exercise tests.

Demonstration Case Study 2.10

Exercise Testing Termination Criteria

Pamela is an exercise specialist working for a strength and conditioning facility. Her primary job responsibility is to conduct maximal cardiorespiratory fitness tests on aspiring endurance athletes. Her first test of the day is on Juan, a local track star. Prior to the test, Pamela gathers all necessary information about Juan. Pamela discovered that Juan has type I diabetes mellitus. Despite this diagnosis, Juan would not need a medical exam prior to exercise testing.

Pamela begins the exercise test and monitors Juan's heart rate, ratings of perceived exertion, blood pressure, and any general perceptions about the exercise bout. Stages one through four go well without any abnormal events, as heart rate and blood pressure rose adequately. In stage five, Juan becomes noticeably fatigued. Juan insists he is fine and wants to continue the test. Juan reaches stage six and then starts to stumble and experience some uncontrolled and uncoordinated movements. Pamela correctly decides to terminate the test because of what appears to be ataxia, and ataxia is an absolute indication for terminating an exercise test.

Demonstration Case Study 2.11

Exercise Testing Termination Criteria

Garell is an exercise professional working for a local health-fitness facility. Garell is responsible for conducting exercise tests and writing exercise prescriptions for clients with preexisting medical conditions. His newest client is Gale. Gale has controlled type II diabetes mellitus and is a survivor of breast cancer. Gale is regularly active and came to the clinic after having been cleared for exercise by both her oncologist and primary care physician.

Garell decides to conduct a submaximal cycle cardiorespiratory fitness test on Gale. Given Gale's age of 62 years old, Garell wants to terminate the test at 85 percent of Gales age-predicted maximal heart rate. Therefore, a heart rate of 135 bpm is chosen as the predetermined end point. Garell records the following data throughout the test: stage one—heart rate 98 bpm, blood pressure 122/78, ratings of perceived exertion 8/20, and no major signs or symptoms; stage two—heart rate 112 bpm, blood pressure 134/78, ratings of perceived exertion 10/20, and no major signs or symptoms; stage 3— heart rate 132 bpm, blood pressure 148/78, ratings of perceived exertion 13/20, and no major signs or symptoms; and stage four—heart rate 141 bpm, blood pressure 164/80, ratings of perceived exertion 15/20, and no major signs or symptoms. Given normal hemodynamic responses and no major signs or symptoms, Garell correctly continues the test to completion when the heart rate passes 135 bpm.

EXERCISE TEST INTERPRETATION

Following the completion of exercise testing, exercise professionals must interpret the results. This process is nearly identical to exercise test interpretation for apparently healthy adults. Exercise test interpretation involves analyzing all collected data and then recording directly measured maximal values or predicting maximal workloads. The results of exercise tests are used to set initial exercise prescriptions, track clients' progress, and client education. Thus the results of exercise tests need to be rigidly evaluated and compared to normative data. In this section, overviews for interpreting cardiorespiratory fitness, muscle fitness, body composition, and flexibility tests will be provided.

Cardiorespiratory Fitness Test Interpretation

The hallmark of cardiorespiratory fitness tests is to obtain a client's maximal oxygen consumption ($\dot{V}O_{2max}$). There are several methods for interpreting cardiorespiratory fitness tests. The simplest interpretation is recording a $\dot{V}O_{2max}$ value from a maximal effort test using open-circuit spirometry. Here an exercise physiologist will determine whether a true $\dot{V}O_{2max}$ was achieved by analyzing if the client achieved three of the following criteria: (1) plateau in $\dot{V}O_2$ between two stages, (2) maximal heart rate was within ten beats per minute of age predicted maximal heart rate, (3) respiratory exchange ratio was 1.15 or higher, (4) the client's perceived exertion was at least an 18 out of 20 on the Borg scale, and (5) blood lactate levels were at least 8 millimoles or more.[12] However, when serving clients with chronic diseases, it is often not advisable or feasible to conduct such tests. Therefore, exercise professionals often rely on mathematical calculations, graphs, and nomograms to predict a client's $\dot{V}O_{2max}$ from submaximal work rates. Therefore, this section of the text will review interpretation techniques using submaximal effort cardiorespiratory fitness test data.

Submaximal cycle protocols are often the preferred cardiorespiratory fitness tests of choice for exercise professionals serving clients with chronic diseases. This is in part because of deconditioning, previous sedentary behavior, and orthopedic limitations. Two common cycle protocols are the YMCA and Astrand-Rhyming cycle tests. The YMCA cycle test consists of three-minute stages in which the intensity increases from one stage to the next based on the heart rate response found in stage one. The Astrand-Rhyming cycle test, on the other hand, is a single-stage, six-minute test.

To interpret the YMCA cycle test, exercise professionals will obtain two heart rates from two separate stages in which the heart rate exceeds 110 beats per minute. These heart rates are graphed over the work rate that elicited the heart rates. Then a line is extrapolated from those two heart rates to the client's age-predicted maximal heart rate. From here a line is drawn from the point where the extrapolated line intersects the age-predicted maximal heart rate down to the x-axis. Where this second line intersects the x-axis provides exercise professionals with an estimate of the client's estimated maximal work rate. The estimated maximal work rate is then entered in the leg-cycling equation to estimate the client's $\dot{V}O_{2max}$.[13]

Interpreting the Astrand-Rhyming cycle test is less intensive than interpreting the YMCA cycle test. The Astrand-Rhyming cycle test is a single-stage, six-minute test where the goal for the exercise professional is to obtain heart rates over the final two minutes between 125 and 170 beats per minute. The average of these two heart rates is used in the modified Astrand-Rhyming nomogram.[14] Upon completion of the nomogram, the estimated $\dot{V}O_{2max}$ is multiplied by a correction factor based on the client's age.[15] The ACSM publishes these correction factors in their *Guidelines for Exercise Testing and Prescription.*[16]

Estimating $\dot{V}O_{2max}$ from submaximal treadmill tests involves recording treadmill speed and incline and then using them in mathematical equations. There are several treadmill equations available; however, the most common are the running and walking equations published by the ACSM. In these equations, it is important for exercise physiologists to know that the speed is in meters per minute and the incline is the decimal form of a percentage.

Exercise professionals have several treadmill protocols available for selection. One of the more common tests is the Bruce protocol. The Bruce protocol is designed in a manner to fatigue clients and patients quickly. Therefore, the protocol emphasizes incline and large MET (metabolic equivalent) increases from one stage to the next. When working with clients who have chronic diseases, especially those with extreme deconditioning, exercise professionals may consider selecting the less demanding modified Bruce protocol. Regardless of the treadmill protocol chosen, when exercise professionals decide to conduct a submaximal treadmill test, they need to establish a predetermined end point. Typically, the end point of 85 percent of age-predicted maximal heart rate is selected. However, for mathematical ease and accuracy, 70 percent of the client's heart rate reserve is a better end point. Once the client reaches 70 percent of the client's heart rate reserve (HRR), the test is terminated, and the speed and incline are recorded. Next, $\dot{V}O_2$ is estimated using the walking or running equations, which are both provided next. Once this $\dot{V}O_2$ is recorded, the $\dot{V}O_{2max}$ is estimated by solving the following equation:

$$\text{Pred } \dot{V}O_{2max} = \frac{\dot{V}O_2 \text{ at 70\% HRR}}{0.7}$$

Walking Equation

$\dot{V}O_2$ = (0.1 x speed in meters · minute) + (1.8 x speed in meters · minute x percent incline) + 3.5

Running Equation

$\dot{V}O_2$ = (0.2 x speed in meters · minute) + (0.9 x speed in meters · minute x percent incline) + 3.5

When serving clients with chronic diseases, exercise professionals must monitor the client's hemodynamic and perceptual responses to exercise. Therefore, throughout an exercise test heart rate, blood pressure, perceived exertion, and signs and symptoms must be recorded in each stage of the test. Should a client have an abnormal response, exercise professionals must note the abnormality and make sure to prescribe exercise at intensities less than the exercise intensity that elicited the abnormal response.

Demonstration Case Study 2.12

Cardiorespiratory Fitness Test Interpretation: YMCA Cycle Test

Justin is an exercise physiologist working for a diabetes management program at his local hospital. His primary responsibility is to conduct and interpret exercise tests for patients with type I or II diabetes. His newest client is Jon. Jon is a 50-year-old, 270-pound man with type II diabetes, and a BMI of 38 kg/m², and he hasn't exercised in 20 years. Justin rightfully chooses not to conduct a maximal effort test given Jon's deconditioned, obesity, and disease status. Jon selects the YMCA cycle test to estimate Jon's $\dot{V}O_{2max}$. Justin records the following data throughout Jon's test (Figure 2.1).

Figure 2.1 This table contains hypothetical cardiorespiratory fitness test data from a YMCA cycle test

Stage	Kp	Kpm/min	Heart Rate	Blood Pressure	RPE
Resting	o o		77	118/66	N/A
I	0.5	150	101	122/68	8
II	1.0	300	111	128/66	11
III	1.5	450	125	136/66	13
Recovery 1 min	o o		87	126/66	N/A
Recovery 5 min	o o		78	120/66	N/A
Recovery 10 min	o o		77	120/66	N/A

Justin records Jon's heart rate in stages two and three and graphs them over the work rate in kilopond meters per minute (kpm/min). Justin draws a straight line connecting the two heart rates on the graph and extends the line to the point where it intersects the graph at Jon's age-predicted maximal heart rate of 170 bpm. Justin then draws another line from this intersection point down to the x-axis. This line intersects the x-axis at approximately 932.5 kp · m · min. Therefore, Justin enters this maximal predicted work rate into the leg cycling equation and solves for Jon's $\dot{V}O_{2max}$, which is 20.67 mL/kg · min. For educational purposes, Justin informs Jon that his $\dot{V}O_{2max}$ is very poor. Justin's work is provided in Figure 2.2.

Figure 2.2 This table contains the hypothetical cardiorespiratory fitness test data in graphical form in which $\dot{V}O_{2max}$ is estimated from a YMCA cycle test

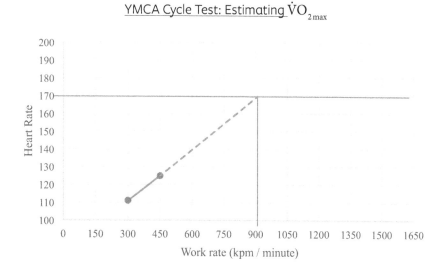

YMCA Cycle Test: Estimating $\dot{V}O_{2max}$

Max Work Rate = 932.5 kpm/min

$\dot{V}O_{2max}$ = (1.8 x 932.5/122.72 kg) + 7

$\dot{V}O_{2max}$ = 20.67 mL/kg · min

Demonstration Case Study 2.13

Cardiorespiratory Fitness Test Interpretation: Astrand-Rhyming Cycle Test

Leigh works as an exercise specialist at a senior-citizen facility. She specializes in serving residents with multiple chronic diseases. Her most recent client is Jane. Jane is a 65-year-old who weighs 175 pounds and has metabolic syndrome. Jane has not exercised in 30 years, and she wants to exercise to improve her health and independence. Following pre-participation screening and evaluation, Leigh determines that an exercise test is safe, and no medical exam is warranted. Leigh selects the Astrand-Rhyming cycle test to evaluate Jane's cardiorespiratory fitness. She makes this decision because Jane has been sedentary and feels that a single-stage test would be the most comfortable for Jane. Leigh set the constant intensity at 300 kpm/min. The test was completed without complication. Leigh recorded a heart rate of 141 beats per minute in the final 30 seconds of minute five and a heart rate of 139 in the final 30 seconds of minute six. Leigh averaged these two heart rates (140 bpm) and then used the modified Astrand-Rhyming nomogram to estimate Jane's $\dot{V}O_{2max}$. Leigh determines that Jane's $\dot{V}O_{2max}$ from the nomogram is 2.2 L/min. Then Leigh makes the age correction from the table (2.2 x .65), resulting in 1.43 L/min, which is then converted to a relative value by dividing by her weight in kilograms (1.43/79.5). She finds Jane's $\dot{V}O_{2max}$ is 0.01797 L/kg or 17.97mL/kg · min. For educational purposes, Leigh informs Jane that her cardiorespiratory fitness level for her age is poor.

Demonstration Case Study 2.14

Cardiorespiratory Fitness Test Interpretation: Submaximal Treadmill Test

Casey is a personal trainer who specializes in serving clients with stable health conditioning. His newest client is Urban. Urban is a 60-year-old recently retired basketball coach who wants to stay active in his retirement. Urban was diagnosed with prostate cancer in 2015 and is now in remission. Urban lost a lot of his cardiorespiratory fitness during his treatment but tried to go for light-paced walks every day. Casey determined a medical exam was not warranted and then moved on to select a submaximal treadmill test to evaluate Urban's cardiorespiratory fitness. Casey selected this test because Urban is accustomed to regular walking but did not want to subject him to a maximal effort test. To conduct the test, Casey had to set an end point. Casey chose 70 percent of Urban's HRR. To calculate HRR reserve, Casey had to record Urban's resting heart rate, which was 70 bpm. Casey then determined that 70 percent of Urban's HRR was 133 beats per minute. Casey conducted the test without complications. He recorded the following data (Figure 2.3).

Figure 2.3 This table contains the hypothetical cardiorespiratory fitness test data from a submaximal treadmill test

Stage	Speed/MPH	Grade %	Heart Rate	Blood Pressure	RPE
Resting	0	0	70	110/76	N/A
1	1.7	10.0	90	122/78	8
2	2.5	12.0	110	136/78	13
3	3.4	14.0	136	148/78	15
Immediate	0	0	164	154/78	17
Recovery 1 min	0	0	124	138/78	N/A
Recovery 5 min	0	0	75	112/76	N/A

Following the test, Casey had to perform some mathematical calculations. First, Casey used the walking equation to estimate Urban's $\dot{V}O_2$ at the time of test termination, which was 33.20 mL/kg · min. Second, Casey set up a proportion to solve for $\dot{V}O_2$ at 100 percent of Urban's HRR, which is equal to $\dot{V}O_{2max}$. Casey calculated Urban's $\dot{V}O_{2max}$ as 47.43 mL/kg · min. For education purposes, Casey informed Urban that his cardiorespiratory fitness level was excellent for his age and condition.

Demonstration Case Study 2.15

Cardiorespiratory Fitness Test Interpretation: Maximal Treadmill Protocol

Taryl is a strength and conditioning specialist working for a facility intended to return cancer survivors to recreational athletics or advanced exercise. Taryl's most recent client is Kenneth. Kenneth, 52-year-old, is a survivor of non-Hodgkin's lymphoma, was an avid marathoner prior to his cancer diagnosis, and currently weighs 142 pounds. Taryl's facility has all the necessary equipment and personnel for conducting maximal treadmill tests with open-circuit spirometry. Moreover, Taryl realized that Kenneth's previous fitness habits and current exercise goals would warrant a maximal treadmill test. The test was completed without complications and the following data were recorded (Figure 2.4).

Figure 2.4 This table contains the hypothetical cardiorespiratory fitness test data from a maximal treadmill test

Stage	Time (min)	Speed (mph)	Grade %	$\dot{V}O_2$ (ml/kg/min)	RER	Blood Lactate (mmol)	RPE	Heart Rate (bpm)
Resting		0	0	4.7	0.7	0.5	NA	67
Warm-Up		2	0	7	0.75	0.8	NA	72
1	2:00	2.5	0	15.4	0.77	1.5	7	90

(Continued)

Figure 2.4 This table contains the hypothetical cardiorespiratory fitness test data from a maximal treadmill test (Continued)

Stage	Time (min)	Speed (mph)	Grade %	$\dot{V}O_2$ (ml/ kg/min)	RER	Blood Lactate (mmol)	RPE	Heart Rate (bpm)
2	4:00	5.5	0	18.1	0.80	2.6	10	107
3	6:00	6.0	2	22.9	0.89	4.5	12	137
4	8:00	6.5	3	30.4	0.99	5.1	15	146
5	10:00	6.5	5.5	38.1	1.12	7.9	16	159
6	12:00	6.5	7.5	43.6	1.16	8.5	18	170
Immediate	N/A	2	0	43.1	1.15	8.1	NA	168
Recovery 1 min	N/A	2	0	32.5	0.95	4.7	NA	151
Recovery 5 min	N/A	2	0	12.3	0.81	2.3	NA	120

Following the test, Taryl determined that Kenneth's $\dot{V}O_{2max}$ was 46.6 mL/kg · min. Taryl also correctly stated that Kenneth achieved a true $\dot{V}O_{2max}$, as Kenneth's max heart rate was within ten beats per minute of his age-predicted maximal heart rate; his blood lactate was greater than 8 millimoles; his perceived exertion was at least 18 out of 20; his respiratory exchange ratio was greater than 1.15. Taryl also notes that only three of those criteria were needed to verify that Kenneth reached a true $\dot{V}O_{2max}$.

Muscular Fitness Test Interpretation

As previously discussed, muscular fitness tests can assess a client's muscular strength, endurance, or power. When serving clients with chronic diseases, attention is usually paid to assessments of muscular strength and endurance. With muscular strength assessments, the objective is to obtain enough data to predict or directly measure the amount of force that can be generated by a given muscle group. Endurance tests, on the other hand, emphasize the successful completion of repetitions or the amount of time a muscle group spends under contraction.

Direct measures of strength obtained via 1RM tests are the most accurate. However, when training clients with chronic diseases, these tests can pose an unnecessary risk of injury or further detriment of a health condition. It is for this reason that muscular strength tests seek to predict maximal strength using mathematical equations. The Lander equation is a commonly used formula to predict strength.[17] Here the weight and amount of successful repetitions of an exercise are recorded and entered into the Lander equation. The goal should be to find resistance by the third trial that the client can overcome three to five times. This is accomplished by having a client perform an initial trial with an amount of weight he or she believes to be 50 to 70 percent of the best 1RM. From here, the exercise professional will add 5 to 10 percent more weight for upper body exercises for each subsequent trial and 10 to 20 percent for lower body exercises.

In addition to the Lander equation, exercise professionals can use dynamometers to measure strength. The handgrip dynamometer is a fairly common modality used to assess muscular strength for the purpose of comparison to normative data. Unfortunately, these tests do not provide enough useful data for formulating an exercise prescription. To conduct a handgrip strength test, exercise professionals will instruct their clients to hold the dynamometer at their side, squeeze hard while exhaling, and repeat three times for each hand. The sum of the results for each hand is determined and compared to normative data.

Demonstration Case Study 2.16

Muscular Strength Testing: Chest Press

Karen is an exercise physiologist working for an orthopedic facility. Karen oversees the "Exercise and Arthritis" program. In this role, Karen performs all pre-exercise participation and evaluation screenings and exercise testing procedures. The program's newest member is Robert. Robert is a 42-year-old male who weighs 255 pounds and reported to the clinic with moderate osteoarthritis in his elbow and knee joints. Robert, like all clients, was cleared to participate by the supervising physician. Robert listed his exercise goals as improving his upper and lower body strength.

Staying in line with the principle of specificity, Karen chose to conduct a 3-5RM strength test on both the chest press and leg press modalities. For the leg press, Karen had Robert do a light warm-up and then become familiar with the leg press. She then had Robert select an initial load that he felt represented 50 percent of his 1RM. Given the ease of Robert's first trial, Karen added 20 percent more weight during each of the next two trials. Karen recorded Robert's best trial and entered the amount of weight and number of successful repetitions into the Lander equation. Karen repeated this process for the chest press except for increasing the amount of weight each trial by 10 percent. Robert's 3-5RM strength test results are provided in Figures 2.5 and 2.6, along with the Lander equation.

Figure 2.5 This is a table that depicts hypothetical leg press muscular strength data from a 3–5RM test. These data will be used to estimate maximal strength using the Lander equation

Robert's Leg Press Strength Test

Trial 1	_____5_____ repetitions _____200_____ weight
Trial 2	_____3_____ repetitions _____240_____ weight
Trial 3	_____3_____ repetitions _____288_____ weight
Best Trial	_____3_____ repetitions _____288_____ weight

<u>Lander Equation</u>

1RM = (100 x weight lifted in pounds)/(101.3 – (2.67123 x repetitions))

<u>Robert's Leg Press Strength Calculations</u>

1RM = (100 x 288)/(101.3 – (2.67123 x 3))

1RM = 308.73 pounds

Figure 2.6 This is a table that depicts hypothetical chest press muscular strength data from a 3–5RM test. These data will be used to estimate maximal strength using the Lander equation

Robert's Leg Press Strength Test

Trial 1	5	repetitions
	125	weight
Trial 2	3	repetitions
	140	weight
Trial 3	3	repetitions
	155	weight
Best Trial	3	repetitions
	155	weight

<u>Robert's Chest Press Strength Calculations</u>

1RM = (100 x 155)/(101.3 – (2.67123 x 3))

1RM = 166.16 pounds

Karen determined that Robert's 1RM leg press was 308.73 pounds. When Karen recorded a leg press to body weight ratio (308.73/255=1.21), she established that Robert's lower body strength was well below average for his age. For the chest press, Karen determined that Robert's 1RM chest press was 166.16 pounds. When Karen recorded a chest press to body weight ratio (166.16/255=0.65), she established that Robert's lower body strength was very poor for his age.

Body Composition Test Interpretation

There are numerous methods for estimating a client's body composition. Methods range from costly, yet accurate, tests, such as air displacement plethysmography, and inexpensive, but still reliable, tests, such as skinfolds, girth measurements, and bioelectrical impedance. Tests such as air displacement plethysmography and bioelectrical impedance are very simple to interpret, as the Bod Pod's software and most bioelectrical impedance devices will calculate body fat percentage. Tests such as skinfolds and girth measurements do require some calculations to interpret a client's body composition. Therefore, this section will focus on interpreting skinfold and anthropomorphic assessments.

Interpreting skinfold tests requires the use of predictive equations to estimate body density.[18] Body density equations are different for males and females and for three- versus seven-site skinfold assessments. To use the body density equations, exercise professionals will need to take an average of three trials, and each site should be recorded. These averages are then summed and entered into site- and sex-related predictive equations for estimating body density. It is important for exercise professionals to understand that the body density derived from these equations must be between 0.9 and 1.1 kilograms per liter (kg/L). Following the calculation of body density, body fat percentage is calculated using the Siri equation.[19] The body density formulas and the Siri equation are provided next:

Seven-Site Body Density Equations

> *Women* Density = $1.097 - (0.00046971 \times X1) + (0.00000056 \times X1^2) - (0.00012828 \times X2)$,

> *Men* Density = $1.112 - (0.00043499 \times X1) + (0.00000055 \times X1^2) - (0.00028826 \times X2)$,

where X1 = sum of triceps, subscapula, chest, abdomen, suprailiac, midaxillary, and thigh skinfolds and X2 = age in years.

Three-Site Body Density Equations

> *Women* Density = $1.089733 - (0.0009245 \times X1) + (0.0000025 \times X1^2) - (0.0000979 \times X2)$,

where X1 = sum of triceps, suprailium, and abdomen skinfolds and X2 = age in years.

> *Men* Density = $1.1125025 - (0.0013125 \times X1) + (0.0000055 \times X1^2) - (0.0002440 \times X2)$,

where X1 = sum of chest, triceps, and subscapula skinfolds and X2 = age in years.

Siri Equation

> Body Fat Percentage = $(495/\text{density}) - 450$

Girth measurements, also known as anthropomorphic tests, are an excellent method for assessing body composition when serving special populations, as improvements in girth measurements have a profound influence on overall health and disease management. This is particularly true when serving obese clients, as skinfold and other assessments may be inaccurate or not warranted. Girth measurements are typically taken at the waist and the hips and measured in either centimeters or inches. With this information, data can be compared to normative data and monitored throughout an exercise program.

Demonstration Case Study 2.17

Caroline is an exercise physiologist working for an executive wellness program. Caroline specializes in serving clients with chronic diseases. As a part of her responsibilities, she conducts exercise tests on new clients. Most recently, she tested Marla. Marla is a 62-year-old patient with type II diabetes and is in some need to lose body fat. Marla has a BMI of 29.3 kg/m^2, which is overweight, but Marla does not have excessive central adiposity. Therefore, Caroline decided it was acceptable to conduct a seven-site skinfold assessment. The following data were collected from Marla's test (Figure 2.7).

Figure 2.7 This table contains hypothetical seven-site skinfold data from a female subject

Site	Trial 1	Trial 2	Trial 3	Average
Triceps	20	21	21	20.66 mm
Subscapular	19	19	19	19 mm
Chest	17	16	17	16.66 mm
Abdominal	25	27	27	26.33 mm
Suprailiac	29	31	31	28.33 mm
Midaxillary	28	28	28	28 mm
Thigh	34	34	36	35.33 mm

Caroline summed the averages of each skinfold site to get a value of 174.31. She then used this value and Marla's age to solve the seven-site skinfold equation for females. Caroline calculated a body density of 1.0242 kg/L. She then entered body density in the Siri equation to solve for body fat percentage. Caroline determined that Marla's body fat percentage was 33.3 percent. This value indicated that Marla's body composition is poor for her age. Caroline's work is provided next.

$$\text{Density} = 1.097 - (0.00046971 \times 174.31) + (0.00000056 \times 174.31^2) - (0.00012828 \times 62)$$

$$\text{Density} = 1.0242 \text{ kg/L}$$

$$\text{Body Fat Percentage} = (495/1.0242) - 450$$

$$\text{Body Fat Percentage} = 33.30 \text{ percent}$$

Demonstration Case Study 2.18

Tony is an exercise physiologist working for a weight-loss clinic. Tony is responsible for conducting body composition tests on new clients. Most recently, he tested James.

James is a 51-year-old and needs to lose body fat to ward off the development of more serious chronic diseases. James is not yet classified as obese but is a bit skeptical of having a seven-site skinfold test performed. Therefore, Tony decided it was acceptable to conduct a three-site skinfold assessment for accuracy and the comfort of the client. The following data were collected from James' test (Figure 2.8).

Figure 2.8 This table contains hypothetical three-site skinfold data from a male subject

Site	Trial 1	Trial 2	Trial 3	Average
Triceps	15	17	17	16.33 mm
Subscapular	20	20	20	20 mm
Chest	16	16	18	16.66 mm

Tony summed the averages of each skinfold site to get a value of 52.99. He then used this value and James's age to solve the three-site skinfold equation for males. Tony calculated a body density of 1.046 kg/L. He then entered body density in the Siri equation to solve for body fat percentage. Tony determined that James's body fat percentage was 23.23 percent. This value indicated that James's body composition is fair for his age. Tony's work is provided next.

Density = 1.1125025 − (0.0013125 x 52.99) + (0.0000055 x 52.99²) − (0.0002440 x 51)

Density = 1.046 kg/L

Body Fat Percentage = (495/1.046) − 450

Body Fat Percentage = 23.23 percent

Demonstration Case Study 2.19

Girth Measurements

Gregg is an exercise physiologist working for his hospital's outpatient weight management clinic. As a part of his responsibilities, Gregg performs body composition assessments on the patients. Given that the program is intended for weight management, the majority of the patients are obese. Gregg correctly avoids the skinfold assessment, as they would not be accurate on individuals with excess central adiposity. He instead chooses to conduct anthropomorphic measurements, particularly waist circumferences. Gregg's most recent male patient had a waist circumference of 49 inches. Gregg used these data to educate this patient about his health, stating that his waist circumference put him at a very high risk for developing chronic health conditions.

Flexibility Test Interpretation

Flexibility testing is somewhat tricky, as tests must be joint specific. To date, there is not a single assessment that can evaluate a client's whole-body flexibility. However, exercise professionals can conduct a series of flexibility assessments, one for each major joint or musculotendon group. Unless exercise professionals are serving clients or patients with a specific need to improve range of motion at specific joints, the flexibility test of choice is generally the sit-and-reach test. To interpret the sit-and-reach test, exercise professionals simply read the maximal achieved reach at the client's fingertips. It is important for exercise professionals to note the "zero" point on a sit-and-reach box, as normative data are based on the "zero" point being at different values.

Demonstration Case Study 2.20

Flexibility Test Interpretation: Sit-and-Reach

Sean is an exercise physiologist who serves clients with stable peripheral artery disease. Sean is a firm believer in designing comprehensive fitness plans that are aimed at improving all components of health-related physical fitness, which includes flexibility. The flexibility assessment of choice for Sean is the sit-and-reach test. Sean's sit-and-reach box has the "zero" point at 23 centimeters. His most recent client was Allen, a 63-year-old male. On Allen's third trial, he achieved a reach of 19 centimeters. Sean had to subtract three from Allen's score to compare his results to normative data. According to normative data, Allen has poor lower body flexibility.

EXERCISE PRESCRIPTION

Exercise prescriptions are designed in a systematic manner using all possible data available. Above all, exercise prescriptions must be individualized to a client's needs, goals, fitness, and health status. The more individualized an exercise prescription, the more effective and safer an exercise program will be at achieving a client's goals. Exercise professionals design exercise prescriptions according to the FITT-VP principle. FITT-VP is an acronym that stands for frequency, intensity, time, type, volume, and progression. When working with special populations, exercise professionals will modify the frequency, intensity, time, type, volume, and progression of an exercise program based on the health condition and capabilities of the client. This section of the text reviews the basic principles of exercise prescription for improving cardiorespiratory fitness, muscular fitness, and flexibility. Special considerations for various special populations will be provided later in the text.

Cardiorespiratory Exercise Prescription

The ACSM publishes recommendations for improving cardiorespiratory fitness.[20] These recommendations suggest that healthy adults should perform cardiorespiratory exercises three to five days per week at a moderate intensity for 30 to 60 minutes per day. This can be thought of as the initial reference when constructing an exercise prescription.

As it pertains to frequency, cardiorespiratory endurance exercises should be performed three to five times per week. The rationale for this is that there is little improvement in $\dot{V}O_{2max}$ when cardiorespiratory endurance exercises are performed less than three days per week. Moreover, performing more than five days of cardiorespiratory endurance exercise offers little additional benefit while posing a risk for overtraining, injury, and muscle soreness. Thus when serving special populations, exercise professionals should seek to improve cardiorespiratory fitness while limiting the likelihood for injury, soreness, or early dropout. The frequency of cardiorespiratory exercise varies according to the intensity of exercise to be performed. For instance, if a client were to exercise at vigorous intensities, then the frequency would be three days per week as opposed to four or five.

Prescribing intensity for cardiorespiratory endurance exercises is the most important aspect of the FITT-VP principle. Exercise professionals should note that the results of an exercise program are largely driven by the intensity at which exercise is performed. When serving special populations, exercise professionals must be cautious as overprescribing intensity can result in early dropout or detriments to a client's given health status. There are several methods for prescribing cardiorespiratory endurance exercise intensity. The two most accurate methods are the HRR and $\dot{V}O_2$ reserve ($\dot{V}O_2R$) methods. Both HRR and $\dot{V}O_2R$ take into account clients' resting values. By doing this, HRR and $\dot{V}O_2R$ make exercise intensity more individualized, and thus the results are more likely to be optimal. The HRR is calculated by subtracting a client's resting heart rate from his or her maximal heart rate. The $\dot{V}O_2R$ is calculated by subtracting one MET, which is equal to 3.5 mL/kg · min, from a client's $\dot{V}O_{2max}$. Intensity can also be quantified based on a client's perceptual response to exercise, kilocalories expended, and percentages of maximal heart rate and $\dot{V}O_{2max}$.

The general recommendation for prescribing intensity for cardiorespiratory endurance exercises is to set an initial intensity between 40 and 60 percent of HRR and $\dot{V}O_2R$.[21] This is modified for various special populations. By establishing an initial cardiorespiratory endurance exercise intensity, exercise professionals can use mathematical equations to make exercise specific to various modalities beyond simply providing a recommended heart rate range. For instance, an exercise professional can set an initial exercise intensity of 60 percent of $\dot{V}O_2R$ and determine that a client would need to walk at a certain speed and incline to elicit that specific $\dot{V}O_2$. These mathematical equations, known as metabolic equations, exist for walking, running, leg cycling, arm cycling, and stepping and are provided next with conversion factors.[22] Additional equations are available for rowing, use of handrails during treadmill exercise, and exercise on the Schwinn Airdyne cycle are beyond the scope of this text.

Metabolic Equations

Walking Equation (4 mph or less):

$$\dot{V}O_2 \text{ mL/kg} \cdot \text{min} = (0.1 \text{ x speed meters} \cdot \text{min}) + (1.8 \text{ x speed meters} \cdot \text{min x grade}) + 3.5$$

Running Equation:

$$\dot{V}O_2 \text{ mL/kg} \cdot \text{min} = (0.2 \times \text{speed meters} \cdot \text{min}) + (0.9 \times \text{speed meters} \cdot \text{min} \times \text{grade}) + 3.5$$

Stepping Equation:

$$\dot{V}O_2 \text{ mL/kg} \cdot \text{min} = (0.2 \times \text{steps} \cdot \text{min}) + (1.33 \times 1.8 \times \text{step height meters} \times \text{steps} \cdot \text{min}) + 3.5$$

Leg Cycling (Monark Cycle):

$$\dot{V}O_2 \text{ mL/kg} \cdot \text{min} = (1.8 \times \text{revolutions/min} \times \text{resistance in kg} \times 6/\text{body weight in kg}) + 7$$

Arm Cycling (Monark Arm Ergometer):

$$\dot{V}O_2 \text{ mL/kg} \cdot \text{min} = (3 \times \text{revolutions/min} \times \text{resistance in kg} \times 2.4/\text{body weight in kg}) + 3.5$$

Conversion Factors

1 inch = 2.54 centimeters

1 mph = 26.8 meters/min

1 pound = 2.2 kg

The ACSM recommends that cardiorespiratory endurance exercise be performed 30 to 60 minutes per exercise session.[23] It should be noted that improvements in $\dot{V}O_{2max}$ can be observed in as little as ten minutes per day, especially among deconditioned or previously sedentary clients.[24] When serving special populations, exercise professionals should set an initial exercise time based on the client's current fitness level, exercise history, and health status. Individuals with some history of exercise who are not deconditioned should be able to tolerate 30 minutes per exercise session with the goal of progressing to 60 minutes per exercise session. With highly deconditioned clients, ten-minute bouts of exercise per day accumulating 30 total minutes would be sufficient for exercise time. Remember, exercise time is tied to exercise intensity, where with greater exercise intensities the less time is required.

The type of cardiorespiratory endurance exercise necessary for improving $\dot{V}O_{2max}$ is called aerobic exercise. Aerobic exercise by definition is any type of exercise involving continuous movements consisting of large muscle mass contractions, which act to stress the cardiopulmonary system and oxidative phosphorylation. Therefore, several exercises could be considered an aerobic exercise. Examples of aerobic exercise include walking, jogging, cycling, dancing, rowing, swimming, and step aerobics. When serving special populations, it is important to select aerobic exercises that clients find enjoyable, are specific to client goals, and are regarded as safe.

Exercise volume is the product of frequency, time, and type. Thus the exercise volume can be increased or decreased by manipulating these variables. There are numerous methods for quantifying exercise volume. These methods include daily or weekly caloric expenditure, MET minutes, or weekly time. Weekly time is often the preferred method when serving special populations given its simplicity. The goal of a cardiorespiratory endurance program should be to accumulate 150 minutes of moderate intensity aerobic exercise per week or 75 minutes of vigorous intensity aerobic exercise per week. These values, of course, are modified for special populations.

For clients to reach their goals, the dose of exercise must be systematically and gradually increased. Failure to do so will result in a "plateau" of positive exercise adaptations. This falls in line with the principle of progressive overload and Wolff's law, which suggests that the body will adapt to imposed stresses. The ACSM recommends that exercise professionals manipulate exercise time and frequency before increasing exercise intensity.[25] A biweekly increase in exercise volume of 5 to 10 percent is a general recommendation for progressing a client's cardiorespiratory endurance exercise. In general, exercise professionals should increase a client's exercise volume slowly and as tolerated.

Demonstration Case Study 2.21

Cardiorespiratory Exercise Prescription

Rick is an exercise physiologist who specializes in serving clients with chronic diseases. His most recent client is Mick. Mick's profile is provided next.

Mick is a 54-year-old male, 220 pounds, with no major cardiac signs or symptoms and has never been diagnosed with a cardiovascular, metabolic, or renal disease. Medical history reveals a diagnosis of osteoarthritis of both knees. The client's previous physical activity was limited because of his knee pain, but he did run five miles regularly until his diagnosis of osteoarthritis. A submaximal cycle test was completed without symptoms. The client's resting heart rate was 60 beats per minute, and his estimated $\dot{V}O_{2max}$ was 40 mL/kg · min. The client is open to any exercise so long as it does not exacerbate his knee pain.

Rick is tasked with providing a cardiorespiratory endurance exercise prescription for Mick. Rick begins by selecting exercise frequency. Because of Mick's recent pattern of sedentary behavior and knee pain, Rick sets Mick's exercise frequency at three days per week. Next, Rick needs to prescribe an initial exercise intensity. Rick wants to be precise, so he uses both the HRR and $\dot{V}O_2R$ method for quantifying exercise intensity. Rick chooses an exercise intensity equal to 40 to 60 percent of HRR/$\dot{V}O_2R$. His calculations are shown next.

HRR = age-predicted maximal heart rate – resting heart rate

HRR = (220 – 54) – 60 beats per minute

HRR = 106

40 percent of HRR = (106 x 0.4) + 60 beats per minute

40 percent of HRR = 103 beats per minute

60 percent of HRR = (106 x 0.6) + 60 beats per minute

60 percent of HRR = 124 beats per minute

HRR range = 103 – 124 beats per minute

$\dot{V}O_2R = \dot{V}O_{2max} - 3.5$ mL/kg · min

$\dot{V}O_2R = 40$ mL/kg · min – 3.5 mL/kg · min

$\dot{V}O_2R = 36.5$ mL/kg · min

40 percent of $\dot{V}O_2R$ = (36.5 mL/kg · min x 0.4) + 3.5 mL/kg · min

40 percent of $\dot{V}O_2R$ = 18.1 mL/kg · min

60 percent of $\dot{V}O_2R$ = (36.5 mL/kg · min x 0.6) + 3.5 mL/kg · min

60 percent of $\dot{V}O_2R$ = 25.4 mL/kg · min

$\dot{V}O_2R$ range = 18.1 – 25.4 mL/kg · min

To further improve the quality of Mick's exercise prescription, Rick decides to use metabolic equations to give Mick specific modality settings to elicit a desired intensity. Rick uses the walking, leg cycling, arm cycling, and stepping. Rick's work is provided next.

Walking Calculations:
Rick believes that a steeper incline would help reduce the impact on Mick's knees. Therefore, he sets an incline of 10 percent and then solves the walking equation for speed in miles per hour (mph) to elicit 60 percent of Mick's $\dot{V}O_2R$.

25.4 mL/kg · min = (0.1 x speed) + (1.8 x speed x 0.10) + 3.5

Speed = 78.21 meters · minute

Speed = 2.9 mph

Leg Cycling Calculations:
Rick feels that Mick can comfortably peddle at 75 revolutions per minute. Therefore, Rick uses the leg cycling equation to solve for resistance in kiloponds (kp) to be placed on the flywheel of a Monark cycle to elicit 60 percent of Mick's $\dot{V}O_2R$.

25.4 mL/kg · min = (1.8 x 75 x resistance x 6/100 kg) + 7

Resistance = 2.16 kp

Arm Cycling Calculations:
Rick believes that arm cycling would be a sufficient cardiorespiratory exercise alternative should Mick's knee pain be too great for lower body involvement. Rick also believes that Mick can arm cycle with a resistance of 2.5 kp on the Monark arm cycle. Therefore, Rick uses the arm cycling equation to solve for revolutions per minute (rpm) to elicit 60 percent of Mick's $\dot{V}O_2R$.

25.4 mL/kg · min = (3 x revolutions per minute x 2.5 x 2.4/100 kg) + 3.5

Revolutions per minute = 122 rpm

<u>Stepping Calculations:</u>

Lastly, Rick would like Mick to occasionally perform stepping exercises. In Rick's facility, he has access to a 50-centimeter step (0.5 meters). Rick uses the stepping equation to determine a stepping rate that would elicit 60 percent of Mick's $\dot{V}O_2R$.

$$25.4 \text{ mL/kg} \cdot \text{min} = (0.2 \text{ x steps} \cdot \text{min}) + (1.33 \text{ x } 1.8 \text{ x } 0.5 \text{ x steps} \cdot \text{min}) + 3.5$$

$$\text{Stepping rate} = 15.6 \text{ steps} \cdot \text{min}$$

After prescribing exercise intensity and exercise settings, Rick moves on to prescribing exercise time, type, and volume. Rick previously chose to set initial exercise time at 30 minutes per day because of Mick's recent sedentary lifestyle and to avoid exacerbating his knee pain. Rick wants to keep Mick interested in cardiorespiratory endurance exercise; therefore, he provides a variety of exercise modalities. Rick suggests that Mick perform walking, cycling, arm cycling, and stepping throughout the program. As for volume, Rick starts Mick at accumulating 90 minutes of cardiorespiratory exercise per week with the goal of progressing to 150 total minutes.

Lastly, Rick constructs an initial progression plan. With Mick's knee pain, Rick wants to start Mick at a lower dose of exercise and progress slowly. Rick designs a plan to increase Mick's exercise time by five minutes per day each week to the point of 60 minutes of exercise time per session. After this, Rick plans to add one day per week of exercise each week until Mick is exercising five days per week. At this time, Rick plans to increase exercise intensity 5 to 10 percent per week as tolerated.

Muscular Fitness Exercise Prescription

Muscle fitness training offers a myriad of benefits for clients with chronic diseases. These benefits include cardiometabolic profile, reduced fall risk, and improved capacity to carry out activities of daily living.[26] Therefore, it is highly recommended that special populations include muscle fitness exercise, also known as resistance exercise, in their exercise program. Like cardiorespiratory exercise, the ACSM publishes recommendations for improving muscular fitness.[27] These recommendations state that healthy adults should perform resistance exercises two to three days per week at a moderate intensity (60–70 percent 1RM) targeting each major muscle group. Each exercise session should consist of two to four sets of eight to ten exercises with each set consisting of eight to 12 repetitions. This initial prescription can and should be modified based on a client's goals, needs, health status, exercise history, and likes and dislikes.

Special populations should seek to perform resistance exercises at least two or three days per week. These exercise sessions should consist of eight to ten exercises that target each major muscle group of the body. For simplicity, exercise professionals can emphasize exercises that stress the skeletal muscles of the abdomen, chest, upper and lower back, lumbo-pelvic hip complex, and shoulders, which would encompass virtually all major muscle groups. Exercise professionals must keep in mind that resistance exercise targeting the same muscles should not be performed on consecutive days. At least 48 hours should separate training sessions targeting the same muscle group. Exercise professionals can implement "split" sessions in which resistance exercise is performed four or more days per week. In this scenario, different muscle groups are targeted on different days.

The intensity of resistance exercises is typically prescribed from a client's estimated 1RM. Here exercise professionals will prescribe a percentage of 1RM for each primary exercise. The intensity of resistance exercise is largely based on a client's goals and needs (i.e., muscular strength or endurance). To elicit gains in strength, exercise professionals would prescribe an intensity of 60–70 percent of 1RM. For improvements in muscular endurance, exercise professionals would set an initial intensity of 40–50 percent of 1RM. Beginning or previously sedentary clients would typically start at 40–50 percent of 1RM. In cases of lengthy sedentary behavior or severe deconditioning, resistance bands and body weight can be used to prescribe exercise intensity.

For resistance training, exercise time is prescribed according to sets and repetitions. Like resistance exercise intensity, exercise time is set based on a client's goals and needs. Whenever a client seeks to improve muscular strength, the amount of repetitions is decreased, and the amount of sets is increased. A starting point for improving muscular strength is two to four sets of eight to 12 repetitions. Whenever a client seeks to improve muscular endurance, the amount of repetitions is increased, and the amount of sets is decreased. A starting point for improving muscular endurance is one to two sets of 15 to 25 repetitions. Sets and repetitions can and should be modified further based on a client's exercise history and health status.

There are several types of resistance exercise. Generically, exercise professionals could classify resistance exercise types as strength, endurance, or power exercises. However, as with cardiorespiratory exercise, it is beneficial for exercise professionals to be as specific as possible. Therefore, exercise professionals can direct their clients to perform body weight, resistance band, machine-based, or free-weight exercise and then further specify the exercise to be performed, such as chest press or leg press. Free-weight multijoint exercises are preferred, as the benefits are more amplified. However, this is not suitable for every population. Beginning or deconditioned clients would be more suited to starting with resistance bands, body weight, or machine-based weight exercise with the goal of progressing to free-weight exercises. Exercise professionals should always use good judgment when selecting resistance exercises and keep selections specific to client goals, needs, and health status.

Like cardiorespiratory exercise, resistance training volume is the product of frequency, intensity, and time. It is more customary for resistance training volume to be reported in research. Thus exercise professionals should focus on correctly setting resistance exercise frequency, intensity, and time, which will in turn make the volume correct. Also, like cardiorespiratory exercise, the dose of resistance exercise must be progressively increased to elicit the benefits desired. To progress clients with chronic diseases, exercise professionals should gradually increase repetitions and sets before considering increasing intensity. When exercise professions serve special populations, they should increase resistance exercise intensity as tolerated.

Demonstration Case Study 2.22

Emily is an exercise physiologist specializing in training clients with chronic diseases. Her newest client is Betsy. Betsy is a 55-year-old female who was recently diagnosed with metabolic syndrome. Betsy is overweight, previously sedentary, isn't severely deconditioned, and is interested in beginning an exercise program to improve her health. She was medically cleared prior to reporting to Emily's facility. Emily correctly asserts that Betsy would benefit from resistance exercise, as it would help her control her blood glucose and assist in weight loss. Therefore, Betsy performed a number of strength tests and found the following: (1) 1RM chest press = 120 pounds, (2) 1RM leg press = 150 pounds, (3) 1RM leg extension = 50 pounds, (4) 1RM leg curl = 50 pounds, (5) 1RM seated row = 60 pounds, (6) 1RM shoulder press = 45 pounds, and (7) seated crunch = 40 pounds. From these data, Emily established the following resistance exercise prescription:

Frequency:
Emily suggested that Betsy perform resistance exercises two days per week. Emily's rationale was that Betsy is sedentary, and she did not want to induce excessive muscle soreness in the client, which could lead to Betsy's early dropout. In addition, Emily wanted to be sure she elicited enough of a stimulus to improve Betsy's metabolic profile.

Intensity:
Given that Betsy is sedentary and has not had experience with resistance training, Emily chose a low starting intensity. Emily selected 40 percent of Betsy's 1RM as the starting intensity.

Time:
Similar to exercise intensity, since Betsy is sedentary, Emily started Betsy with less time for resistance exercise. Emily suggested that Betsy complete one set for each exercise prescribed and perform 15 repetitions for each set.

Type:
Because of Betsy's sedentary behavior and inexperience with resistance exercise, Emily chose machine-based and resistance band modalities. She specifically suggested that Betsy perform the following exercises and resistances: (1) chest press with 48 pounds, (2) leg press with 60 pounds, (3) seated row with 24 pounds, (4) seated shoulder press with 18 pounds, (5) leg extensions with 20 pounds, (6) leg curls with 20 pounds, and (7) seated crunches with 10 pounds. In addition, Emily recommended biceps curls and triceps extensions using resistance bands.

Progression:

Emily wanted to progress Betsy slowly. Emily recommended adding two repetitions for each exercise each week until 25 repetitions can be completed. At this point, Emily recommended adding another set for each exercise and reducing the repetitions for each set to 15. Next, Emily suggested slowly adding resistance as tolerated.

Flexibility Exercise

Flexibility exercises are recommended as a part of any general exercise program. Flexibility exercise becomes important with age, as range of motion at given joints decreases with age.[28] In addition, flexibility exercise can improve balance and posture.[29] The ACSM suggests that flexibility exercises be performed two to three days per week.[30] Exercise professionals should design a flexibility regimen in which each major muscle-tendon group is targeted two to four times per exercise session. Each flexibility exercise (stretch) should be held from ten to 30 seconds. "The recent ACSM recommendations suggest that static stretches should not be held for longer than 60 seconds as this may lead to deleterious effects.[31] Further, older adults should hold static stretches longer than general healthy adults, but not to exceed 60 seconds.[32] There are several types of flexibility exercises, such as static, dynamic, proprioceptive neuromuscular facilitation, and ballistic. Any type of flexibility is sufficient for improving joint range of motion in clients with chronic diseases. However, ballistic exercises should be avoided in these populations so as not to evoke a stretch reflex that could lead to injury. As a part of a general exercise program, flexibility exercises are most effective when performed at the end of an exercise session when the muscles are warmer. All variables of flexibility exercise can and should be modified to meet a client's goals.

Student Case Study 2.1

Exercise Test Selection

An exercise specialist is working for a hospital's chronic disease management clinic and is responsible for providing exercise testing, prescriptions, and supervisory services for the patients. The newest client is Blane. Blane's profile is provided next:

Demographics: (1) male and (2) 60 years old

Family History: (1) father died of heart failure at age 72, (2) mother had coronary angioplasty at age 70, and (3) all grandparents died of natural causes

Biometrics: (1) resting heart rate = 60 beats per minute; (2) resting blood pressure = 120/80 mmHg; (3) LDL-c = 106 mg/dL, HDL-c = 44 mg/dL, total cholesterol = 180 mg/dL; (4) glycosylated hemoglobin = 6.0 percent; and (5) weight = 285 lbs, BMI = 40 kg/m²

Medical Diagnoses: (1) obesity and (2) hypertension

Medications: (1) lisinopril, (2) lovastatin, and (3) aspirin

<u>Symptoms:</u> (1) fatigue associated with poor physical fitness

<u>Exercise History:</u> (1) hiking, 15 years ago; (2) manufacturing; and (3) doesn't like cycling

<u>Exercise Goals and Needs:</u> (1) weight loss and (2) reduction of cholesterol medication

1. Should the exercise specialist conduct a maximal or submaximal cardiorespiratory fitness test? In four to five sentences, indicate why based on the client's profile.
2. Which cardiorespiratory fitness test should be conducted? In four to five sentences, indicate why based on the client's profile.
3. Given limitless resources, which body composition test should be selected? In four to five sentences, provide a defense for the selection based on the client's profile.
4. Given minimal resources with a small budget, which body composition test should be selected? In four to five sentences, provide a defense for the decision based on the client's profile.
5. Specific to this case, which body composition test would be preferred? In four to five sentences, provide a defense for the decision based on the client's profile.
6. To assess muscular fitness, should one conduct muscular endurance assessments or muscular strength assessments, or both? In four to five sentences, provide a defense for the decision based on the client's profile.
7. Provide a list of four specific muscular fitness tests to conduct on the client. Then provide a four- to five-sentence defense supporting the selections.
8. To assess flexibility, which muscle-tendon group or joint(s) should be assessed? Provide a brief defense for the decision.

Student Case Study 2.2

Exercise Test Selection

An exercise physiologist is working for a hospital's diabetes management program. There, she is responsible for overseeing all exercise-related aspects of the program. Her newest client is Leigh. Leigh's profile is provided next:

<u>Demographics:</u> (1) female and (2) 40 years old

<u>Family History:</u> (1) both parents are living and neither has had surgery or a diagnosis of cardiovascular, metabolic, or renal diseases; (2) grandfather passed away at age 71 from lung cancer; (3) grandmother passed away from a myocardial infarction at the age of 64; and (4) other two grandparents passed away of natural causes

<u>Biometrics:</u> (1) resting heart rate = 71 beats per minute; (2) resting blood pressure = 118/70 mmHg; (3) LDL-c = 120 mg/dL, HDL-c = 55 mg/dL, total cholesterol = 191 mg/dL; (4) glycosylated hemoglobin = 6.4 percent; and (5) weight = 145 lbs, BMI = 23 kg/m^2

Medical Diagnoses: (1) type I diabetes mellitus

Medications: (1) Lantus

Symptoms: none

Exercise History: (1) jogging, daily; (2) swimming, three days per week in the summer; and (3) doesn't like stepping exercise

Exercise Goals and Needs: (1) improved diabetes management and (2) improved muscle mass

1. Should she conduct a maximal or submaximal cardiorespiratory fitness test? In four to five sentences, provide a defense for the decision based on the client's profile.
2. Which cardiorespiratory fitness test should she conduct? In four to five sentences, provide a defense for the decision based on the client's profile.
3. Given limitless resources, which body composition test should be selected? In four to five sentences, provide a defense for the selection based on the client's profile.
4. Given minimal resources with a small budget, which body composition test should be selected? In four to five sentences, provide a defense for the decision based on the client's profile.
5. Specific to this case, which body composition test would be preferred? In four to five sentences, provide a defense for the decision based on the client's profile.
6. To assess muscular fitness, should one conduct muscular endurance assessments or muscular strength assessments, or both? In four to five sentences, provide a defense for the decision based on the client's profile.
7. Provide a list of four specific muscular fitness tests to conduct on the client. Then provide a four- to five-sentence defense supporting the selections.

Student Case Study 2.3

Exercise Test Selection

An exercise professional working for an employee wellness program. She is responsible for serving employees with elevated risk for chronic diseases and those with chronic diseases. She performs several exercise tests per day. The newest client is Marcus, and his profile is provided next:

Demographics: (1) male and (2) 48 years old

Family History: (1) father had a myocardial infarction at age 52, (2) mother was diagnosed with chronic obstructive pulmonary disease at the age of 60, (3) all grandparents passed away from natural causes

Biometrics: (1) resting heart rate = 84 beats per minute; (2) resting blood pressure = 152/88 mmHg; (3) LDL-c = 145 mg/dL, HDL-c = 38 mg/dL, total cholesterol = 236 mg/dL; (4) glycosylated hemoglobin = 6.7 percent; and (5) weight = 300 lbs, BMI = 44 kg/m^2

Medical Diagnoses: (1) metabolic syndrome and (2) radicular low back pain

Medications: (1) atorvastatin, (2) aspirin, and (3) gabapentin

Symptoms: (1) low back pain and (2) fatigue because of poor fitness

Exercise History: (1) football player, college (2) working on cars, biweekly, and (3) doesn't like treadmill exercise

Exercise Goals and Needs: (1) weight loss, (2) improved metabolic health, and (3) medication reduction

1. Should she conduct a maximal or submaximal cardiorespiratory fitness test? In four to five sentences, provide a defense for the decision based on the client's profile.
2. Which cardiorespiratory fitness test should she conduct? In four to five sentences, provide a defense for the decision based on the client's profile.
3. Given limitless resources, which body composition test should be selected? In four to five sentences, provide a defense for the selection based on the client's profile.
4. Given minimal resources with a small budget, which body composition test should be selected? In four to five sentences, provide a defense for the decision based on the client's profile.
5. Specific to this case, which body composition test would be preferred? In four to five sentences, provide a defense for the decision based on the client's profile.
6. To assess muscular fitness, should one conduct muscular endurance assessments or muscular strength assessments, or both? In four to five sentences, provide a defense for the decision based on the client's profile.
7. Provide a list of four specific muscular fitness tests to conduct on the client. Then provide a four- to five-sentence defense supporting the selections.

Student Case Study 2.4

Exercise Test Selection: Critical Thinking

An exercise physiologist is working for a vascular rehabilitation program. Specifically within this program, she is responsible for providing direct supervision for patients exercising with peripheral artery disease. This includes conducting exercise tests. Nelson is the newest client, and his profile is provided next:

Demographics: (1) male and (2) 53 years old

Family History: (1) father had a fatal myocardial infarction at age 60, (2) mother had deep vein thrombosis and suffered a fatal pulmonary embolism at the age of 63, and (3) all grandparents passed away from heart disease in their mid-60s

Biometrics: (1) resting heart rate = 101 beats per minute; (2) resting blood pressure = 142/94 mmHg; (3) LDL-c = 122 mg/dL, HDL-c = 42 mg/dL, total cholesterol = 209 mg/dL; (4) glycosylated hemoglobin = 6.6 percent; and (5) weight = 244 lbs, BMI = 35 kg/m²

Medical Diagnoses: (1) bilateral peripheral artery disease, popliteal artery and (2) coronary artery disease

Medications: (1) atenolol, (2) simvastatin, (3) lisinopril, (4) CoQ10, and (5) clopidogrel

Symptoms: (1) claudication with walking, relieved by rest

Exercise History: (1) phase II cardiovascular rehabilitation and (2) does not like walking or running because it causes lower leg pain

Exercise Goals and Needs: (1) improved claudication threshold and (2) improved cardiovascular disease risk profile

1. Which cardiorespiratory fitness test should she conduct? In four to five sentences, provide a defense for the decision based on the client's profile.
2. Should she consider conducting a treadmill test? In four to five sentences, provide a defense for the decision based on the client's profile.
3. Specific to this case, which body composition test should she conduct? In four to five sentences, provide a defense for the decision based on the client's profile.
4. Provide a list of four specific muscular fitness tests she should conduct on the client. Then provide a four- to five-sentence defense supporting the selections.

Student Case Study 2.5

Contraindications for Exercise Testing

A self-employed exercise specialist serves clients with chronic diseases. As a part of the job, he gathers relevant medical information, conducts exercise tests, writes exercise prescriptions, and supervises exercise programs. His newest client is Tonya. Tonya's medical history is provided next:

Demographics: (1) female and (2) 61 years old

Family History: (1) mother, father, and grandparents all passed away from natural causes in their 70s and 80s and (2) sister was diagnosed with a dissecting aortic aneurysm at the age of 67

Biometrics: (1) resting heart rate = 68 beats per minute; (2) resting blood pressure = 170/116 mmHg; (3) LDL-c = 113 mg/dL, HDL-c = 44 mg/dL, total cholesterol = 212 mg/dL; (4) glycosylated hemoglobin = 6.5 percent; and (5) weight = 189 lbs, BMI = 34 kg/m²

Medical Diagnoses: (1) coronary artery disease, coronary angioplasty, 2017; (2) atrial fibrillation, uncontrolled; (3) dissecting aortic aneurysm, surgery, 2015; (3) hypercholesterolemia; and (4) sleep apnea

Medications: (1) atenolol, (2) simvastatin, (3) lisinopril, (4) CoQ10, and (5) clopidogrel

Symptoms: (1) substernal chest pain, occasionally relieved by rest

1. Should he conduct a cardiorespiratory fitness test on this client? Succinctly defend the answer.
2. List all present contraindications the client has for exercise testing.
3. Research each present contraindication and provide a four- to five-sentence response to explain how performing an exercise test may present an immediate danger to the client's health (four to five sentences for each contraindication).
4. Does the client have any contraindications for exercise testing in which the benefit of conducting an exercise test would outweigh the risks? If so, provide the contraindication(s).

Student Case Study 2.6

Contraindications for Exercise Testing

An exercise professional who specializes in serving clients with chronic diseases. The newest client is Scott. Scott's profile is provided below

Demographics: (1) male and (2) 59 years old

Family History: (1) mother passed away at age 81 from emphysema, (2) father passed away at age 50 from a farm accident

Biometrics: (1) resting heart rate = 59 beats per minute; (2) resting blood pressure = 108/66 mmHg; (3) LDL-c = 98 mg/dL, HDL-c = 40 mg/dL, total cholesterol = 177 mg/dL; (4) glycosylated hemoglobin = 6.4 percent; and (5) weight = 180 lbs, BMI = 27 kg/m^2

Medical Diagnoses: (1) ischemic stroke, 2017; (2) heart failure, decompensated, 2016; (3) second-degree atrioventricular block; and (4) hyperthyroidism

Medications: (1) digitalis, (2) atorvastatin, (3) telmisartan, (4) CoQ10, and (5) Coumadin

Symptoms: (1) fatigue associated with poor fitness and (2) occasional palpitations

1. Should the exercise professional conduct a cardiorespiratory fitness test on this client? Succinctly defend the answer.
2. List all present contraindications the client has for exercise testing.
3. Research each present contraindication and provide a four- to five-sentence response to explain how performing an exercise test may present an immediate danger to the client's health (four to five sentences for each contraindication).
4. Does the client have any contraindications for exercise testing in which the benefit of conducting an exercise test would outweigh the risks? If so, provide the contraindication(s).

Student Case Study 2.7

Contraindications for Exercise Testing: On Your Own

You are an exercise specialist responsible for overseeing exercise testing procedures on clients with chronic diseases. You have a licensed physician who provides medical clearance and supervision for all exercise tests. In your role, you encounter cases where exercise testing can pose a threat to immediate health. You also encounter cases in which the benefits of an exercise test outweigh the risks. In this exercise, provide two instances where exercise testing should not be conducted. Then provide a four- to five-sentence response explaining how exercise would pose immediate danger to health. Next, provide two instances when the benefits of exercise testing would outweigh the risks and provide a four- to five-sentence response explaining why the benefits would outweigh the risks.

Student Case Study 2.8

Exercise Test Termination

An exercise physiologist is working for a local hospital. His job is to oversee all exercise tests conducted on clients with chronic diseases. Within this job, he must be knowledgeable of normal and abnormal physiological responses to exercise and make the judgment when to terminate an exercise test. The following cycle test (Figure 2.9) was recently conducted on a 55-year-old female with type II diabetes with a predetermined end point 85 percent of the client's age-predicted maximal heart rate.

Figure 2.9 This table depicts hypothetical data from a cycle test. Students should use these data to answer the questions in Student Case Study 2.8

Stage	Kpm/ min	Heart Rate	Blood Pressure	RPE	ECG	Symptoms/Comments
Resting	0	60	118/78	NA	Sinus	No symptoms
I	150	85	128/78	7	Sinus	No symptoms
II	300	102	138/78	9	Sinus	Sweating
III	450	115	156/78	11	Sinus	Fatigue
IV	600	117	146/78	15	Sinus	Pale skin, sweating
V	750	140	146/78	16	Sinus	Pale skin, sweating
Immediate	0	140	140/78	NA	Sinus	Pale skin, breathlessness
Recovery 1 min	0	133	138/78	NA	Sinus	Breathlessness
Recovery 5 min	0	85	122/78	NA	Sinus	No symptoms

1. Calculate the predetermined end point heart rate.
2. Should this exercise test have been terminated prior to completion? Why or why not?
3. In five to six complete sentences, thoroughly explain either why it was physiologically safe or unsafe to complete the exercise test.
4. Explain how an exercise professional can make sure that all exercise tests are conducted safely. Specifically, address issues related to knowledge, skills, and test supervision.

Student Case Study 2.9

Exercise Test Termination

An exercise physiologist works in a stress testing lab. Her job is to conduct stress tests on clients with chronic diseases. In this role, she must be very knowledgeable of normal and abnormal exercise responses. The following test (Figure 2.10) was recently conducted on a 47-year-old male suffering from metabolic syndrome. The predetermined end point was 70 percent of the client's HRR.

Figure 2.10 This table depicts hypothetical data from a YMCA cycle test. Students should use these data to answer the questions in Student Case Study 2.11

Stage	Speed (mph)	Grade %	Heart Rate	Blood Pressure	RPE	ECG	Symptoms
Resting	0	0	71	120/82	NA	Sinus	No symptoms
I	1.7	10.0	99	130/82	8	Sinus	No symptoms
II	2.5	12.0	119	142/80	11	Sinus	No symptoms
III	3.4	14.0	129	158/80	15	Sinus	No symptoms
IV	4.2	16.0	188	166/80	17	Ventricular Tachycardia	Breathlessness, palpitations
Immediate	0	0	180	160/80	NA	Ventricular Tachycardia	Breathlessness, palpitations
Recovery 1 min	0	0	172	134/80	NA	Sinus Tachycardia	Breathlessness
Recovery 5 min	0	0	110	122/80	NA	Sinus Tachycardia	Breathlessness

1. Calculate the predetermined end point heart rate.
2. Should this exercise test have been terminated prior to completion? Why or why not?
3. In five to six complete sentences, thoroughly explain either why it was physiologically safe or unsafe to complete the exercise test.

4. Explain how an exercise professional can make sure that all exercise tests are conducted safely. Specifically, address issues related to knowledge, skills, and test supervision.

Student Case Study 2.10

Exercise Test Termination: On Your Own

You are an exercise specialist responsible for overseeing exercise testing procedures on clients with chronic diseases. You were recently tasked with training a new exercise specialist to conduct exercise tests. One of the most important objectives is to ensure that the trainee is fully knowledgeable of the normal physiological responses to exercise and test termination criteria. Explain the normal heart rate, cardiac output, stroke volume, and blood pressure responses to exercise. Then provide a list of all test termination criteria not present in Case Studies 2.8 and 2.9, and fully explain why continuing a test under those circumstances would be a danger to immediate health.

Student Case Study 2.11

Exercise Test Interpretation: YMCA Cycle Test

An exercise physiologist specializes in serving clients with chronic diseases. He just completed a YMCA cycle test on a 53-year-old male client with peripheral artery disease who weighs 190 pounds. The results of the test are provided in Figure 2.11. After reading the results use the graph and leg cycling equation to interpret the results and answer the questions.

Figure 2.11 This table depicts hypothetical data from a YMCA cycle test. Students should use these data to answer the questions in Student Case Study 2.11

Stage	Kpm/ min	Heart Rate	Blood Pressure	RPE	ECG	Symptoms/ Comments
Resting	0	68	122/74	NA	Sinus	No symptoms
I	150	95	130/74	7	Sinus	No symptoms
II	450	112	138/74	11	Sinus	No symptoms
III	600	128	148/76	13	Sinus	No symptoms
Immediate	0	126	140/74	NA	Sinus	No symptoms
Recovery 1 min	0	103	120/76	NA	Sinus	No symptoms
Recovery 5 min	0	85	118/72	NA	Sinus	No symptoms

1. Using graph paper (Figure 2.12), estimate the maximal work rate (kpm/min). Then insert the estimated maximal work rate into the following equation to estimate $\dot{V}O_{2\,max}$:

   $\dot{V}O_2$ max mL/kg $\cdot$ min = (1.8 x estimated maximal work rate/kg body weight) + 7.

2. Given that this was a submaximal cardiorespiratory test, there are factors that exercise professionals must control. List and explain three factors that can limit the accuracy of a submaximal cardiorespiratory fitness test.

3. Given the results of the test, compare the results to normative data.

Figure 2.12 Students may use these gridlines to graph data from the YMCA cycle test

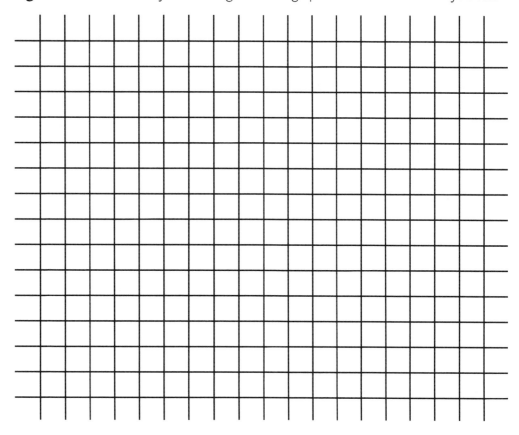

Student Case Study 2.12

Exercise Test Interpretation: YMCA Cycle Test

An exercise physiologist specializes in serving clients with chronic diseases. She just completed a YMCA cycle test on a 47-year-old male client with osteoarthritis who weighs 200 pounds. The results of the test are provided in Figure 2.13. After reading the results, use the graph and leg cycling equation to interpret the results and answer the questions.

Figure 2.13 This table depicts hypothetical data from a YMCA cycle test. Students should use these data to answer the questions in Student Case Study 2.12

Stage	Kpm/ min	Heart Rate	Blood Pressure	RPE	ECG	Symptoms/ Comments
Resting	0	56	116/70	NA	Sinus	No symptoms
I	150	75	122/70	7	Sinus	No symptoms
II	750	122	140/72	10	Sinus	No symptoms
III	900	134	152/72	13	Sinus	No symptoms
Immediate	0	130	148/70	NA	Sinus	No symptoms
Recovery 1 min	0	114	126/70	NA	Sinus	No symptoms
Recovery 5 min	0	67	120/70	NA	Sinus	No symptoms

1. Using graph paper, estimate maximal work rate (kpm/min). Then insert the estimated maximal work rate into the following equation to estimate $\dot{V}O_{2max}$:

$\dot{V}O_2$ max mL/kg · min = (1.8 x estimated maximal work rate/kg body weight) + 7

2. Assuming this client consumed a cup of coffee and smoked a cigarette prior to the test how might the results have been influenced?
3. Given the results of the test compare the results to normative data.

Figure 2.14 Students may use these gridlines to graph data from the YMCA cycle test

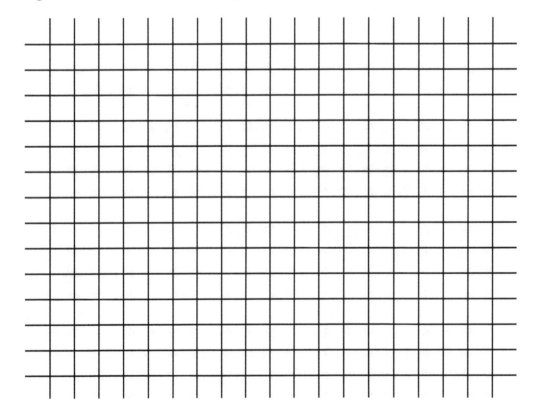

Exercise Test Interpretation: Astrand-Rhyming Cycle Test

An exercise physiologist specializes in serving clients with chronic diseases. He just completed an Astrand-Rhyming cycle test on a deconditioned, 227-pound, 40-year-old male client with dyslipidemia. The results of the test are provided in Figure 2.15. After reading the results, use the modified Astrand-Rhyming to interpret the results and answer the questions.

Figure 2.15 This table depicts hypothetical data from an Astrand-Rhyming cycle test. Students should use these data to answer the questions in Student Case Study 2.13

Stage/Minute	Kpm/m	Heart Rate	Blood Pressure	RPE	ECG	Symptoms
Resting		80	132/86	NA	Sinus	No symptoms
I	300	130	160/86	10	Sinus	No symptoms
II	300	130	160/86	11	Sinus	No symptoms
III	300	130	162/86	11	Sinus	No symptoms
IV	300	131	166/88	11	Sinus	No symptoms
V	300	133	166/86	12	Sinus	No symptoms
VI	300	135	170/86	12	Sinus	No symptoms
Immediate	150	130	168/86	NA	Sinus	No symptoms
Recovery 1 min	150	115	144/84	NA	Sinus	No symptoms
Recovery 5 min	75	108	140/80	NA	Sinus	No symptoms

1. Using the Astrand-Rhyming nomogram, estimate $\dot{V}O_{2max}$ in L · min. Be sure to multiply by a correction factor. Then convert $\dot{V}O_{2max}$ to mL/kg · min.
2. If this client were a female who was previously active, how might one modify the Astrand-Rhyming protocol from the aforementioned test?
3. Compare the client's $\dot{V}O_{2max}$ to normative data.

Exercise Test Interpretation: Astrand-Rhyming Cycle Test

An exercise physiologist specializes in serving clients with chronic diseases. He just completed an Astrand-Rhyming cycle test on a well-conditioned, 132-pound, 40-year-old female client with osteoarthritis. The results of the test are provided in Figure 2.16. After reading the results, use the modified Astrand-Rhyming to interpret the results and answer the questions.

Figure 2.16 This table depicts hypothetical data from an Astrand-Rhyming cycle test. Students should use these data to answer the questions in Student Case Study 2.14

Stage/Minute	Kpm/m	Heart Rate	Blood Pressure	RPE	ECG	Symptoms
Resting		60	118/76	NA	Sinus	No symptoms
I	600	125	128/74	9	Sinus	No symptoms
II	600	125	134/76	10	Sinus	No symptoms
III	600	126	134/76	11	Sinus	No symptoms
IV	600	127	134/74	11	Sinus	No symptoms
V	600	127	136/74	11	Sinus	No symptoms
VI	600	128	136/76	12	Sinus	No symptoms
Immediate	300	126	134/76	NA	Sinus	No symptoms
Recovery 1 min	150	85	124/74	NA	Sinus	No symptoms
Recovery 5 min	75	75	120/74	NA	Sinus	No symptoms

1. Using the Astrand-Rhyming nomogram, estimate $\dot{V}O_{2max}$ in L · min. Be sure to multiply by a correction factor. Then, convert $\dot{V}O_{2max}$ to mL/kg · min.
2. If this client were a female who was deconditioned, how might one modify the Astrand-Rhyming protocol from the aforementioned test?
3. Compare the client's $\dot{V}O_{2max}$ to normative data.

Student Case Study 2.15

Exercise Test Interpretation: Submaximal Treadmill Test

An exercise physiologist specializes in serving clients with chronic diseases. She just completed a submaximal treadmill test on a 56-year-old male client with hypertension. The test was terminated at a heart rate equal to 70 percent of the client's HRR. The results of the test are provided in Figure 2.17. After reading the results, use the walking or running equation and a proportion equation to interpret the results and answer the questions.

Figure 2.17 This table depicts hypothetical data from a submaximal treadmill test. Students should use these data to answer the questions in Student Case Study 2.15

Stage	Speed (mph)	Grade %	Heart Rate	Blood Pressure	RPE	ECG	Symptoms
Resting	0	0	85	130/82	NA	Sinus	No symptoms
I	1.7	10.0	100	142/82	8	Sinus	No symptoms
II	2.5	12.0	129	156/80	11	Sinus	No symptoms
III	3.4	14.0	144	168/80	15	Sinus	No symptoms

(Continued)

Figure 2.17 This table depicts hypothetical data from a submaximal treadmill test. Students should use these data to answer the questions in Student Case Study 2.15 (Continued)

Stage	Speed (mph)	Grade %	Heart Rate	Blood Pressure	RPE	ECG	Symptoms
Immediate	0	0	180	168/82	NA	Sinus	No symptoms
Recovery 1 min	0	0	172	142/80	NA	Sinus	No symptoms
Recovery 5 min	0	0	110	132/80	NA	Sinus	No symptoms

1. Using one of the following two equations, estimate $\dot{V}O_2$ for the last completed stage:

   Walking: $\dot{V}O_2$ = (0.1 x speed in m/min) + (1.8 x speed in m/min x grade) + 3.5
   Running: $\dot{V}O_2$ = (0.2 x speed in m/min) + (0.9 x speed in m/min x grade) + 3.5
   Find $\dot{V}O_2$ in last stage in mL/kg · min
   Find estimated $\dot{V}O_{2max}$ in mL/kg · min

2. How might one modify the protocol used if the client was deconditioned?
3. Compare the client's $\dot{V}O_{2max}$ to normative data.

Student Case Study 2.16

Exercise Test Interpretation: Submaximal Treadmill Test

An exercise physiologist specializes in serving clients with chronic diseases. The exercise physiologist just completed a submaximal treadmill test on a 62-year-old female client who is a survivor of cancer. The test was terminated at a heart rate equal to 70 percent of the client's HRR. The results of the test are provided in Figure 2.18. After reading the results, use the walking or running equation and a proportion equation to interpret the results and answer the questions.

Figure 2.18 This table depicts hypothetical data from a submaximal treadmill test. Students should use these data to answer the questions in Student Case Study 2.16

Stage	Speed (mph)	Grade %	Heart Rate	Blood Pressure	RPE	ECG	Symptoms
Resting	0	0	74	108/62	NA	Sinus	No symptoms
1	1.7	0.0	110	118/62	8	Sinus	No symptoms
2	1.7	5.0	122	130/62	11	Sinus	No symptoms
3	1.7	10.0	133	144/62	15	Sinus	No symptoms
Immediate	0	0	130	140/62	NA	Sinus	No symptoms
Recovery 1 min	0	0	110	118/60	NA	Sinus	No symptoms
Recovery 5 min	0	0	81	106/60	NA	Sinus	No symptoms

1. Using one of the following two equations, estimate $\dot{V}O_2$ for the last completed stage:

    Walking: $\dot{V}O_2 = (0.1 \times \text{speed in m/min}) + (1.8 \times \text{speed in m/min} \times \text{grade}) + 3.5$

    Running: $\dot{V}O_2 = (0.2 \times \text{speed in m/min}) + (0.9 \times \text{speed in m/min} \times \text{grade}) + 3.5$

    Find $\dot{V}O_2$ in last stage in mL/kg · min

    Find estimated $\dot{V}O_{2\,max}$ in mL/kg · min

2. If the client used the handrails during the test, how might that influence the accuracy of the estimate?

3. Compare the client's $\dot{V}O_{2\,max}$ to normative data.

Student Case Study 2.17

Exercise Test Interpretation: Maximal Treadmill Test

An exercise physiologist specializes in serving clients with chronic diseases. She just completed a maximal treadmill test on a 42-year-old male client who has asthma. The results of the test are provided in Figure 2.19. After reading the results, interpret them and answer the questions.

Figure 2.19 This table depicts hypothetical data from a maximal treadmill test. Students should use these data to answer the questions in Student Case Study 2.17

Stage	Time	Speed (mph)	Grade %	$\dot{V}O_2$ (mL/ kg · min)	$\dot{V}O_2$ (L · min)	Blood Lactate (mmol)	RPE	Heart Rate
Resting	NA	0	0	4.7	0.39	NA	NA	72
Warm-Up	NA	2	0	7	0.57	NA	NA	85
I	2:00	2.5	0	15.4	1.26	0.5	7	108
II	4:00	5.5	0	18.1	1.48	1.6	9	133
III	6:00	6.0	2	32.9	2.69	2.2	13	147
IV	8:00	6.5	3	40.4	3.30	4.8	16	168
V	10:00	6.5	5.5	52.1	4.31	7.5	17	177
VI	12:00	6.5	7.5	53.6	4.39	8.6	18	179
Immediate	NA	3	0	52.1	NA	NA	NA	175
Recovery 1 min	NA	2.5	0	35.7	NA	NA	NA	160
Recovery 5 min	NA	1.5	0	12.3	NA	NA	NA	97

1. After analyzing the data, what is the client's $\dot{V}O_{2\,max}$ in mL/kg · min?
2. Did this client achieve a true $\dot{V}O_{2\,max}$? Thoroughly explain why or why not.
3. Compare this client's results to normative data.

An exercise physiologist specializes in serving clients with type II diabetes mellitus. The newest client is a 54-year-old male who weighs 255 pounds. The exercise physiologist wants to prescribe this client a resistance training program to help him better control his blood glucose. Therefore, she conducts a series of muscular strength tests and collects the following data (Figure 2.20).

Figure 2.20 This table depicts hypothetical data from 3–5RM tests. Students should use these data to answer the questions in Student Case Study 2.18

Leg Press Strength Test

Trial 1	5 repetitions
	225 weight
Trial 2	3 repetitions
	240 weight
Trial 3	3 repetitions
	255 weight
Best Trial	3 repetitions
	255 weight

Chest Press Strength Test

Trial 1	5 repetitions
	165 weight
Trial 2	3 repetitions
	180 weight
Trial 3	3 repetitions
	200 weight
Best Trial	3 repetitions
	200 weight

1. Use the Lander equation to predict the client's maximal leg press strength.
2. Calculate a weight pushed to body weight ratio and compare the client's results to normative data.

3. Use the Lander equation to predict the client's maximal chest press strength.
4. Calculate a weight pushed to body weight ratio and compare the client's results to normative data.

Student Case Study 2.19

Muscular Strength

An exercise physiologist specializes in serving clients with cardiometabolic diseases. The newest client is a 60-year-old female who weighs 165 pounds. The client suffers from metabolic syndrome, and the exercise physiologist wants to prescribe the client a resistance training program to help her improve her blood pressure and blood lipids. Therefore, the exercise physiologist conducts a series of muscular strength tests and collects the following data (Figure 2.21).

Figure 2.21 This table depicts hypothetical data from 3–5RM tests. Students should use these data to answer the questions in Student Case Study 2.19

Leg Press Strength Test

Trial 1	5 repetitions 145 weight
Trial 2	3 repetitions 165 weight
Trial 3	3 repetitions 180 weight
Best Trial	3 repetitions 180 weight

Chest Press Strength Test

Trial 1	5 repetitions 100 weight
Trial 2	3 repetitions 120 weight
Trial 3	3 repetitions 140 weight
Best Trial	5 repetitions 140 weight

1. Use the Lander equation to predict the client's maximal leg press strength.

2. Calculate a weight pushed to body weight ratio and compare the client's results to normative data.
3. Use the Lander equation to predict the client's maximal chest press strength.
4. Calculate a weight pushed to body weight ratio and compare the client's results to normative data.

Student Case Study 2.20

Body Composition Test Interpretation: Skinfolds

An exercise specialist is responsible for interpreting body composition assessments conducted on special populations. He was recently presented with the following skinfold and anthropomorphic data from a 237-pound, 43-year-old male cancer survivor. Analyze the results to interpret body composition (Figure 2.22) and answer the questions.

Figure 2.22 This table depicts hypothetical data from a seven-site skinfold assessment. Students should use these data to answer the questions in Student Case Study 2.20

Site	Trial 1	Trial 2	Trial 3	Average
Triceps	13	15	14	mm
Subscapular	9	11	11	mm
Chest	20	22	20	mm
Abdominal	26	27	25	mm
Suprailiac	30	33	32	mm
Midaxillary	18	17	17	mm
Thigh	13	13	15	mm
Waist Circumference	42 inches			

1. Using the seven-site skinfold body density equation for men, calculate body density.
2. Using the Siri equation, estimate the client's body fat percentage.
3. Calculate the client's fat and nonfat weight in pounds.
4. Compare the results to normative data.
5. Using the three-site skinfold body density equation for men, calculate body density.
6. Using the Siri equation, estimate the client's body fat percentage.
7. Calculate the client's fat and nonfat weight in pounds.
8. Was there a difference between the seven- and three-site skinfold calculations for body density and body fat? If there was a difference, why would the difference exist?
9. Classify the client's waist circumference according to disease risk.

Body Composition Test Interpretation: Skinfolds

An exercise specialist is responsible for interpreting body composition assessments conducted on special populations. She was recently presented with the following skinfold and anthropomorphic data from a 173-pound, 54-year-old female with type I diabetes. Analyze the results to interpret body composition (Figure 2.23) and answer the questions.

Figure 2.23 This table depicts hypothetical data from a seven-site skinfold assessment. Students should use these data to answer the questions in Student Case Study 2.21

Site	Trial 1	Trial 2	Trial 3	Average
Triceps	20	22	21	mm
Subscapular	19	21	23	mm
Chest	19	19	18	mm
Abdominal	22	24	24	mm
Suprailiac	16	19	18	mm
Axilla	22	25	23	mm
Thigh	29	28	29	mm
Waist Circumference	38 inches			

1. Using the seven-site skinfold body density equation for women, calculate body density.
2. Using the Siri equation, estimate the client's body fat percentage.
3. Calculate the client's fat and nonfat weight in pounds.
4. Compare the results to normative data.
5. Using the three-site skinfold body density equation for women, calculate body density.
6. Using the Siri equation, estimate the client's body fat percentage.
7. Calculate the client's fat and nonfat weight in pounds.
8. Was there a difference between the seven- and three-site skinfold calculations for body density and body fat? If there was a difference, why would the difference exist?
9. Classify the client's waist circumference according to disease risk.

Exercise Prescription: Cardiorespiratory Endurance

An exercise professional specializes in serving clients with metabolic disorders. The newest client is a 67-year-old man with type II diabetes who weighs 235 pounds. The exercise professional just conducted a graded exercise test, completed without complications, and the client achieved an estimated $\dot{V}O_{2max}$ of 32 mL/kg · min. Prior to the test, the client's resting heart rate was 69 beats per minute. The client was previously sedentary and does not like cycling exercise because of discomfort.

1. Calculate a heart rate range based on HRR that the client should maintain during aerobic exercise.
2. Calculate a $\dot{V}O_2$ range based on $\dot{V}O_2$ reserve that the client should maintain during aerobic exercise.
3. Provide an exercise type (be specific), frequency, and time at the $\dot{V}O_2$ range found in question number 1 for the client to improve his cardiorespiratory fitness.
4. Suggest four possible aerobic exercises that would be appropriate for this client. Then explain the rationale for each selection.
5. Use the walking equation to calculate a walking speed (in mph) for the client that elicits 60 percent of the $\dot{V}O_2$ reserve. The percent grade of the treadmill is 12 percent.
6. Use the stepping equation to calculate a stepping rate for the client that elicits 40 percent of his $\dot{V}O_2$ reserve. The height of the step is 25 centimeters.
7. Use the arm cycle equation to calculate a resistance to be placed on the flywheel for the client that elicits 50 percent of the $\dot{V}O_2$ reserve. The client turns the arm crank at 70 rpm.
8. Suggest a progression scheme to advance the client toward a goal of improving the $\dot{V}O_{2max}$ by 20 percent.
9. How could the exercise prescription be modified if this client had orthopedic limitations?

Student Case Study 2.23

Exercise Prescription: Cardiorespiratory Endurance

An exercise specialist is responsible for designing exercise prescriptions for clients with chronic diseases. The most recent client is a 270-pound, 47-year-old, obese male. The exercise specialist conducted a submaximal cycle test without complications and estimated a $\dot{V}O_{2max}$ of 24 mL/kg · min. Prior to the test, a resting heart rate of 78 beats per minute was recorded. The client is deconditioned, has not exercised in 20 years, and does not like running or stepping.

1. Calculate a heart rate range based on HRR that the client should maintain during aerobic exercise.
2. Calculate a $\dot{V}O_2$ range based on $\dot{V}O_2$ reserve that the client should maintain during aerobic exercise.
3. Provide an exercise type (be specific), frequency, and time at the $\dot{V}O_2$ range found in question number 1 for the client to improve his cardiorespiratory fitness.
4. Suggest four possible aerobic exercises that would be appropriate for this client. Then explain the rationale for each selection.

5. Use the walking equation to calculate a walking speed (in mph) for the client that elicits 55 percent of his $\dot{V}O_2$ reserve. The percent grade of the treadmill is 10 percent.
6. Use the leg cycling equation to calculate a peddling frequency for the client that elicits 45 percent of his $\dot{V}O_2$ reserve. The resistance on the flywheel is 2 kiloponds.
7. Use the arm cycle equation to calculate a resistance to be placed on the flywheel of a Monark ergometer for the client that elicits 40 percent of his $\dot{V}O_2$ reserve. The client turns the arm crank at 80 rpm.
8. Suggest a progression scheme to advance the client to meet his weight loss goal.
9. How could the exercise prescription be modified if this client were previously active and not deconditioned?

Student Case Study 2.24

Exercise Prescription: Muscular Strength

A corporate health specialist who serves employees of a large company specializes in chronic diseases. As a part of his responsibilities, he designs all exercise plans. He was recently presented with the following data: (1) 40-year-old client with type I diabetes, (2) exercises regularly, (3) goal to improve blood glucose and improve muscular strength, (4) no orthopedic limitations, (5) chest press 1RM = 200 pounds, (6) leg press 1RM = 275 pounds, and (7) open to any resistance exercise program.

1. Provide a range for weight that the client should chest press.
2. Provide a range for weight that the client should leg press.
3. Provide a resistance exercise prescription for frequency, number of exercises, sets, and repetitions to improve muscular strength.
4. Suggest at least four specific resistance training exercises that are appropriate for this client.
5. Suggest a progression scheme to advance the client toward the goal of improving overall muscular strength by 20 percent.
6. How would one modify the exercise prescription if this client's goal were to improve muscular endurance?

Student Case Study 2.25

Exercise Prescription: Muscular Endurance

A clinical exercise physiologist in a phase III cardiovascular rehabilitation program is responsible for overseeing all exercise programs for the patients with multiple chronic diseases. One of the patients is ready to begin a resistance training program. She is a 70-year-old female who weighs 165 pounds. The patient has never performed resistance training. Prior to prescribing exercise, the exercise physiologist conducts a modified push-up test and the patient completes five successful repetitions.

1. Provide a resistance exercise prescription for frequency, intensity, number of exercises, sets, and repetitions to improve muscular endurance.
2. Suggest at least four specific resistance training exercises that are appropriate for this client.
3. Suggest a progression scheme to advance the client toward the goal of improving overall muscular fitness.
4. How would one modify the exercise prescription if this client had experience with resistance training?

Student Case Study 2.26

Exercise Testing and Prescription: Comprehensive Case Study

An exercise physiologist is working for a health-fitness facility specializing in serving special populations. She thoroughly collected the following data from her most recent client:

Demographics: (1) male and (2) 61 years old

Family History: (1) father passed away of natural causes at the age of 83, (2) mother passed away of an ischemic stroke at the age of 64, (3) oldest brother was diagnosed with coronary artery disease at the age of 54, and (4) youngest sister was diagnosed with type II diabetes mellitus at the age of 60

Biometrics: (1) resting heart rate = 83 beats per minute; (2) resting blood pressure = 134/86 mmHg; (3) LDL-c = 131 mg/dL, HDL-c = 39 mg/dL, total cholesterol = 220 mg/dL; (4) glycosylated hemoglobin = 6.7 percent; and (5) weight = 256 lbs, BMI = 35.2 kg/m^2

Medical Diagnoses: (1) metabolic syndrome, (2) obesity, and (3) bilateral knee joint osteoarthritis

Medications: (1) atorvastatin, (2) lisinopril, and (3) naproxen

Symptoms: Knee pain when climbing stairs and walking uphill

Exercise History: (1) daily static stretching, (2) doesn't like to walk uphill or climb stairs

Exercise Goals and Needs: (1) lose body fat, (2) increase fat-free mass to assist in weight loss, and (3) improve capacity function with arthritis.

1. Should she conduct a maximal or submaximal cardiorespiratory fitness test? In four to five sentences, provide a defense for the decision based on the client's profile.
2. Which cardiorespiratory fitness test should she conduct? In four to five sentences, provide a defense for the decision based on the client's profile.
3. Given limitless resources, which body composition test would she conduct? In four to five sentences, provide a defense for the decision based on the client's profile.

4. Given minimal resources with a small budget, which body composition test should she conduct? In four to five sentences, provide a defense for the decision based on the client's profile.
5. Specific to this case, which body composition test should she conduct? In four to five sentences, provide a defense for the decision based on the client's profile.
6. To assess muscular fitness, should she conduct muscular endurance assessments or muscular strength assessments, or both? In four to five sentences, provide a defense for the decision based on the client's profile.
7. Provide a list of four specific muscular fitness tests she should conduct on the client. Then provide a four- to five-sentence defense supporting the selections.
8. Based on the answer for questions one and two, calculate the client's $\dot{V}O_{2\,max}$ from the most appropriate of the following cardiorespiratory fitness tests (Figures 2.24–2.28).

Figure 2.24 This table depicts hypothetical data from a YMCA cycle test

YMCA Cycle Test

Stage	Kpm/min	Heart Rate	Blood Pressure	RPE	ECG	Symptoms/ Comments
Resting	0	83	134/86	NA	Sinus	No symptoms
I	150	107	148/84	7	Sinus	No symptoms
II	300	121	162/84	13	Sinus	No symptoms
III	450	133	180/86	15	Sinus	No symptoms
Immediate	0	140	178/86	NA	Sinus	No symptoms
Recovery 1 min	0	133	152/82	NA	Sinus	No symptoms
Recovery 5 min	0	85	140/84	NA	Sinus	No symptoms

Figure 2.25 Students may use these gridlines to graph data from the YMCA cycle test

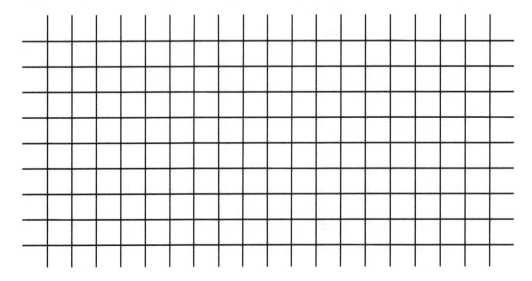

Figure 2.26 This table depicts hypothetical data from an Astrand-Rhyming cycle test

Astrand-Rhyming Cycle Test

Stage/Minute	Kpm/min	Heart Rate	Blood Pressure	RPE	ECG	Symptoms
Resting		83	134/86	NA	Sinus	No symptoms
I	300	132	152/86	10	Sinus	No symptoms
II	300	133	152/86	11	Sinus	No symptoms
III	300	134	154/84	11	Sinus	No symptoms
IV	300	134	154/84	12	Sinus	No symptoms
V	300	134	156/84	12	Sinus	No symptoms
VI	300	135	156/86	12	Sinus	No symptoms
Immediate	150	133	152/84	NA	Sinus	No symptoms
Recovery 1 min	75	100	140/84	NA	Sinus	No symptoms
Recovery 5 min	50	92	138/86	NA	Sinus	No symptoms

Figure 2.27 This table depicts hypothetical data from a maximal cycle test

Maximal Cycle Test

Stage	Time	Kpm/min	Heart Rate	Blood Pressure	RPE	$\dot{V}O_2$ (mL/ kg · min.)	RER	Blood Lactate (mmol)	ECG
Resting		0	83	134/86	NA	4.2	0.7	NA	Sinus
I	2:00	600	122	142/86	11	10.3	0.87	1.2	Sinus
II	4:00	900	142	160/86	14	20.1	0.99	3.3	Sinus
III	6:00	1200	152	178/88	16	29.6	1.12	5.2	ST-seg depress
IV	8:00	1500	161	200/88	18	34.7	1.17	8.9	ST-seg depress
Immediate	NA	300	160	190/86	NA	34.4	1.15	NA	ST-seg depress
Recovery 1 min	NA	150	140	162/84	NA	26.5	1.0	NA	ST-seg depress
Recovery 5 min	NA	75	101	140/84	NA	12.6	0.92	NA	Sinus

Comments: Chest pain, 3/4 on anginal pain scale in stage 3

Figure 2.28 This table depicts hypothetical data from a maximal treadmill test

Maximal Treadmill Test

Stage	Time	Speed (mph)	Grade %	Blood Pressure	$\dot{V}O_2$ (mL/ kg · min)	Blood Lactate (mmol)	RPE	Heart Rate	RER
Resting	NA	0	0	134/86	4.5	NA	NA	83	0.7
Warm-Up	NA	2	0	138/86	13.0	NA	NA	88	0.75
I	2:00	2.5	0	144/86	15.1	0.6	10	111	0.8
II	4:00	5.5	0	158/84	18.6	1.8	12	120	0.92
III	6:00	6.0	2	170/86	22.7	2.9	14	127	0.99
IV	8:00	6.5	3	152/86	28.9	5.2	16	149	1.08
V	10:00	6.5	5.5	150/86	35.9	8.4	19	166	1.15
Immediate	NA	3	0	150/86	52.1	NA	NA	160	1.14
Recovery 1 min	NA	2.5	0	140/84	35.7	NA	NA	140	1.01
Recovery 5 min	NA	1.5	0	138/84	12.3	NA	NA	91	0.99

Comments: ECG monitor went blank at the beginning of the test. Client complained of palpitations and breathlessness in stage 4.

9. For the cardiorespiratory fitness test chosen to interpret for question eight, should the test have been terminated prior to completion? Explain why or why not.

10. Assuming she selected the skinfold assessment for the body composition test, calculate body fat percentage from the following seven-site skinfold data (Figure 2.29).

Figure 2.29 This table depicts hypothetical data from a seven-site skinfold assessment

Site	Trial 1	Trial 2	Trial 3	Average
Triceps	20	22	22	mm
Subscapular	27	27	26	mm
Chest	29	29	29	mm
Abdominal	28	28	28	mm
Suprailiac	35	37	37	mm
Midaxillary	23	22	21	mm
Thigh	18	21	21	mm

11. If the client's waist circumference were 50 inches, what would be the risk classification?

12. Assuming she chose to assess muscular strength, interpret and classify the client's leg and chest press strength from the following data (Figure 2.30).

Figure 2.30 This table depicts hypothetical data from a 3–5RM test

Leg Press Strength Test

Trial 1	_____5_____ repetitions _____150_____ weight
Trial 2	_____3_____ repetitions _____170_____ weight
Trial 3	_____3_____ repetitions _____190_____ weight
Best Trial	_____3_____ repetitions _____190_____ weight

Chest Press Strength Test

Trial 1	_____5_____ repetitions _____120_____ weight
Trial 2	_____3_____ repetitions _____140_____ weight
Trial 3	_____3_____ repetitions _____160_____ weight
Best Trial	_____3_____ repetitions _____160_____ weight

13. Calculate a heart rate range based on the HRR that the client should maintain during aerobic exercise.
14. Calculate a $\dot{V}O_2$ range based on $\dot{V}O_2$ reserve that the client should maintain during aerobic exercise.
15. Provide an exercise type (be specific), frequency, and time at the $\dot{V}O_2$ range found in question number 14 for the client to improve their cardiorespiratory fitness.
16. Suggest four possible aerobic exercises that would be appropriate for this client.
17. Provide a walking speed and grade for the client to maintain on the treadmill to elicit the lower end of the $\dot{V}O_2$ range listed in question 14.
18. Provide a resistance and peddle frequency for leg cycling to elicit the lower end of the $\dot{V}O_2$ range listed in question 14.
19. Provide a resistance and peddle frequency for arm cycling to elicit the lower end of the $\dot{V}O_2$ range listed in question 14.

20. Provide a range for weight that the client should chest press.
21. Provide a range for weight that the client should leg press.
22. Provide a resistance exercise prescription for frequency, number of exercises, sets, and repetitions to improve muscular strength.
23. Suggest at least four specific resistance training exercises that are appropriate for this client.
24. Suggest a progression scheme to help the client improve overall muscular fitness.
25. Provide a frequency, intensity, number of stretches, sets, and the amount of time each stretch should be to help improve the client's flexibility.

REFERENCES

1. B. R. A. Wilson and M. D. McCabe, *Exercise Prescription Case Studies for Health Adults* (San Diego: Cognella Publishing, 2019).

2. American College of Sports Medicine, *ACSM's Guidelines for Exercise Testing and Prescription*, 11th ed. (Philadelphia: Wolters Kluwer Health, 2022).

3. Wilson and McCabe, *Exercise Prescription*.

4. P. O. Astrand and I. Rhyming, "A Nomogram for Calculation of Aerobic Capacity from Pulse Rate during Sub-Maximal Work," *Journal of Applied Physiology* 7, no. 2 (1954): 218–21.

5. American College of Sports Medicine, *ACSM's Guidelines*.

6. W. E. Siri, "Body Composition from Fluid Spaces and Density: Analysis of Methods," *Nutrition* 9, no. 5 (1993): 480–91.

7. A. S. Jackson and M. L. Pollock, "Practical Assessment of Body-Composition," *The Physician and Sports Medicine* 13 (1985): 76–90.

8. American College of Sports Medicine, *ACSM's Guidelines*.

9. ibid.

10. ibid.

11. ibid.

12. E. T. Howley, D. R. Bassett, and H. G. Welch, "Criteria for Maximal Oxygen Uptake: Review and Commentary," Medicine and Science in Sports and Exercise 27, no. 9 (1995):1292–1301.

13. American College of Sports Medicine, *ACSM's Guidelines*.

14. Astrand and Rhyming, "A Nomogram for Calculation."

15. P. O. Astrand, "Aerobic Work Capacity in Men and Women with Special Reference to Age," *Acta Physiologica Scandinavica* 49, no. 169 (1960): 45–60.

16. American College of Sports Medicine, *ACSM's Guidelines*.

17. J. Lander, "Maximum Based on Reps," *NSCA Journal* 6, no. 6 (1985): 60–1.

18. Jackson and Pollock, "Practical Assessment."

19. Siri, "Body Composition."

20. American College of Sports Medicine, *ACSM's Guidelines*.

21. ibid.

22. ibid.

23. ibid.

24. ibid.

25. ibid.

26. M. L. Pollock, B. A. Franklin, G. J. Balady, et al., "Resistance Exercise in Individuals with and without Cardiovascular Disease: Benefits, Rationale, Safety, and Prescription an Advisory from the Committee on Exercise, Rehabilitation, and Prevention, Council on Clinical Cardiology," *Circulation* 101, no. 7 (2000): 828–33.

27. American College of Sports Medicine, *ACSM's Guidelines*.

28. C. E. Garber, B. Blissmer, M. R. Deschenes, et al., "Quantity and Quality of Exercise for Developing and Maintaining Cardiorespiratory, Musculoskeletal, and Neuromotor Fitness in Apparently Healthy Adults: Guidance for Prescribing Exercise," *Medicine and Science in Sports and Exercise* 43, no. 7 (2011): 1334–59.

29. ibid.

30. American College of Sports Medicine, *ACSM's Guidelines*.

31. ibid

32. ibid

Exercise Testing and Prescription for Clients with Diabetes Mellitus

INTRODUCTION

D IABETES MELLITUS IS a group of metabolic diseases marked by a chronic state of elevated blood glucose concentration. Diabetes mellitus stems from the body's inability to produce sufficient amounts of insulin or to effectively use insulin for glucose metabolism. There are two primary forms of diabetes mellitus: type I and type II. Type I diabetes mellitus accounts for about 5 percent of all diabetes cases and is an autoimmune condition in which the body's immune system degrades the beta cells of the pancreas. This limits the ability of the pancreas to produce enough insulin to sustain adequate glucose metabolism. The most common and most preventable form of diabetes mellitus is type II diabetes. Type II diabetes results from the impairment of insulin-mediated glucose uptake in peripheral tissues coupled with the inability of pancreatic beta cells to produce and secrete sufficient amounts of insulin to elicit glucose transport across cellular membranes.[1]

Diabetes mellitus is associated with numerous adverse health consequences. Among the top of these consequences is the development of cardiovascular disease.[2] The insufficient production of insulin or insulin resistance characteristics of diabetes mellitus is linked to inefficiencies of specific physiological and metabolic pathways that maintain appropriate blood pressure, blood lipids, vascular function, and autonomic control.[3,4] These inefficiencies, in part, account for an elevated risk for developing cardiovascular disease in persons with diabetes mellitus. For these reasons, it is critical that therapeutic interventions be aimed at improving glycosylated hemoglobin (*A1C*) and cardiovascular disease risk factors in persons with diabetes mellitus.

Acute exercise provides a powerful stimulus for the body to uptake glucose from the blood independent of insulin. When exercise is accumulated over time, *A1C* and cardiovascular disease risk factors are significantly reduced in individuals with diabetes mellitus.[5] Furthermore, regular exercise has been shown to slow the pathophysiology of type II diabetes, reduce medication requirements, and decrease diabetes-related health risks.[6,7]

Currently, the ACSM and the American Diabetes Association recommends that adults with diabetes mellitus perform aerobic exercise for at least 150 minutes per week at an intensity of 40 to 60 percent of $\dot{V}O_2R$.[8,9] More specifically, the type of diabetes can have an influence on exercise prescription. For instance, persons with type I diabetes mellitus may perform more vigorous exercise and thus the option of 75 minutes of vigorous and moderate intensity aerobic exercise can be considered. In addition, the ACSM recommends that adults with diabetes mellitus complete resistance exercise for each major muscle group, two to four sets of eight to 12 repetitions, two to three days per week, at an intensity of 60 to 70 percent of 1RM.

Although the general exercise prescription for persons with diabetes mellitus seems simple, there are several safety considerations that exercise professionals must take into account, such as symptoms of hypo/hyperglycemia and medication timing. Further, exercise professionals must be able to modify and individualize exercise prescriptions to make them more effective. This chapter outlines exercise test selection and interpretation, FITT-VP modification, and safety considerations for serving clients with diabetes mellitus.

The purpose of this chapter is to teach students how to apply their knowledge of diabetes, exercise testing, and exercise prescription. Upon completion of the case studies, students will be able to achieve the following:

1. Differentiate between type I and type II diabetes and their medical management
2. Commit to working memory the normal and abnormal glucometabolic responses to exercise in clients with diabetes mellitus
3. Identify safety measures involved in exercise test selection and special considerations for exercise test interpretation
4. Apply the cardiorespiratory, muscular fitness, and flexibility FITT-VP recommendations and modifications to clients with type I or type II diabetes mellitus
5. Identify and understand safety considerations for training clients with diabetes mellitus

GLUCOMETABOLIC RESPONSES TO EXERCISE

During an acute bout of exercise, several hormones increase in their production and secretion. One such hormone is glucagon. Glucagon is produced in and released from the pancreas when blood glucose concentration is low. Glucagon signals for a process called glycogenolysis in the liver and the muscles. In addition, epinephrine is increased in its production and secretion during exercise, which also increases the rate of glycogenolysis. The combination of glucagon and epinephrine effectively acts to increase the glucose available for energy use and blood glucose concentration. Insulin, on the other hand, an anabolic hormone that signals for the uptake of blood glucose, decreases in its production and secretion during exercise. Nevertheless, glucose is continuously removed from the blood during exercise and used for adenosine triphosphate production in skeletal muscle cells. The reason for the continued glucose disposal is that contracting skeletal muscles stimulate calcium-mediated GLUT 4 translocation, which allows glucose uptake to occur independently of insulin.

Exercise professionals can think of the glucometabolic response to exercise as a competition between the influence of glucagon, epinephrine, and calcium-mediated GLUT 4 translocation. Typically, blood glucose concentration will decrease slightly during exercise. In addition, blood glucose disposal will remain amplified up to 24 hours postexercise.[10] For these reasons, exercise professionals should monitor blood glucose for clients with diabetes before, during, and after exercise. The rationale for this is that if a person with diabetes administers a glucose-lowering medication prior to exercise, the result could be a dangerous drop in blood glucose. Furthermore, if the blood glucose level is low prior to exercise (<70 mg/dL), then exercise may evoke a further decrease in blood glucose. On the other end of this spectrum is hyperglycemia, specifically in type I diabetes. Clients with diabetes reporting to a facility with a blood glucose concentration of 250 mg/dL or more should be evaluated for ketones to determine if exercise is safe. Although exercise-induced hyper/hypoglycemia is rare, exercise professionals must remain cautious and assure safety first and foremost.

TYPE I DIABETES MELLITUS

Type I diabetes mellitus is characterized by limited concentration of plasma insulin. Further, type I diabetes is marked by the failure of pancreatic beta cells to respond to stimuli to produce insulin. In most cases of type I diabetes, the pancreatic beta cells are damaged by autoimmune responses. Therefore, type I diabetes is not a disease to which individuals have a high degree of control in its prevention. Typically, type I diabetes is diagnosed in younger individuals and was previously termed juvenile diabetes.

The medical management of type I diabetes, like all cases of diabetes mellitus, is complex. Given that the pancreas is unable to produce enough insulin, the medical management of type I diabetes centers on synthetic insulin injection. This treatment poses specific challenges for exercise professionals, as insulin injection prior to exercise can lead to a hypoglycemic response. Other treatment strategies for managing type I diabetes include patient education, diet modification, and monitoring of cardiovascular and renal disease risk factors.

Exercise is an important lifestyle modification for type I diabetes. Although exercise cannot reverse or slow the progression of type I diabetes, exercise through skeletal muscle contractions can aid in glucose disposal and better blood glucose management. Moreover, through regular exercise, people with type I diabetes may be able to reduce their exogenous insulin requirements.[11] Throughout an exercise program, it is imperative that exercise professionals monitor clients with type I diabetes for symptoms associated with hypo/hyperglycemia and new and developing sores and blisters by doing everything possible to reduce the likelihood of new and developing sores. Prior to exercise participation, those with type I diabetes will need to be medically cleared for participation under three scenarios: (1) previously sedentary, (2) regularly active participants seeking an increase to vigorous exercise intensity, or (3) the presence of major signs or symptoms suggestive of cardiovascular, metabolic, or renal disease.[12]

TYPE II DIABETES MELLITUS

Individuals with type II diabetes, unlike those with type I diabetes, have a high degree of control in its prevention. Approximately 21 million Americans have a diagnosis of type II diabetes. In addition, with physical inactivity and obesity on the rise, it is projected that nearly 21 percent of the adult population in the United States will have a type II diabetes diagnosis by the year 2050.[13] These statistics indicate that exercise professionals are highly likely to encounter clients with type II diabetes during their careers. This means that exercise professionals must be familiar with normal glucose metabolism, glucometabolic responses to exercise, how to modify the FITT-VP of an exercise prescription for clients with type II diabetes, and how to ensure safety throughout an exercise program.

The pathogenesis of type II diabetes is complex and involves multiple factors. Generally, type II diabetes begins with a decrease in insulin sensitivity, which is the inability of skeletal muscle and fat cells to respond to insulin and uptake glucose from the blood. The decrease in insulin sensitivity then leads to high fasting blood glucose, and over time, this alters the ability of the pancreas to properly function. Further, high blood glucose over time leads to micro and macro blood vessel and nerve tissue damage, which contributes to the development of atherosclerosis, kidney disease, and various neuropathies. In years past, type II diabetes was thought to be the form of diabetes mellitus nearly exclusive to older adults. However, type II diabetes now affects individuals of all ages.

Like the treatment of type I diabetes, the treatment of type II diabetes is very complex. Depending on the severity of type II diabetes, patients may be prescribed any combination of insulins and oral medications intended to reduce the plasma concentration of glucose. These combinations of medications have many possible side effects, mainly the risk of hypoglycemia. Like with type I diabetes, exercise professionals must be able to recognize and monitor signs and symptoms associated with hypoglycemia. Further, prior to exercise participation, patients with type II diabetes will need to be medically cleared for participation under three scenarios: (1) previously sedentary, (2) regularly active participants seeking an increase to vigorous exercise intensity, or (3) the presence of major signs or symptoms suggestive of cardiovascular, metabolic, or renal disease.[14]

Demonstration Case Study 3.1

Differentiating Diabetes Mellitus

CJ is an exercise physiologist working for a health-fitness facility. CJ's newest client is Barry. Barry is 50 years old and presents to CJ's facility with the following medical description: (1) class two obesity, (2) A1C = 6.8 percent, (3) new symptoms of hyperglycemia, (4) physically inactive, and (5) no previous medical diagnoses. CJ takes this information into account. CJ determines that Barry possibly has type II diabetes given his A1C is high coupled with his obesity and physical inactivity. Moreover, CJ is concerned about training Barry without a physician's approval. CJ correctly recommends that Barry see a physician for not only a possible type II diabetes diagnosis but also medical clearance to exercise.

EXERCISE TESTING FOR CLIENTS WITH DIABETES

Exercise testing is a very useful set of tools for gathering client data and establishing individualized exercise prescriptions. The selection of appropriate exercise tests, test termination criteria, and test interpretation for clients with diabetes is like those for healthy adults and individuals with chronic diseases. Thus exercise professionals can opt to conduct any appropriate health-related fitness test, including submaximal or maximal cardiorespiratory tests, muscular strength or endurance tests, body composition assessments, and flexibility tests.

Although the contraindications for exercise testing are the same for those with diabetes as with healthy populations, exercise professionals should use sound judgment before initiating an exercise test. With diabetes, there are several potential health-related issues that exercise professionals must consider, aside from hypo and hyperglycemic responses. These concerns are centered on the influence of sustained high blood glucose on the nervous system, cardiac, and vascular function. Specific issues include the presence of silent ischemia, exaggerated pressor responses to movement, presence of peripheral and central neuropathy, possibility of retinopathy, and open sores.[15]

Silent ischemia, abnormal blood pressure response to movement, and chronotropic incompetence stem from central nervous system damage as a result of high blood glucose. Silent ischemia refers to an individual's reduced capacity to sense ischemic pain. The classic symptom of ischemia is angina pectoris. With diabetes, sustained elevated blood glucose concentration can interfere with cardiac afferents, thus limiting their capacity to sense ischemia and experience typical angina.[16] Therefore, exercise professionals should consider the use of electrocardiography when conducting cardiorespiratory fitness tests on clients with diabetes to detect ST-segment changes indicative of myocardial ischemia, especially if the client is previously sedentary and seeking a vigorous-intensity exercise program.[17] Further, damage to cardiac-specific nerve cells can result in augmented and attenuated exercise blood pressures. Thus exercise professionals must monitor blood pressure throughout cardiorespiratory fitness tests on patients with diabetes. Also, nerve damage can influence the heart rate at rest, during an exercise test, and immediately following exercise. Exercise professionals should closely monitor heart rate responses as the failure of the heart rate to properly rise during an exercise test will result in insufficient oxygen transport.[18] Moreover, chronotropic incompetence may result in the prolonged elevation of the heart rate after an exercise test. The normal heart rate recovery should be a reduction in the heart rate by 12 beats per minute in the first minute of recovery and 22 beats per minute by the second minute. If the heart rate does not recover in this manner, exercise professionals can consider recommending that their client seek medical consultation.

Neuropathy not only interferes with cardiovascular exercise responses; it can also interfere with proprioception, vision, and ability to sense and heal open wounds. Exercise professionals should consider avoiding exercise tests, which require significant skill if clients with diabetes are suspected of having peripheral neuropathy. Exercise professionals should also consider the influence of diabetes on vision health. Patients with diabetes are at risk of diabetic retinopathy and visual impairments. As such, exercise professionals should avoid having these clients perform the Valsalva maneuver during exercise testing, as this could cause further damage to vision health and visual acuity. Prior to exercise testing and training, exercise professionals need to consider evaluating these clients' feet for blisters and open wounds and to the best of their ability help them to avoid developing new blisters or wounds. This can be accomplished by suggesting dry and proper footwear.

Exercise-induced hypoglycemia and hyperglycemia always need to be a concern for exercise professionals when conducting exercise tests on clients with diabetes. The ACSM suggests that these client's blood glucose be 70 mg/dL or higher prior to exercise in any capacity.[19] However, some clients may have specific blood glucose ranges deemed safe by a physician supervising their care. In these cases, exercise professionals should adhere to such ranges. Should a client's blood glucose level be below 100 mg/dL, an exercise professional can recommend carbohydrate consumption prior to exercise or exercise testing. Further, exercise professionals should not conduct exercise tests within three hours of insulin injection, especially fast-acting insulin injections.[20]

Demonstration Case Study 3.2

Exercise Testing and Diabetes Mellitus

Shelia is an exercise physiologist working for a local hospital. Shelia is responsible for overseeing the diabetes exercise program. Her newest client is a sedentary 57-year-old Elijah. Elijah has type I diabetes, weighs 200 pounds with a BMI of 29.8 kg/m². He wants to exercise to better manage his blood glucose. Elijah's endocrinologist cleared him to exercise and provided Shelia with a safe blood glucose range of 100 to 300 mg/dL for Elijah to exercise. Elijah reports to the facility three hours post insulin injection with a resting heart rate of 98 beats per minute, a resting blood pressure of 138/84 mmHg, and a blood glucose level of 92 mg/dL. In addition to these resting measures, Elijah has known peripheral neuropathy, low visual acuity, and a history of hypertensive responses to exercise. Shelia wants to make sure that she prescribes the most effective exercise program as possible, so she wants to conduct a series of exercise tests. Shelia wants to conduct a cardiorespiratory fitness test, a muscular fitness test, a body composition test, and a flexibility test as safely as possible.

Given Elijah's initial blood glucose level is less than 100 mg/dL, Shelia recommends that Elijah consume a light complex carbohydrate snack prior to exercise testing. This snack caused Elijah's blood glucose level to rise above 100 mg/dL. Then Shelia considers Elijah's history with peripheral neuropathy and selects cardiorespiratory fitness and a muscular fitness tests that do not involve complicated movements. So Shelia selects the Astrand-Rhyming cycle test, the modified push-up test, and the body squat test. Prior to testing, Shelia exams Elijah's feet for open wounds and finds none. Shelia instructs Elijah not to hold his breath during the muscular fitness tests so as not to cause further disturbances in vision and chooses to monitor blood pressure, heart rate, and electrocardiographic activity closely during the Astrand-Rhyming cycle test because of Elijah's history of autonomic neuropathy. For body composition testing, Shelia chooses a seven-site skinfold assessment and waist measurement since Elijah is not considered obese. Lastly, for flexibility, Shelia chooses the sit-and-reach test.

Demonstration Case Study 3.3

Exercise Testing and Diabetes Mellitus

Walter is an exercise physiologist working for a diabetes management clinic. Walter is responsible for overseeing all exercise programs at his clinic. His newest client is 62-year-old Maryse. Maryse is sedentary, has type II diabetes, weighs 186 pounds with a BMI of 33.4 kg/m², and wants to exercise to better manage her blood glucose and body weight. Maryse's endocrinologist cleared her to exercise but did not provide a safe exercise blood glucose range. Maryse is prescribed Metformin and Lantus to control her blood glucose. She reports to the facility having injected Lantus 30 minutes prior, with a resting heart rate of 90 beats per minute, a resting blood pressure of 120/82 mmHg, and a blood glucose level of 65 mg/dL. In addition to these resting measures, Maryse has known peripheral neuropathy and has a history of slow healing open wounds on her feet. Walter wants to make sure that he prescribes the most effective exercise program as possible, so he wants to conduct a series of exercise tests. Walter wants to conduct a cardiorespiratory fitness test, a muscular fitness test, a body composition test, and a flexibility test as safely as possible.

Walter is first disturbed by Maryse's blood glucose level and her recent injection of Lantus. In addition, Walter is concerned about Maryse's history of slow healing feet wounds. Walter decides to examine Maryse's feet and finds newer wounds. Given Maryse's low blood glucose, recent Lantus injection, and new open wounds on her feet, Walter correctly decides exercise testing is not safe and does not move to initiate testing. Instead, Walter calls Maryse's endocrinologist, reports his findings, and Maryse's endocrinologist recommends an immediate office visit.

Demonstration Case Study 3.4

Exercise Testing and Diabetes Mellitus

Audrey is an exercise physiologist working for a diabetes exercise program. Audrey is responsible for overseeing all exercise and education programs. Her newest client is 53-year-old Rusty. Rusty is sedentary, has type II diabetes, weighs 261 pounds with a BMI of 37.7 kg/m², and wants to exercise to better manage his blood glucose and body weight. Rusty was recently diagnosed with type II diabetes, and his endocrinologist cleared him to exercise and suggested his blood glucose be between 150 and 350 mg/dL. Rusty is prescribed a myriad of blood glucose–lowering medications, including a fast-acting insulin. Rusty reports to the facility having injected his fast-acting insulin four hours prior, with a resting heart rate of 88 beats per minute, a resting blood pressure of 132/78 mmHg, and a blood glucose level of 166 mg/dL. Audrey wants to make sure that she prescribes the most effective exercise program as possible, so she wants to conduct a series of exercise tests. Audrey wants to conduct a cardiorespiratory fitness test, a muscular fitness test, a body composition test, and a flexibility test as safely as possible.

Audrey analyzes Rusty's profile and correctly determines that it is safe to conduct exercise tests. Just to be safe, prior to exercise, Audrey examines Rusty's feet for open sores. Since Rusty has no history with neuropathy but is sedentary, Audrey decides to conduct a submaximal Bruce treadmill test. To err on the side of caution, Audrey chooses to closely monitor heart rate, blood pressure, and electrocardiographic changes. For muscular fitness testing, Audrey chooses to conduct 3RM testing on the chest press and leg press modalities, although she instructed Rusty to not hold his breath during the tests. For body composition assessment, Audrey chooses to perform simple anthropomorphic (circumference) measures because of Rusty's obesity, which would make skinfold assessments inaccurate. For flexibility testing, Audrey chooses the sit-and-reach test.

EXERCISE PRESCRIPTION FOR THE CLIENT WITH DIABETES

Regular exercise is extraordinarily important for managing diabetes. With regular exercise, patients with diabetes can see marked improvement in *A1C*, cardiovascular disease risk factors, muscular strength and/or endurance, and cardiorespiratory endurance.[21,22] Importantly, the muscular contractions associated with exercise stimulate calcium-mediated GLUT 4 translocation, thereby allowing glucose uptake independent of insulin. This potent effect of exercise lasts up to 48 hours postexercise. Therefore, people with diabetes should be prescribed an exercise program of which there are no more than two consecutive nonexercise days. In total, those with diabetes benefit from cardiorespiratory, muscular fitness, and flexibility exercise. Exercise professionals must account for the pathology of diabetes, individual fitness and health status, physician orders, and client goals when modifying the FITT-VP. This section explains these modifications for cardiorespiratory, muscular fitness, and flexibility exercise for clients with diabetes.

Cardiorespiratory Exercise Prescription

The general exercise recommendations discussed in Chapter 2 apply to clients with diabetes. However, some modifications to these recommendations are suggested. The ACSM recommends an initial cardiorespiratory exercise prescription for diabetes that consists of three to seven days per week at a moderate intensity accumulating 150 minutes each week.[23]

It is recommended that those with diabetes perform cardiorespiratory endurance exercises three to seven times per week. As discussed in Chapter 2, the minimum frequency should be three days per week because there is little improvement in $\dot{V}O_{2max}$ when cardiorespiratory endurance exercises are performed less than three days per week. More specifically for diabetes, three days per week can be considered a minimum for cardiorespiratory endurance exercise because of glucose uptake being amplified 48 hours postexercise and no more than two consecutive nonexercise days should be prescribed. Also discussed in Chapter 2, performing more than five days of cardiorespiratory endurance exercise offers little additional improvement in $\dot{V}O_{2max}$ while posing a risk for injury and soreness. However, with diabetes, cardiorespiratory endurance exercises performed up to seven days per week is quite beneficial. Not only do the accumulated exercise sessions help those with diabetes manage blood glucose but also the accumulated exercise promotes continued caloric expenditure and fat metabolism. These two benefits also aid in managing or preventing other comorbidities, such as obesity, dyslipidemia, and hypertension. Like exercise prescription for apparently healthy adults, the frequency of cardiorespiratory exercise varies according to the intensity of the prescribed exercise. With higher frequency, the intensity of cardiorespiratory exercise is reduced.

The prescription of intensity for cardiorespiratory endurance exercise remains the most important aspect of the FITT-VP principle, even with diabetes. As with serving all special populations, exercise professionals must be cautious about overprescribing intensity. Not only can overprescribing cardiorespiratory endurance exercise intensity result in early dropout of clients with diabetes, but it can cause either an excessive decrease or increase in blood glucose. Thus a start low and progress slow approach is usually warranted. Further, blood glucose, along with blood pressure, should be carefully monitored before, during, and after cardiorespiratory endurance exercise. The methods for prescribing cardiorespiratory endurance exercise intensity largely remain the same when serving clients with diabetes. However, given that those with diabetes may have autonomic neuropathy, heart rate is not the most reliable method for quantifying intensity. Thus when serving clients with diabetes, $\dot{V}O_2R$ is the most accurate method for prescribing cardiorespiratory endurance exercise. When $\dot{V}O_2R$ is not a plausible method for quantifying intensity, RPE can be used. The starting cardiorespiratory endurance intensity for patients with diabetes should be 40–60 percent $\dot{V}O_2R$ or an RPE of 11 to 12. Vigorous intensity, 60 to 89 percent of $\dot{V}O_2R$, or RPE of 14 to 17, can be prescribed if a client with diabetes has been previously active and has the capacity to perform vigorous-intensity exercise. The use of the metabolic equations in Chapter 2 is recommended for prescribing highly specific exercise intensities.

The ACSM recommends that people with diabetes accumulate 150 minutes of cardiorespiratory endurance exercise per week.[24] This translates to approximately 30 to 60 minutes of cardiorespiratory exercise per session. In general, people with diabetes benefit from more exercise time, as this assists in glucometabolic control and the management of other comorbidities. Thus an exercise professional should encourage continued progression in daily or weekly exercise time. It is not uncommon for patients with diabetes to be highly deconditioned, especially with type II diabetes. In these instances, bouts of ten minutes or less can be completed to accumulate at least 30 minutes of exercise per session. Like with healthy and other special populations, exercise professionals should set an initial exercise time based on the client's current fitness level, exercise history, and health status.

The type of cardiorespiratory endurance exercise that should be prescribed for patients with diabetes is the same required for improving health in apparently healthy adults and other special populations. Exercise professionals should select cardiorespiratory endurance exercises that require the participation of several muscle groups contracting to perform the exercise. The rationale with this is that more muscles contracting would augment total glucose metabolism thereby enhancing blood glucose control. When serving clients with diabetes, exercise professionals should select exercises based on their clients' likes, goals, effectiveness of the exercise, and safety.

Clients with diabetes should be systematically progressed through a cardiorespiratory endurance program. Exercise professionals can modify exercise frequency, intensity, and time to accomplish adequate progression. A biweekly increase in exercise volume of 5 to 10 percent remains the general recommendation for progressing patients with diabetes. Exercise frequency and time should be increased before intensity. Of special note, those with diabetes should be encouraged to eventually progress to high-intensity interval training if possible, as such training has been shown to have a profound influence on *A1C* and cardiovascular disease risk factors.[25,26,27]

Demonstration Case Study 3.5

Cardiorespiratory Exercise Prescription and Diabetes Mellitus

Noel is an exercise physiologist who specializes in serving clients with diabetes mellitus. Her most recent client is Emmanuel. Emmanuel's profile is provided: 48-year-old male, type II diabetes, 275 pounds, and sedentary. Emmanuel's only diabetic-related complication is peripheral neuropathy. Emmanuel takes Lantus and Glucozide to control his blood glucose. Noel found no new or developing sores on Emmanuel's feet. A YMCA cycle test was completed without symptoms. The client's resting heart rate was 94 beats per minute, resting blood pressure was 142/86, and estimated $\dot{V}O_{2max}$ was 29 mL/kg · min. The client is open to any exercise.

After analyzing Emmanuel's profile, Noel, begins to write a cardiorespiratory exercise prescription. Noel first selects an exercise frequency. Noel wants to have Emmanuel exercise five or more days per week, but because of Emmanuel's sedentary lifestyle, she initially selects three days per week with no more than 48 hours of inactivity between exercise sessions. Next, Noel selects an exercise time of 30 minutes per exercise session. After that, Noel calculates the appropriate exercise intensity. She wants to be precise and specific, so she uses the $\dot{V}O_2R$ method to quantify the intensity and select corresponding workloads on several modalities. Noel chooses a narrow intensity range equal to 40 to 45 percent of $\dot{V}O_2R$. Noel chooses the lower end of a moderate-intensity range because of Emmanuel's sedentary lifestyle. Noel's calculations are shown next.

$$\dot{V}O_2R = \dot{V}O_{2max} - 3.5 \text{ mL/kg} \cdot \text{min}$$

$$\dot{V}O_2R = 29 \text{ mL/kg} \cdot \text{min} - 3.5 \text{ mL/kg} \cdot \text{min}$$

$$\dot{V}O_2R = 25.5 \text{ mL/kg} \cdot \text{min}$$

$$40 \text{ percent of } \dot{V}O_2R = (25.5 \text{ mL/kg} \cdot \text{min} \times .4) + 3.5 \text{ mL/kg} \cdot \text{min}$$

$$40 \text{ percent of } \dot{V}O_2R = 13.7 \text{ mL/kg} \cdot \text{min}$$

$$45 \text{ percent of } \dot{V}O_2R = (25.5 \text{ mL/kg} \cdot \text{min} \times .45) + 3.5 \text{ mL/kg} \cdot \text{min}$$

$$45 \text{ percent of } VO \dot{V}O_2R\,_2R = 14.9 \text{ mL/kg} \cdot \text{min}$$

$$\dot{V}O_2R \text{ range} = 13.7 - 14.9 \text{ mL/kg} \cdot \text{min}$$

Noel chooses to have Emmanuel perform walking, stepping, and leg cycling. Therefore, Noel decided to provide specific workloads for each modality using the metabolic equations. Noel's work is provided next.

Walking Calculations:

Noel believes Emmanuel can walk comfortably at 3.0 mph. Therefore, she solves for incline using the walking equation that would elicit 40 percent of Emmanuel's $\dot{V}O_2R$.

$$13.7 \text{ mL/kg} \cdot \text{min} = (0.1 \times 3.0 \times 26.8) + (1.8 \times 3.0 \times 26.8 \times \text{incline}) + 3.5$$

$$\text{Incline} = 1.5\,\%$$

Leg Cycling Calculations:

Given Emmanuel's poor cardiorespiratory fitness, Noel feels that Emmanuel should stick with 50 revolutions per minute when leg cycling. Therefore, Noel uses the leg cycling equation to solve for resistance, in kiloponds (kp), to be placed on the flywheel of a Monark cycle to elicit 40 percent of Emmanuel's $\dot{V}O_2R$.

$$13.7 \text{ mL/kg} \cdot \text{min} = (1.8 \times 50 \times \text{resistance} \times 6/125 \text{ kg}) + 7$$

$$\text{Resistance} = 1.55 \text{ kp}$$

Stepping Calculations:

Lastly, Noel believes Emmanuel should perform stepping exercises because of its incorporation of larger muscle masses. Noel feels Emmanuel can step comfortably at a rate of ten steps per minute. Noel uses the stepping equation to determine a step height in centimeters that would elicit 40 percent of Emmanuel's $\dot{V}O_2R$.

$$13.7 \text{ mL/kg} \cdot \text{min} = (0.2 \times 10) + (1.33 \times 1.8 \times \text{step height} \times 10) + 3.5$$

$$\text{Step height in meters} = 0.19 \text{ meters}$$

$$\text{Step height in centimeters} = 19 \text{ centimeters}$$

The last issue Noel addresses is exercise progression. Noel designs a progression plan that involves a slow increase in exercise dose each week. First, Noel will add five minutes of exercise time to each session each week until Emmanuel is exercising 60 minutes each session. Then each week, Noel plans to increase the frequency one day per week each week until Emmanuel is exercising 60 minutes per day seven days per week. At this point, Noel will increase exercise intensity by 5 percent each week and reduce exercise frequency to five days per week. Once Emmanuel can exercise five days per week, 60 minutes per day, at an intensity equal to 60 percent of his $\dot{V}O_2R$, Noel will move on to high-intensity interval training.

Demonstration Case Study 3.6

Cardiorespiratory Exercise Prescription and Diabetes Mellitus

Hilda is an exercise physiologist who specializes in serving clients with diabetes mellitus. Her most recent client is Stephen. Stephen's profile is as follows: 58-year-old male, type I diabetes, 220 pounds, regularly performs cardiorespiratory endurance exercise.

Despite Stephen's physically active lifestyle, he has numerous diabetes-related complications. Stephen has documented autonomic neuropathy, peripheral neuropathy, slow healing feet wounds, and visual disturbances. Stephen has an insulin pump to control his blood glucose. Hilda recommended new dry socks prior to exercise testing and conducted a submaximal Bruce treadmill test without complications. Stephen's resting heart rate was 87 beats per minute, resting blood pressure was 136/76, and estimated $\dot{V}O_{2max}$ was 42 mL/kg · min. The client enjoys any exercise except cycling.

After analyzing Stephen's profile, Hilda, begins to write a cardiorespiratory exercise prescription. Hilda first selects an exercise frequency. Given Stephen's exercise history, Hilda selects five days per week as the starting frequency. Next, Hilda selects an exercise time. With Stephen's physically active lifestyle, she feels Stephen should exercise 60 minutes per day. After that, Hilda calculates the appropriate exercise intensity. To be precise and specific, Hilda uses the $\dot{V}O_2R$ method to quantify the intensity and select workloads on several modalities. Hilda chooses a narrow intensity range equal to 55 to 60 percent of $\dot{V}O_2R$. Hilda chooses the higher end of a moderate-intensity range because of Stephen's active lifestyle. The following are Hilda's calculations.

$\dot{V}O_2R = \dot{V}O_{2max} - 3.5$ mL/kg · min

$\dot{V}O_2R = 42$ mL/kg · min $- 3.5$ mL/kg · min

$\dot{V}O_2R = 38.5$ mL/kg · min

55 percent of $\dot{V}O_2R = (38.5$ mL/kg · min x .55) + 3.5 mL/kg · min

55 percent of $\dot{V}O_2R = 24.6$ mL/kg · min

60 percent of $\dot{V}O_2R = (38.5$ mL/kg · min x .6) + 3.5 mL/kg · min

60 percent of $\dot{V}O_2R = 26.6$ mL/kg · min

$\dot{V}O_2R$ range $= 24.6 - 26.6$ mL/kg · min

Hilda choosess to have Stephen perform walking, running, and stepping. Therefore, Hilda decided to provide specific workloads for each modality using the metabolic equations. Hilda's work is provided next.

Walking Calculations:

Hilda believes Stephen can walk comfortably at 3.5 mph. Therefore, she solves for incline using the walking equation that would elicit 60 percent of Stephen's $\dot{V}O_2R$.

$$26.6 \text{ mL/kg} \cdot \text{min} = (0.1 \times 3.5 \times 26.8) + (1.8 \times 3.5 \times 26.8 \times \text{incline}) + 3.5$$

$$\text{Incline} = 8.1 \%$$

Running Calculations:

Given Stephen's experience with cardiorespiratory exercise, Hilda feels that he is perfectly capable of running, so long as it doesn't exacerbate current feet wounds or induce new feet wounds. Also, Hilda plans to monitor Stephen carefully during running exercises in case his peripheral neuropathy interferes with his ability to safely run on the treadmill. Hilda believes that Stephen can run up a modest incline of 1.5 percent. Therefore, Hilda solves for speed using the running equation to elicit 60 percent of Stephen's $\dot{V}O_2R$.

$$26.6 \text{ mL/kg} \cdot \text{min} = (0.2 \times \text{speed}) + (0.9 \times \text{speed} \times 0.015) + 3.5$$

$$\text{Speed} = 108.1 \text{ meters} \cdot \text{min}$$

$$\text{Speed} = 4.03 \text{ mph}$$

Stepping Calculations:

Lastly, Hilda believes Stephen should perform stepping exercises because she feels it will increase long-term glucose disposal. Hilda's facility has a 20-centimeter step, and therefore she solves for a stepping rate to elicit 60 percent of Stephen's $\dot{V}O_2R$.

$$26.6 \text{ mL/kg} \cdot \text{min} = (0.2 \times \text{stepping rate}) + (1.33 \times 1.8 \times 0.20 \times \text{stepping rate}) + 3.5$$

$$\text{Stepping rate} = 34 \text{ steps per minute}$$

The last issue Hilda addresses is exercise progression. With Stephen's history of cardiorespiratory exercise, Hilda wants to be a little more aggressive with her progression scheme. She plans to add one exercise session each week until Stephen is exercising daily. Then Hilda wants to move Stephen to high-intensity interval training two days per week and three steady state exercise days.

Muscular Fitness Exercise Prescription

Resistance training offers numerous benefits for clients with diabetes, such as enhanced blood glucose control and muscular strength. Moreover, resistance training can help clients with diabetes combat other comorbidities, such as obesity, dyslipidemia, and hypertension. Therefore, exercise professionals should encourage them to perform resistance exercises in addition to cardiorespiratory exercises. It should be noted that not all patients with diabetes should perform resistance training. Conditions such as uncontrolled hypertension, severe retinopathy, and recent ocular surgeries would exclude patients with diabetes from performing resistance training exercises.[28]

The recommended muscular fitness exercise prescription for diabetes is like the muscular fitness exercise for apparently healthy adults. The difference really lies with the initial repetition scheme. It is recommended that people with diabetes perform one to three sets of moderate-intensity resistance exercises (50–70 percent 1RM) and complete 10 to 15 repetitions per set. Exercise professionals should prescribe at least eight resistance exercises, emphasizing multiple joints, per resistance exercise session. As with healthy adults, those with diabetes should perform resistance exercises two to three days per week.

Patients with diabetes should be gradually progressed through a resistance training program. They should begin a resistance training program by performing 10 to 15 repetitions per exercise and then repetitions can be reduced as resistance is added once clients can successfully complete 15 repetitions per set to fulfill the aforementioned prescription. This process should continue until they can perform eight to ten repetitions per set.[29]

Exercise professionals need to continue to ensure safety. Those with diabetes would benefit from free-weight resistance exercises, although resistance bands and machine-based modalities may be more appropriate for deconditioned or inexperienced clients. The Valsalva maneuver should always be avoided regardless of the presence of retinopathy or hypertension. In addition, the complexity of exercises must suit the capability of clients, as neuropathies can interfere with proprioception. Exercise professionals must be mindful of the influence of elevated blood glucose on connective tissue and avoid subjecting those with diabetes to musculoskeletal injury.[30]

Demonstration Case Study 3.7

Muscular Fitness Exercise Prescription and Diabetes Mellitus

Brian is an exercise physiologist specializing in training clients with diabetes mellitus. His newest client is Lynn. Lynn is a 50-year-old female with type I diabetes. Lynn is overweight, weighing 190 pounds, only walks at a light pace for exercise, has no experience with resistance exercise, and is interested in beginning a resistance exercise program to improve her glucose control and reduce her insulin requirements. Lynn does not have retinopathy but does have peripheral neuropathy. Lynn was medically cleared to participate in resistance exercise.

Given Lynn's inexperience with resistance exercise, Brian decided to conduct two muscular endurance tests just to assess Lynn's capacity for resistance training. Lynn was able to successfully complete eight body squats correctly before fatigue and seven modified push-ups. From this information, Brian put together a muscular fitness exercise prescription, which is provided next.

Frequency:

Brian suggested that Lynn perform resistance exercises two days per week. Brian's rationale was that Lynn has no previous experience with resistance exercise, and he doesn't want to discourage Lynn by causing muscle soreness.

Intensity:

Given Lynn has no experience with resistance exercise and did not perform well on her muscular endurance tests, Brian selects resistance bands as the modality and thus the intensity is very light.

Time:

Brian chooses to have Lynn perform one set of 15 repetitions per each prescribed exercise. Brian chooses this starting point because of Lynn's inexperience with resistance exercise.

Type:

Because of Lynn's inexperience with resistance exercise, Brian chooses resistance band exercises. He chooses the following exercises: (1) curl press, (2) resistance band squats, (3) lateral lunges, (4) chest press, (5) upright rows, (6) seated rows, (7) leg curls, and (8) shoulder flies. Brian chooses these exercises for their simplicity and to target the major muscle groups.

Progression:

Brian decides to choose a slow progression scheme. His plan is to have Lynn add one set per each of the aforementioned exercises until Lynn can successfully complete three sets of 15 repetitions. At this point, Brian will increase the resistance, still using resistance bands, and decrease repetitions. Once Lynn can complete three sets of ten repetitions using the most challenging resistance bands, Brain will reassess Lynn's strength and prescribe an individualized exercise plan using machine-based weight.

Flexibility Exercise Prescription

Flexibility exercises are recommended as a part of any general exercise program, including exercise programs for those with diabetes.[31] The flexibility prescription remains the same for diabetes as apparently healthy adults. This means people with diabetes should perform flexibility exercises at least two to three days per week targeting each major muscle-tendon group two to four times each day.[32] Exercise professionals should instruct clients with diabetes to perform each flexibility exercise 10 to 30 seconds. Whichever frequency and time is chosen, the client should perform each stretch for a total of 60 seconds. Any type of flexibility exercise is acceptable except for ballistic stretches. In addition, complex dynamic exercises should be avoided if clients with diabetes have peripheral neuropathy interfering with proprioception. Further, they should be instructed to avoid pain during flexibility exercise and not to hold their breath. Clients with diabetes should be progressed slowly and in accordance with their goals and needs.

Exercise Safety Considerations

A major concern for exercise professionals when serving clients with diabetes is the risk of exercise-induced hypoglycemia because of the combination of glucose-lowering medication coupled with exercise's influence on GLUT-4 translocation. Therefore, knowing the signs and symptoms of hypoglycemia and monitoring blood glucose before, during, and after exercise is recommended. Exercise professionals should not allow a client with diabetes to begin an exercise training session if the client's blood glucose concentration is below 70 mg/dL without physician approval.[33,34] If clients report to training with a blood glucose concentration between 70 and 100 mg/dL, exercise professionals should consider having the client consume carbohydrates prior to exercise. To further prevent exercise-induced hypoglycemia, exercise professionals should be aware of the timing and type of insulin or glucose-lowering medication clients administer. Although exercise-induced hypoglycemia is more likely to occur with short-acting insulins, exercise professionals should practice caution and regularly monitor clients' blood glucose levels if they administer any insulin or glucose-lowering medication within three hours of exercise.

When serving clients with type I diabetes, exercise professionals need to be concerned with exercise-induced hyperglycemia, as well as hypoglycemia. So, knowing the signs and symptoms of hyperglycemia is important for exercise professionals working with this population. Type I diabetes is more likely to cause exercise hyperglycemic events when the blood glucose concentration is 250 mg/dL or higher. Should a client with type I diabetes report to training with a blood glucose concentration of 250 mg/dL or higher, exercise professionals should encourage the client to check for urinary ketones, and if ketones are present exercise, should not be performed.[35] Further, those with type I diabetes are prone to exercise-induced hyperglycemia, particularly during high-intensity training. Therefore, exercise professionals should monitor these clients' blood glucose during and after high-intensity exercise, and the client should be encouraged to continuously check blood glucose after exercise and adjust insulin administration as needed.[36]

Neuropathies are also a concern for exercise professionals serving clients with diabetes. Autonomic neuropathy can impair a client's cardiovascular response to exercise. Therefore, exercise professionals should regularly monitor client's heart rate, blood pressure, and signs of poor perfusion during exercise. Further, exercise professionals should avoid "spikes" in their clients' blood pressure by having them avoid performing the Valsalva maneuver and only prescribing vigorous exercise intensities once a predictable pressor response is established. Given the likelihood for having cardiovascular risk factors is high, exercise professionals should monitor for signs and symptoms of silent ischemia such as dyspnea.

Peripheral neuropathy can cause disturbances in proprioception and wound-healing ability. Thus exercise professionals should carefully monitor clients with diabetes during exercise to ensure that movements are being completed correctly and without noticeable strain. Exercise professionals can also ensure safety by selecting exercises that are well-suited to a client's physical capabilities. Also, with peripheral neuropathy, exercise professionals should be cautious not to create new wounds, particularly on the client's feet. Exercise professionals should occasionally inspect the feet of clients with diabetes and recommend dry socks and proper footwear.

Occasionally, people with diabetes have microvascular conditions, such as retinopathy and nephropathy. Retinopathy results in the impairment of visual acuity. To ensure safety, exercise professionals should not prescribe exercises for which a high degree of reliance is placed on vision. Next, exercise should educate their clients to avoid the Valsalva maneuver. If clients have nephropathy, exercise professionals should encourage continued exercise at low to moderate intensities and stay within any physician orders.

Demonstration Case Study 3.8

Safety Considerations for Clients with Diabetes

Dan is an exercise physiologist specializing in serving clients with diabetes. Dan is currently training Valerie. Valerie has had type II diabetes for ten years and has been training with Dan for the past five weeks. Valerie's medications have been altered numerous times over the last ten years. Recently, her endocrinologist prescribed her a sulfonylurea medication to enhance her production of insulin. Valerie also administers a basal insulin daily. Valerie recently reported to Dan's facility having consumed her sulfonylurea drug one-hour prior. Dan checked Valerie's blood glucose, and it was 102 mg/dL. Since this was "in range" Dan proceeded to allow Valerie to exercise. Ten minutes into Valerie's exercise, she started to feel fatigued and developed a headache. Dan was alerted and decided to check her blood glucose again. Valerie's blood glucose had dropped to 68 mg/dL, and Dan immediately stopped Valerie's exercise session. He recommended that she consume some carbohydrates. Twenty minutes later, Valerie's blood glucose rose to 85 mg/dL, and Dan called her endocrinologist for further guidance.

Demonstration Case Study 3.9

Safety Considerations for Clients with Diabetes

Mollie is an exercise physiologist specializing in serving clients with diabetes. Mollie's current client is Judy, and she has been training Judy for ten weeks. Judy has had type I diabetes for 30 years. As such, Judy injects insulin regularly to control her blood glucose. Mollie recently prescribed high-intensity interval training for Judy. Judy really enjoyed that form of training and requested more for the next training session. Judy reported for the next training session, and as a part of the routine, she checked her blood glucose. Judy's blood glucose concentration was 260 mg/dL. Mollie correctly asked Judy to check for urinary ketones, none were present, and Mollie proceeded to permit Judy to exercise. However, Mollie correctly decided to not have Judy perform high-intensity interval training, as it might have further elevated Judy's blood glucose.

Demonstration Case Study 3.10

Safety Considerations for Clients with Diabetes

Dakota is an exercise physiologist who trains clients with metabolic disorders. She is currently training Lance. Lance has had type II diabetes for 15 years and is currently obese. Dakota is very cautious with Lance and checks his blood glucose, heart rate, blood pressure, and signs of normal perfusion before, during, and after exercise. During their most recent training session, Dakota noticed something peculiar while Lance was exercising. Dakota noticed perfuse sweating, and Lance complaining of back pain and shortness of breath. Dakota stopped the exercise session and checked Lance's electrocardiogram. Lance's ECG revealed ST-segment depression in the inferior leads. Lance was suffering from silent ischemia, and Dakota called emergency medical services immediately.

Student Case Study 3.1

Exercise Test Selection for Clients with Diabetes

An exercise physiologist at a diabetes management clinic performs several exercise tests per day. The newest client is Lilian. She last took her glucose-lowering medications three hours prior to reporting to the facility, and her profile is provided next.

Demographics: (1) female and (2) 51 years old

Biometrics: (1) resting heart rate = 91 beats per minute; (2) resting blood pressure = 142/82 mmHg; (3) LDL-c = 102 mg/dL, HDL-c = 41 mg/dL, total cholesterol = 198 mg/dL; (4) blood glucose = 104 mg/dL; (5) weight = 180 lbs; and (6) BMI = 29.9 kg/m^2

Medical Diagnoses: (1) type II diabetes (2) peripheral neuropathy

Medications: (1) Lantus and (2) Actos

Symptoms: (1) poor coordination and (2) foot ulcers

Exercise History: (1) 20 minutes of cycling, two days per week, light intensity; (2) gardening; and (3) doesn't like walking or jogging

Exercise Goals and Needs: (1) manage blood glucose and (2) reduce medication requirements

1. Assuming the client has been medically cleared to exercise, would it be safe to conduct exercise testing on this client? In two to three sentences, provide a defense for the answer.
2. Assuming it is safe to test this client, should one conduct a maximal or submaximal cardiorespiratory fitness test? In four to five sentences, provide a defense for the decision based on the client's profile.
3. Assuming it is safe to test this client, which cardiorespiratory fitness test should be conducted? In four to five sentences, provide a defense for the decision based on the client's profile.

4. Specific to this case, which body composition test should one prefer to conduct? In four to five sentences, provide a defense for the decision based on the client's profile.

5. Assuming it is safe to test this client to assess muscular fitness, should one conduct muscular endurance assessments or muscular strength assessments, or both? In four to five sentences, provide a defense for the decision based on the client's profile.

6. Assuming it is safe to test this client, provide a list of four specific muscular fitness tests one could conduct on the client. Then provide a four- to five-sentence defense supporting the selections.

7. List any special considerations that should be considered when choosing exercise tests for this client.

Student Case Study 3.2

Exercise Test Selection for Clients with Diabetes

An exercise physiologist at a diabetes management clinic performs several exercise tests per day. The newest client is Felipe. He last took his glucose-lowering medications 30 minutes prior to reporting to the facility, and his profile is provided next.

Demographics: (1) male and (2) 42 years old

Biometrics: (1) resting heart rate = 87 beats per minute; (2) resting blood pressure = 158/80 mmHg; (3) LDL-c = 109 mg/dL, HDL-c = 39 mg/dL, total cholesterol = 196 mg/dL; (4) blood glucose = 81 mg/dL; (5) weight = 192 lbs; and (6) BMI = 27.1 kg/m^2

Medical Diagnoses: (1) type I diabetes, (2) autonomic neuropathy, and (3) retinopathy

Medications: (1) basal insulin and (2) short-acting insulin

Symptoms: (1) headaches associated with high blood pressure and (2) occasional blurred vision

Exercise History: (1) light walking three days per week, 20 minutes per walk; (2) golf; and (3) doesn't like stepping exercises

Exercise Goals and Needs: (1) manage blood glucose and (2) improve muscle mass

1. Assuming the client has been medically cleared to exercise, would it be safe to conduct exercise testing on this client? In two to three sentences, provide a defense for the answer.

2. Assuming it is safe to test this client, should a maximal or submaximal cardiorespiratory fitness test be conducted? In four to five sentences, provide a defense for the decision based on the client's profile.

3. Assuming it is safe to test this client, which cardiorespiratory fitness test should be conducted? In four to five sentences, provide a defense for the decision based on the client's profile.
4. Specific to this case, which body composition test should be conducted? In four to five sentences, provide a defense for the decision based on the client's profile.
5. Assuming it is safe to test this client, to assess muscular fitness, should one conduct muscular endurance assessments or muscular strength assessments, or both? In four to five sentences, provide a defense for the decision based on the client's profile.
6. Assuming it is safe to test this client, provide a list of four specific muscular fitness tests one could conduct on the client. Then provide a four to five sentence defense supporting the selections.
7. List any special considerations when choosing exercise tests for this client.

Student Case Study 3.3

Exercise Test Selection for Clients with Diabetes

An exercise physiologist at a diabetes management clinic performs several exercise tests per day. The newest client is Gina. She last took her glucose-lowering medications four hours prior to reporting to the facility, and her profile is provided next.

Demographics: (1) female and (2) 53 years old

Biometrics: (1) resting heart rate = 71 beats per minute; (2) resting blood pressure = 118/72 mmHg; (3) LDL-c = 100 mg/dL, HDL-c = 54 mg/dL, total cholesterol = 190 mg/dL; (4) blood glucose = 110 mg/dL; (5) weight = 145 lbs; and (6) BMI = 22.9 kg/m^2

Medical Diagnoses: (1) type I diabetes and (2) peripheral neuropathy

Medications: (1) basal insulin (2) short-acting insulin

Symptoms: (1) new foot ulcer

Exercise History: (1) moderate walking/jogging three days per week, 30 minutes per session; (2) resistance band exercise two days per week; and (3) open to any kind of exercise

Exercise Goals and Needs: (1) manage blood glucose and (2) further improve fitness

1. Assuming the client has been medically cleared to exercise, would it be safe to conduct exercise testing on this client? In two to three sentences, provide a defense for the answer.
2. Assuming it is safe to test this client, should a maximal or submaximal cardiorespiratory fitness test be conducted? In four to five sentences, provide a defense for the decision based on the client's profile.

3. Assuming it is safe to test this client, which cardiorespiratory fitness test should one conduct? In four to five sentences, provide a defense for the decision based on the client's profile.

4. Specific to this case, which body composition test would be preferred? In four to five sentences, provide a defense for the decision based on the client's profile.

5. Assuming it is safe to test this client, to assess muscular fitness, should one conduct muscular endurance assessments or muscular strength assessments, or both? In four to five sentences, provide a defense for the decision based on the client's profile.

6. Assuming it is safe to test this client, provide a list of four specific muscular fitness tests to conduct on the client. Then provide a four- to five-sentence defense supporting the selections.

7. List any special considerations one should consider when choosing exercise tests for this client.

Student Case Study 3.4

Exercise Test Interpretation: YMCA Cycle Test

An exercise physiologist specializes in serving clients with diabetes. She just completed a YMCA cycle test on a 50-year-old with type II diabetes weighing 180 pounds. The results of the test are provided in Figure 3.1. After reading the results, use the graph and leg cycling equation to interpret the results and answer the questions.

Figure 3.1 This table depicts hypothetical data from a YMCA cycle test

Stage	Kpm/min	Heart Rate	Blood Pressure	RPE	ECG	Symptoms/ Comments
Resting	0	95	136/80	NA	Sinus	No symptoms
I	150	107	150/84	10	Sinus	No symptoms
II	300	129	162/84	13	Sinus	No symptoms
III	450	142	174/84	15	Sinus	No symptoms
Immediate	0	140	170/84	NA	Sinus	No symptoms
Recovery 1 min	0	128	160/82	NA	Sinus	No symptoms
Recovery 5 min	0	100	138/72	NA	Sinus	No symptoms

1. Using graph paper (Figure 3.2), estimate the maximal work rate (kpm/min). Then insert the estimated maximal work rate into the following equation to estimate $\dot{V}O_{2max}$:

$$\dot{V}O_2 \text{ max mL/kg} \cdot \text{min} = (1.8 \text{ x estimated maximal work rate/kg body weight}) + 7.$$

2. Assuming this client has autonomic neuropathy, how would an exercise physiologist ensure the safety of the client?

3. Assuming this client has autonomic neuropathy, could the accuracy of this test be limited? Why?
4. What could an exercise physiologist do to further assure the safety of this client during testing?

Figure 3.2 Students may use these gridlines to graph data from the YMCA cycle test

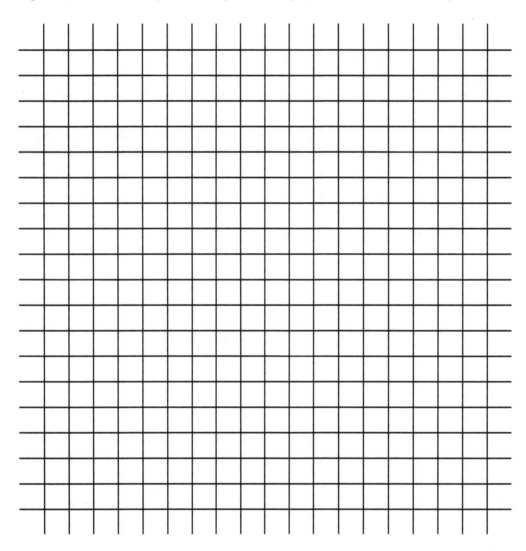

Student Case Study 3.5

Exercise Test Interpretation: Astrand-Rhyming Cycle Test

An exercise physiologist specializes in serving clients with diabetes. He just completed an Astrand-Rhyming cycle test on a 43-year-old female, previously sedentary client with type I diabetes who weighs 221 pounds. The results of the test are provided in Figure 3.3. After reading the results. use the modified Astrand-Rhyming to interpret the results and answer the questions.

Figure 3.3 This table depicts hypothetical data from an Astrand-Rhyming cycle test

Stage/Minute	Kpm/m	Heart Rate	Blood Pressure	RPE	ECG	Symptoms
Resting		101	140/88	NA	Sinus	No symptoms
I	300	135	164/88	13	Sinus	No symptoms
II	300	137	168/88	13	Sinus	No symptoms
III	300	138	170/88	15	Sinus	No symptoms
IV	300	140	172/88	15	Sinus	No symptoms
V	300	141	172/88	15	Sinus	No symptoms
VI	300	141	174/88	16	Sinus	No symptoms
Immediate	150	140	174/88	NA	Sinus	No symptoms
Recovery 1 min	150	131	170/84	NA	Sinus	No symptoms
Recovery 5 min	75	120	152/84	NA	Sinus	No symptoms

1. Using the Astrand-Rhyming nomogram, estimate $\dot{V}O_{2max}$ in L · min. Be sure to multiply by a correction factor. Then convert $\dot{V}O_{2max}$ to mL/kg · min.

   Find estimated $\dot{V}O_{2max}$ in L · min

   Find estimated $\dot{V}O_{2max}$ in mL/kg · min

2. If this client reported to a clinic with a blood glucose concentration of 280 mg/dL, would the exercise physiologist have conducted this test? Why or why not? What if the client did not have any urinary ketones?

3. If this client had autonomic neuropathy, provide two methods to detect silent ischemia?

Student Case Study 3.6

Exercise Test Interpretation: Submaximal Treadmill Test

An exercise physiologist specializes in serving clients with diabetes. She just completed a submaximal treadmill test on a 60-year-old male, moderately physically active, with type II diabetes. The client has known peripheral neuropathy and a tendency to develop open sores on his feet. No other complications are noted. The test was terminated at a heart rate equal to 70 percent of the client's heart rate reserve. The results of the test are provided in Figure 3.4. After reading the results use, the walking or running equation and a proportion equation to interpret the results and answer the questions.

1. Using one of the following two equations, estimate $\dot{V}O_2$ for the last completed stage:

   Walking: $\dot{V}O_2 = (0.1 \times \text{speed in m/min}) + (1.8 \times \text{speed in m/min} \times \text{grade}) + 3.5$,

   Running: $\dot{V}O_2 = (0.2 \times \text{speed in m/min}) + (0.9 \times \text{speed in m/min} \times \text{grade}) + 3.5$.

   Find $\dot{V}O_2$ in last stage in mL/kg · min

   Find estimated $\dot{V}O_{2max}$ in mL/kg · min

2. Given the client's known peripheral neuropathy, what steps can be taken to ensure client safety during a submaximal treadmill test?

Figure 3.4 This table depicts hypothetical data from a submaximal treadmill test

Stage	Speed (mph)	Grade %	Heart Rate	Blood Pressure	RPE	ECG	Symptoms
Resting	0	0	72	120/70	NA	Sinus	No symptoms
I	1.7	10.0	110	122/72	9	Sinus	No symptoms
II	2.5	12.0	122	148/72	12	Sinus	No symptoms
III	3.4	14.0	134	170/74	16	Sinus	No symptoms
Immediate	1.5	0	135	170/70	NA	Sinus	No symptoms
Recovery 1 min	1.5	0	114	152/70	NA	Sinus	No symptoms
Recovery 5 min	1	0	105	128/70	NA	Sinus	No symptoms

Student Case Study 3.7

Muscular Strength Testing for Clients with Diabetes

An exercise physiologist specializes in serving clients with diabetes. The newest client is a 50-year-old male with type I diabetes who weighs 200 pounds. He has mild retinopathy and known autonomic neuropathy. The exercise physiologist wants to prescribe this client a resistance training program to help him better control his blood glucose. Therefore, the exercise physiologist conducts a series of muscular strength tests. The following data were collected (Figure 3.5).

Figure 3.5 This table depicts hypothetical data from a 3–5RM test

Leg Press Strength Test

| Trial 1 | 5 repetitions |
| | 180 weight |

| Trial 2 | 3 repetitions |
| | 190 weight |

| Trial 3 | 3 repetitions |
| | 205 weight |

| Best Trial | 3 repetitions |
| | 205 weight |

Chest Press Strength Test

| Trial 1 | 5 repetitions |
| | 135 weight |

| Trial 2 | 3 repetitions |
| | 145 weight |

(Continued)

Chest Press Strength Test

Trial 3	3	repetitions
	150	weight
Best Trial	3	repetitions
	150	weight

1. Use the Lander equation to predict the client's maximal leg press strength.
2. Calculate a weight pushed to body weight ratio and compare the client's results to normative data.
3. Use the Lander equation to predict the client's maximal chest press strength.
4. Calculate a weight pushed to body weight ratio and compare the client's results to normative data.
5. Because of the client's known retinopathy and autonomic neuropathy, what can be done as an exercise physiologist to ensure safety while gathering the most accurate data?

Student Case Study 3.8

Body Composition Test Interpretation: Skinfolds

An exercise specialist is responsible for interpreting body composition assessments conducted on clients with diabetes. She was recently presented with the following skinfold and anthropomorphic data (Figure 3.6) from a 224-pound, 51-year-old male with type II diabetes. Analyze the results to interpret body composition and answer the questions.

Figure 3.6 This table depicts hypothetical data from a seven-site skinfold assessment

Site	Trial 1	Trial 2	Trial 3	Average
Triceps	20	22	23	mm
Subscapular	23	23	24	mm
Chest	19	18	20	mm
Abdominal	29	28	30	mm
Suprailiac	34	35	36	mm
Midaxillary	23	22.5	21	mm
Thigh	18	18	20	mm
Waist Circumference	43 inches			

1. Using the seven-site skinfold body density equation for men, calculate body density.
2. Using the Siri equation, estimate the client's body fat percentage.
3. Calculate the client's fat and nonfat weight in pounds.
4. Compare the results to normative data.
5. Using the three-site skinfold body density equation for men, calculate body density.

6. Using the Siri equation, estimate the client's body fat percentage.
7. Calculate the client's fat and nonfat weight in pounds.
8. Was there a difference between the seven- and three-site skinfold calculations for body density and body fat? If there were a difference, why would the difference exist?
9. Classify the client's waist circumference according to disease risk.
10. Should a different body composition assessment be used for this client? If so, which assessment(s)? Would these tests be more accurate for this client?
11. Would this client benefit from fat loss? If so, in what way(s)?

Student Case Study 3.9

Exercise Prescription for Clients with Diabetes: Cardiorespiratory Endurance

An exercise professional specializes in serving clients with diabetes. The newest client is a 62-year-old male with type II diabetes who weighs 230 pounds with peripheral and autonomic neuropathy. The client's blood glucose levels range from 90 to 300 mg/dL, depending on the timing of insulin injection. The exercise professional just conducted a YMCA cycle test, completed without complications, and the client achieved an estimated $\dot{V}O_{2max}$ of 27 mL/kg · min. Prior to the test, the client's resting heart rate was 91 beats per minute. The client was previously sedentary and does not like cycling exercise because of discomfort.

1. Calculate a heart rate range based on the heart rate reserve that the client should maintain during aerobic exercise. Should an exercise professional use this heart rate range during exercise training or consider other methods of quantifying exercise intensity? Why or why not?
2. Calculate a $\dot{V}O_2$ range based on $\dot{V}O_2$ reserve that the client should maintain during aerobic exercise.
3. Provide an exercise type (be specific), frequency, and time at the $\dot{V}O_2$ range found in question 2 for the client to improve cardiorespiratory fitness and better manage blood glucose.
4. Suggest four possible aerobic exercises that would be appropriate for this client. Then explain the rationale for each selection.
5. Use the walking equation to calculate a walking speed (in mph) for the client that elicits the lower end of the $\dot{V}O_2$ reserve range found in question 2. The percent grade of the treadmill is 8 percent.
6. Use the stepping equation to calculate a stepping rate for the client that elicits the upper end of the $\dot{V}O_2$ reserve range found in question 2. The height of the step is 20 centimeters.
7. Use the arm cycle equation to calculate a resistance to be placed on the flywheel for the client that elicits the lower end of the $\dot{V}O_2$ reserve range found in question 2. The client turns the arm crank at 80 rpm.

8. Suggest a progression scheme to advance the client toward a goal of improving blood glucose levels.
9. Provide three training considerations to help this client improve blood glucose through cardiorespiratory exercise safely. One consideration must address pre-exercise blood glucose.
10. Provide a list of five signs or symptoms of exercise-induced hypoglycemia.

Student Case Study 3.10

Exercise Prescription for Clients with Diabetes: Cardiorespiratory Endurance

An exercise specialist is responsible for designing exercise prescriptions for clients with diabetes. The most recent client is a 175-pound, 43-year-old male with type I diabetes. The client has a history of autonomic neuropathy, exaggerated blood pressure responses to physical activity, and exercise-induced hyperglycemia. The exercise specialist conducted a submaximal cycle test without complications and estimated a $\dot{V}O_{2max}$ of 30 mL/kg · min. Prior to the test, the exercise specialist recorded a resting heart rate of 87 beats per minute. The client is deconditioned and does not like exercises that involve complex and coordinated movements because of the risk of injury.

1. Calculate a heart rate range based on the heart rate reserve that the client should maintain during aerobic exercise. Should the exercise specialist use this heart rate range during exercise training or consider other methods of quantifying exercise intensity? Why or why not?
2. Calculate a $\dot{V}O_2$ range based on $\dot{V}O_2$ reserve that the client should maintain during aerobic exercise.
3. Provide an exercise type (be specific), frequency, and time at the $\dot{V}O_2$ range found in question 2 for the client to improve cardiorespiratory fitness and better manage blood glucose.
4. Suggest four possible aerobic exercises that would be appropriate for this client. Then explain the rationale for each selection.
5. Use the walking equation to calculate an appropriate walking speed (in mph) and incline for the client that elicits the lower end of the $\dot{V}O_2$ reserve range found in question 2.
6. Use the leg cycling equation to calculate an appropriate peddling frequency and resistance to elicit the upper end of the $\dot{V}O_2$ reserve range found in question 2.
7. Use the arm cycle equation to calculate an appropriate peddle frequency and resistance to be placed on the flywheel for the client that elicits the lower end of the $\dot{V}O_2$ reserve range found in question 2.
8. Suggest a progression scheme to advance the client toward a goal of improving blood glucose levels.

9. Would progressing to high-intensity interval training be appropriate for this client? If so, what cautions should be considered? If not, explain why.

10. Provide three training considerations to help this client improve his blood glucose through cardiorespiratory exercise safely. One consideration must address the client's exaggerated blood pressure responses to exercise.

11. Provide a list of five signs or symptoms of exercise-induced hyperglycemia.

Student Case Study 3.11

Exercise Prescription for Clients with Diabetes: Muscular Fitness

An exercise physiologist specializes in training clients with diabetes. The exercise physiologist was recently presented with the following client data: (1) 55-year-old with type I diabetes, (2) some experience with resistance training, (3) goals to improve blood glucose and muscular strength, (4) history of retinopathy and autonomic neuropathy, (5) chest press 1RM = 220 pounds, (6) leg press 1RM = 255 pounds, and (7) open to any resistance exercise program.

1. Provide a range for weight that the client should chest press.
2. Provide a range for weight that the client should leg press.
3. Provide a resistance exercise prescription for frequency, number of exercises, sets, and repetitions to improve muscular strength.
4. Suggest at least four specific resistance training exercises that are appropriate for this client.
5. Suggest a progression scheme to advance the client toward the goal of improving muscle mass.
6. Provide three training considerations to help this client improve muscle mass through resistance exercise safely. One of the considerations must account for the client's history of retinopathy.

Student Case Study 3.12

Exercise Prescription for Clients with Diabetes: Muscular Fitness

A clinical exercise physiologist specializes in training clients with diabetes. The newest client is a 60-year-old with type II diabetes. He has never performed resistance training but wants to begin a program to better control his blood glucose and cut his medication requirement. The client experiences regular fluctuations in blood glucose that varies according to the timing of insulin injection. In addition, the client has a history of peripheral neuropathy. Prior to prescribing exercise, the exercise physiologist conducted a modified push-up test with the client completing six repetitions and a body squat test with the client completing four repetitions.

1. Provide a resistance exercise prescription for frequency, intensity, number of exercises, sets, and repetitions to improve the client's muscular fitness and manage blood glucose.
2. Suggest at least four specific resistance training exercises that are appropriate for this client.
3. Suggest a progression scheme to advance the client toward the goal of improving overall muscular fitness and manage blood glucose.
4. Provide three training considerations to help this client improve his muscle mass through resistance exercise safely. One of the considerations must account for the client's history of blood glucose fluctuations.

Student Case Study 3.13

Exercise Testing and Prescription: Comprehensive Case Study

An exercise physiologist works for a diabetes rehabilitation clinic. He thoroughly collected the following from the most recent client:

Demographics: (1) female and (2) 56 years old

Family History: (1) parents passed away in their 70s because of diabetic complications and (2) all grandparents passed away in their 70s because of heart disease and diabetic complications

Biometrics: (1) resting heart rate = 97 beats per minute; (2) resting blood pressure = 140/78 mmHg; (3) LDL-c = 142 mg/dL, HDL-c = 37 mg/dL, total cholesterol = 255 mg/dL; (4) glycosylated hemoglobin = 6.6 percent and blood glucose = 167 mg/dL; and (5) weight = 180 lbs., BMI = 30.5 kg/m²

Medical Diagnoses: (1) type II diabetes, (2) autonomic neuropathy, (3) peripheral neuropathy, (4) foot ulcers, (5) mild retinopathy, (6) exaggerated pressor responses to physical activity, and (7) a history with exercise-induced hypoglycemia

Medications: (1) Lantus, (2) NovoLog, and (3) Actos

Symptoms: (1) headaches with hypoglycemia and hypertension, (2) fatigue with chronotropic incompetence, (3) visual disturbances with retinopathy, (4) foot ulcers, and (5) loss of coordination with complex movements

Exercise History: (1) light walking and (2) resistance exercise

Exercise Goals and Needs: (1) increase cardiorespiratory endurance, (2) increase fat-free mass to assist in weight loss and glucose metabolism, and (3) improve neuromotor function.

1. Should the exercise physiologist conduct a maximal or submaximal cardio-respiratory fitness test? In four to five sentences, provide a defense for the decision based on the client's profile.
2. Which cardiorespiratory fitness test should be conducted? In four to five sentences, provide a defense for the decision based on the client's profile.
3. Given limitless resources, which body composition test should the exercise physiologist conduct? In four to five sentences, provide a defense for the decision based on the client's profile.
4. Given minimal resources with a small budget, which body composition test should be conducted? In four to five sentences, provide a defense for the decision based on the client's profile.
5. Specific to this case, which body composition test would be preferred? In four to five sentences, provide a defense for the decision based on the client's profile.
6. To assess muscular fitness, should muscular endurance assessments or muscular strength assessments be conducted, or both? In four to five sentences, provide a defense for the decision based on the client's profile.
7. Provide a list of four specific muscular fitness tests to be conducted on the client. Then provide a four to five sentence defense supporting the selections.
8. Based on the answer for questions one and two, calculate the client's $\dot{V}O_{2max}$ from the most appropriate of the following cardiorespiratory fitness tests (Figures 3.7–3.11).

Figure 3.7 This table depicts hypothetical data from a YMCA cycle test

YMCA Cycle Test

Stage	Kpm/min	Heart Rate	Blood Pressure	RPE	ECG	Symptoms/ Comments
Resting	0	97	140/78	NA	Sinus	No symptoms
I	150	112	168/80	11	Sinus	No symptoms
II	300	130	188/82	15	Sinus	No symptoms
Immediate	100	129	186/82	NA	Sinus	No symptoms
Recovery 1 min	50	120	172/82	NA	Sinus	No symptoms
Recovery 5 min	25	110	162/80	NA	Sinus	No symptoms

Figure 3.8 Students may use these gridlines to graph data from the YMCA cycle test

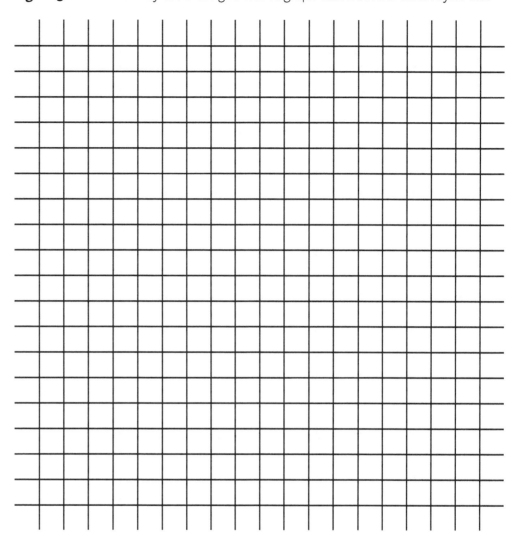

Figure 3.9 This table depicts hypothetical data from an Astrand-Rhyming cycle test

Astrand-Rhyming Cycle Test

Stage/Minute	Kpm/m	Heart Rate	Blood Pressure	RPE	ECG	Symptoms
Resting		97	140/78	NA	Sinus	No symptoms
I	300	130	174/82	10	Sinus	No symptoms
II	300	130	174/82	11	Sinus	No symptoms
III	300	131	176/84	11	Sinus	No symptoms
IV	300	132	178/84	12	Sinus	No symptoms
V	300	134	180/84	12	Sinus	No symptoms
VI	300	134	180/86	12	Sinus	No symptoms
Immediate	150	130	178/84	NA	Sinus	No symptoms
Recovery 1 min	75	117	170/84	NA	Sinus	No symptoms
Recovery 5 min	50	107	142/82	NA	Sinus	No symptoms

Figure 3.10 This table depicts hypothetical maximal cycle test data

Maximal Cycle Test

Stage	Time	Kpm /min	Heart Rate	Blood Pressure	RPE	$\dot{V}O_2$ (mL/kg · min.)	RER	Blood Lactate (mmol)	ECG
Resting		0	97	140/78	NA	4.4	0.75	NA	Sinus
I	2:00	600	122	160/80	11	11.8	0.89	1.2	Sinus
II	4:00	900	142	170/82	14	19.7	1.07	3.3	Sinus
III	6:00	1200	152	184/84	16	23.9	1.11	5.2	Sinus
IV	8:00	1500	161	190/86	18	28.8	1.15	8.9	ST-seg depress
Immediate	NA	300	160	188/86	NA	28.4	1.14	NA	ST-seg depress
Recovery 1 min	NA	150	140	168/84	NA	20.2	1.02	NA	ST-seg depress
Recovery 5 min	NA	75	101	142/84	NA	18.6	0.97	NA	Sinus

Comments: Shortness of breath, 3/4 in stage 4

Figure 3.11 This table depicts hypothetical maximal treadmill test data

Maximal Treadmill Test

Stage	Time	Speed (mph)	Grade %	Blood Pressure	$\dot{V}O_2$ (mL/kg · min)	Blood Lactate (mmol)	RPE	Heart Rate	RER
Resting	NA	0	0	140/78	4.7	NA	NA	97	0.75
Warm-Up	NA	2	0	158/80	13.2	NA	NA	123	0.80
I	2:00	2.5	0	174/80	17.1	0.7	13	147	0.89
II	4:00	3.5	0	192/84	22.6	4.9	15	159	0.99
III	6:00	4.0	2	204/86	28.9	8.2	19	164	1.15
Immediate	NA	1.5	0	200/86	27.6	NA	NA	160	1.14
Recovery 1 min	NA	1.5	0	180/84	20.6	NA	NA	150	1.01
Recovery 5 min	NA	1	0	168/84	18.1	NA	NA	108	0.99

Comments: ECG monitor went blank at the beginning of the test. Client complained of breathless-ness in stage 3

9. For the cardiorespiratory fitness test chosen to interpret for question eight, should the test have been terminated prior to completion? Explain why or why not.

10. Assuming the skinfold assessment for body composition test was selected, calculate body fat percentage from the following seven-site skinfold data (Figure 3.12).

Figure 3.12 This table depicts hypothetical data from a seven-site skinfold assessment

Site	Trial 1	Trial 2	Trial 3	Average
Triceps	17	17	19	mm
Subscapular	25	27	26	mm
Chest	21	22	23	mm
Abdominal	38	38	36	mm
Suprailiac	41	42	43	mm
Midaxillary	28	26	27	mm
Thigh	20	23	24	mm

11. If the client's waist circumference were 47 inches, what would be her risk classification?

12. Assuming muscular strength was selected, interpret and classify the client's leg and chest press strength from the following data (Figure 3.12).

Figure 3.13 This table depicts hypothetical data from a 3–5RM test

Leg Press Strength Test

Trial 1	5	repetitions
	160	weight
Trial 2	3	repetitions
	180	weight
Trial 3	3	repetitions
	200	weight
Best Trial	3	repetitions
	200	weight

Chest Press Strength Test

Trial 1	5	repetitions
	130	weight
Trial 2	3	repetitions
	150	weight
Trial 3	3	repetitions
	170	weight
Best Trial	3	repetitions
	170	weight

13. Calculate a heart rate range based on the heart rate reserve that the client should maintain during aerobic exercise. Is this the most reliable method for quantifying cardiorespiratory endurance exercise? Why or why not?

14. Calculate a $\dot{V}O_2$ range based on $\dot{V}O_2$ reserve that the client should maintain during aerobic exercise.

15. Provide an exercise type (be specific), frequency, and time at the $\dot{V}O_2$ range found in question 14 for the client to improve their cardiorespiratory fitness and manage blood glucose.

16. Suggest four possible aerobic exercises that would be appropriate for this client.
17. Provide a walking speed and grade for the client to maintain on the treadmill to elicit the lower end of the $\dot{V}O_2$ range listed in question 14.
18. Provide a resistance and peddle frequency for leg cycling to elicit the lower end of the $\dot{V}O_2$ range listed in question 14.
19. Provide a resistance and peddle frequency for arm cycling to elicit the lower end of the $\dot{V}O_2$ range listed in question 14.
20. Provide a range for weight that the client should chest press.
21. Provide a range for weight that the client should leg press.
22. Provide a resistance exercise prescription for frequency, number of exercises, sets, and repetitions to improve muscular fitness.
23. Suggest at least four specific resistance training exercises that are appropriate for this client.
24. Suggest a progression scheme to help the client improve overall muscular fitness.
25. Provide a frequency, intensity, number of stretches, sets, and amount of time each stretch should be to help improve the client's flexibility.
26. Provide a list consisting of all safety considerations that should be considered when supervising this client's exercise program.

Student Case Study 3.14

Safety Considerations for Clients with Diabetes

A recent college graduate is interviewing for his or her first job. The job for which he or she is interviewing is a diabetes exercise specialist. The person conducting the interview wants to determine the interviewee's knowledge regarding safety considerations for clients with diabetes. Please thoroughly respond to the following interview questions.

1. What is autonomic neuropathy, and what are the concerns for an exercise physiologist when training clients with diabetes and this condition?
2. What is peripheral neuropathy, and what are the concerns for an exercise physiologist when training clients with diabetes and this condition?
3. Considering a person with type I diabetes with a history of exercise-induced hyperglycemia, what are the considerations regarding high-intensity interval training? What steps are needed to ensure safety during such training?
4. Assuming there are no physician orders specifying a safe blood glucose range for exercise, what would be the "cutoff" range. When would you recommend carbohydrate consumption prior to exercise?
5. How would you reduce the risk of exercise-induced hypoglycemia among all clients with diabetes?
6. When would you be concerned about medication timing? When would you recommend delaying the start of exercise following medication administration?

7. How would you avoid further ocular damage in patients with mild to moderate retinopathy?

8. How would you modify an exercise prescription (both cardiorespiratory endurance and muscular fitness exercise prescriptions) for a patient with diabetes and nephropathy?

9. How would you modify an exercise prescription (both cardiorespiratory endurance and muscular fitness exercise prescriptions) for a patient with diabetes and proprioceptive issues as a result of peripheral neuropathy?

10. How would you reduce the risk of a client with diabetes developing new wounds, particularly feet wounds?

11. What signs and symptoms would indicate a client is experiencing hypoglycemia?

12. What signs and symptoms would indicate a client is experiencing hyperglycemia? When a client reports to the facility with a blood glucose level of 250 mg/dL or more, what steps would you take to ensure safety? In this situation, when is exercise unsafe?

REFERENCES

1. S. E. Kahn, M. E. Cooper, and S. Del Prato, "Pathophysiology and Treatment of Type 2 Diabetes: Perspectives on the Past, Present, and Future," *Lancet* 383, no. 9922 (2014): 1068–83.

2. S. Inzucchi, R. Bergenstal, J. Buse, et al., "Management of Hyperglycemia in Type 2 Diabetes, 2015: A Patient-Centered Approach: Update to a Position Statement of the American Diabetes Association and the European Association for the Study of Diabetes," *Diabetes Care* 38, no. 1 (2015): 140–49.

3. D. Leroith, "Pathophysiology of the Metabolic Syndrome: Implications for the Cardiometabolic Risks Associated with Type 2 Diabetes. *American Journal of the Medical Sciences* 343, no. 1 (2012): 13–16.

4. R. Pop-Busui, "What Do We Know and We Do Not Know about Cardiovascular Autonomic Neuropathy in Diabetes," *Journal of Cardiovascular Translation Research* 5, no. 4 (2012): 463–78.

5. S. R. Colberg, R. J. Sigal, B. Fernhall, et al., "Exercise and Type 2 Diabetes: The American College of Sports Medicine and the American Diabetes Association: A Joint Statement," *Diabetes Care* 33, no. 12 (2010): 147–67.

6. ibid.

7. E. Teixeira-Lemos, S. Nunes, F. Teixeira, et al., "Regular Physical Exercise Training Assists in Preventing Type 2 Diabetes Development: Focus on Its Antioxidant and Anti-Inflammatory Properties," *Cardiovascular Diabetology* 10, no. 12 (2011).

8. American College of Sports Medicine, *ACSM's Guidelines for Exercise Testing and Prescription*, 11th ed. (Philadelphia: Wolters Kluwer Health, 2022).

9. Colberg et al., "Exercise and Type 2 Diabetes."

10. American College of Sports Medicine, *ACSM's Guidelines*.

11. ibid.

12. ibid.

13. E. Selvin, C . M. Parrinello, D. B. Sacks, et al., "Trends in Prevalence and Control of Diabetes in the United States, 1988–1994 and 1999–2010," *Annals of Internal Medicine* 160, no. 8 (2014): 517–25.

14. American College of Sports Medicine, *ACSM's Guidelines*.

15. American College of Sports Medicine, *ACSM's Exercise Management for Persons with Chronic Diseases and Disabilities* (Champaign, IL: Human Kinetics, 2016).

16. A. I. Vinik and D. Ziegler, "Diabetic Cardiovascular Autonomic Neuropathy," *Circulation* 115, no. 3 (2007): 387–97.

17. American College of Sports Medicine, *ACSM's Guidelines*.

18. ibid.

19. ibid.

20. ibid.

21. ibid.

22. Colberg et al., "Exercise and Type 2 Diabetes."

23. American College of Sports Medicine, *ACSM's Guidelines*.

24. ibid.

25. B. B. Gibbs, D. A. Dobrosielski, S. Bonekamp, et al., "A Randomized Trial of Exercise for Blood Pressure Reduction in Type 2 Diabetes: Effect on Flow-Mediated Dilation and Circulating Biomarkers of Endothelial Function," *Atherosclerosis* 224, no. 2 (2012): 446–53.

26. M. P. Jorge, V. N. de Oliveira, N. M. Resende, et al., "The Effects of Aerobic, Resistance, and Combined Exercise on Metabolic Control, Inflammatory Markers, Adipocytokines, and Muscle Insulin Signaling in Patients with Type 2 Diabetes Mellitus," *Metabolism* 60, no. 9 (2011): 1244–52.

27. W. R. Sukala, R. Page, D. S. Rowlands, et al., "South Pacific Islanders Resist Type 2 Diabetes: Comparison of Aerobic and Resistance Training," *European Journal of Applied Physiology* 112, no. 1 (2012): 317–25.

28. American College of Sports Medicine, *ACSM's Guidelines*.

29. ibid.

30. ibid.

31. ibid.

32. ibid.

33. ibid.

34. Colberg et al., "Exercise and Type 2 Diabetes."

35. American College of Sports Medicine, *ACSM's Guidelines*.

36. ibid.

Exercise Testing and Prescription for Clients with Hypertension

INTRODUCTION

HYPERTENSION IS DEFINED as having a resting systolic blood pressure ≥140 mmHg and/or a resting diastolic blood pressure ≥90 mmHg recorded on at least two separate occasions, and it affects nearly 30 percent of the US adult population.[1,2,3] In addition, many more US adults have prehypertension, having a resting systolic blood pressure ≥120 mmHg and/or a resting diastolic blood pressure ≥80 mmHg, which can eventually progress to hypertension. Given the number of adults with hypertension and its propensity for contributing to the development of cardiovascular disease, exercise professionals will almost assuredly serve patients or clients with a need for blood pressure reduction.

Hypertension can be divided into two types: essential and secondary.[4] Essential hypertension accounts for the vast majority of hypertension cases and is linked to a number of preventable factors. Such factors include high alcohol consumption,[5] obesity,[6] chronic distress,[7] tobacco use, and a sedentary lifestyle.[8] Moreover, essential hypertension is highly correlated with the development of cardiovascular diseases, such as coronary artery disease, ischemic and hemorrhagic stroke, and pathologic left ventricular hypertrophy.[9,10] Secondary hypertension arises from primarily renal or adrenal abnormalities, such as chronic kidney disease, renal failure, and pheochromocytoma and is less preventable in nature.[11]

The long-term pathological changes induced by hypertension can be somewhat complex and result in both chemical and structural changes in the vasculature. To keep things simple, from the standpoint of chronic disease development, hypertension can be viewed as the engine that powers the atherosclerotic cascade. Underexposure to increased rates of blood flow, the endothelium is damaged, allowing for the penetration of low-density lipoprotein cholesterol molecules through the endothelium, which ultimately leads to the accumulation of atherosclerotic plaque.[12] Over time, the very function of the endothelium can become compromised, resulting in autoregulatory disfunction and diminishing the capacity of vasodilation leading to further augmentations in long-term blood pressure.[13] Long-term structural changes can occur in response to chronic hypertension. With increased peripheral resistance, a characteristic of hypertension, the heart's left ventricle can undergo hypertrophic remodeling, contributing to possible heart failure.[14] Further, in response to chronic hypertension, structural weaknesses can occur to the vasculature, leading to dissections and aneurysms.[15]

It is common for health professionals to refer to hypertension as the "silent killer." The reason for this is that hypertension often does not induce symptoms until resting blood pressure suddenly "spikes" and or reaches the approximate pressure of 180/120 mmHg indicating a hypertensive crisis.[16] Typically, hypertension progresses over time and with advancing age.[17] Therefore, it is imperative that exercise professionals screen for and encourage regular blood pressure screenings to detect changes and prevent prehypertension from progressing to stage 1 hypertension and beyond.

A multitude of research suggests that regular exercise, both aerobic and resistance training, has the capacity to effectively lower blood pressure in the prevention and/or management of hypertension.[18,19,20,21,22] Research has shown that that regular exercise participation can lower overall blood pressure by 5–7 mmHg.[23] Further, research shows that simple lifestyle interventions, such as increasing walking distance per day, are associated with reductions in the risk.[24] Therefore, exercise professionals serving clients with hypertension or prehypertension should encourage regular exercise participation in addition to increased physical activity beyond a fitness facility setting to better manage and prevent hypertension.

The ACSM recommends that adults with hypertension and prehypertension perform aerobic exercise for 150–210 minutes per week at an intensity of 40 to 60 percent of $\dot{V}O_2R$.[25] In addition, the ACSM recommends that adults with hypertension complete resistance exercise for each major muscle group, two to four sets of eight to 12 repetitions, two to three days per week, at an intensity of 60 to 70 percent of 1RM.[26]

However, exercise professionals must be cautious when serving patients with hypertension, as exercise may induce exaggerated blood pressure responses, unexpected postexercise hypotension because of the influence of antihypertensive medications and exercise and may have existing comorbidities, making exercise difficult. Therefore, exercise professionals must be able to modify and individualize exercise prescriptions to make them safe and effective. This chapter outlines exercise test selection and interpretation, FITT-VP modification, and safety considerations for serving clients with hypertension.

The purpose of this chapter is to teach students how to apply their knowledge of hypertension and prehypertension, exercise testing, and exercise prescription. On completion of the case studies within this chapter, students will be able to achieve the following:

1. Recall the acute and chronic blood pressure responses to exercise to educate clients or patients on the importance of exercise and the underlying risks
2. Recognize individual exercise risks and implement safety measures in exercise test selection and exercise testing procedures
3. Apply the cardiorespiratory, muscular fitness, and flexibility FITT-VP recommendations and modifications to clients or patients with hypertension
4. Identify and understand safety considerations for training clients or patients with hypertension

ACUTE AND CHRONIC BLOOD PRESSURE RESPONSES TO EXERCISE

Exercise professionals should encourage clients with hypertension and prehypertension to participate in regular physical activity to manage and/or prevent long-term high blood pressure. However, in doing so, exercise professionals need to be aware of the acute and chronic influences of exercise on blood pressure. Such information is useful in the safe selection of exercise tests, the prescription of an effective exercise program, and the education of clients or patients.

Blood pressure can be expressed as a mathematical formula. Here blood pressure is equal to the product of flow and resistance. Flow is representative of cardiac output, and thus the pressure exerted against artery walls during ventricular systole—systolic blood pressure. Resistance, on the other hand, is representative of the viscosity and volume of the blood and the radius of peripheral blood vessels. Further, resistance can be thought of as the pressure exerted against artery walls during ventricular diastole—diastolic blood pressure. Both flow and resistance are influenced by acute and chronic exercise training.

At the onset of steady-state exercise, cardiac output increases to meet new metabolic demands, which increases systolic blood pressure. A steady rise in systolic blood pressure with increasing exercise intensity is a normal hemodynamic response. Systolic blood pressure should increase approximately 10 mmHg with each 1 MET increase in exercise intensity until the $\dot{V}O_{2\,max}$ is achieved.[27] Normal increases in systolic blood pressure may be blunted if a client or patient is taking antihypertensive medications, such as beta-blockers and calcium channel blockers. Regardless of medication status, the systolic blood pressure should never decrease with increases in exercise intensity. Should decreases in systolic blood pressure occur, exercise should be terminated to prevent myocardial ischemia because of underlying ischemic heart disease or left ventricular dysfunction.[28] Diastolic blood pressure typically does not change in response to exercise; however, slight decreases or increases can be expected. Should diastolic blood pressure increase more than 10 mmHg or exceed 115 mmHg during an exercise test or exercise session, it is appropriate for an exercise professional to terminate the test or session.

An important consideration concerning the blood pressure response to acute exercise is the influence of local mechanics on skeletal muscle blood flow. As skeletal muscles become more active during exercise, exercise hyperemia, which is when blood flow increases to the active skeletal muscles, occurs.[29] This increase in local blood flow is, in part, the result of autoregulation and the release of local vasodilators, such as prostacyclin and nitric oxide.[30,31] In theory, this vasodilatory effect of exercise would result in an acute decrease in diastolic blood pressure. However, the circulatory system is not capable of supplying enough blood through maximally dilated vessels to large groups of active muscle.[32] Therefore, as more skeletal muscles are activated and the intensity of exercise increases, vasodilation is offset by modest local vasoconstriction and vasoconstriction elsewhere in circulation (i.e., splanchnic blood flow) to maintain mean arterial pressure.[33] Nevertheless, the cumulative vasodilatory effect of acute exercise can last up to 24 hours postexercise, resulting in *temporary* reductions in resting blood pressure.[34] It is for this reason that exercise professionals should recommend repeated exercise bouts throughout the week to reduce blood pressure long term. Moreover, exercise professionals need to consider the combination of exercise and antihypertensive drugs and should discourage abrupt stoppage of an exercise session to avoid postexercise hypotension.

Long-term blood pressure is primarily regulated by the kidneys, particularly via the renin-angiotensin-aldosterone system. Renin is an enzyme that is released by kidneys, which converts the hepatic-produced plasma protein angiotensinogen into angiotensin I. Angiotensin I is then converted to angiotensin II via an enzymatic reaction with angiotensin converting enzyme. Angiotensin II elevates blood pressure by stimulating vasoconstriction and the release of aldosterone, which in turn causes the kidneys to reabsorb sodium and thereby water. With long-term exercise adherence, evidence suggests that plasma renin levels are reduced,[35] which should theoretically lower long-term blood pressure. Other evidence suggests that in response to exercise training, long-term blood pressure may be reduced by a decreased concentration of circulating catecholamine hormones, increased parasympathetic tone at rest, and improvement of other cardiovascular risk factors, such as dyslipidemia and obesity.[36,37] Overall, blood pressure can be expected to decrease 5–7 mmHg over time in response to long-term exercise training.

Demonstration Case Study 4.1

Exercise Responses

Craig is an exercise physiologist working for a risk factor reduction program at a large university. His most recent client is Cooper, a 48-year old male with diagnosed stage 1 hypertension. Cooper resisted his physician's recommendation for antihypertensive medication, suggesting he would rather attempt lifestyle modification first.

Cooper consulted Craig about how exercise could help manage his hypertension. Craig, a recent college graduate, remembers a lecture he had in the fall regarding blood pressure responses to acute and chronic exercise. Craig tells Cooper that acute exercise causes an increase in the rate of blood flow through the arteries. Craig assures Cooper that this is normal and further states that the increase in blood flow induces vascular sheer stress, which signals the release of local vasodilators and permits blood flow with less resistance. Then Craig said this effect lasts up to 24 hours postexercise, which can help decrease resting blood pressure, but only temporarily. For this reason, Craig claimed, exercise should be completed on a near daily basis to effectively lower blood pressure and manage hypertension.

Craig then offered some long-term mechanisms by which regular exercise can lower blood pressure by roughly 5–7 mmHg. Craig claimed that adaptations of the kidneys, parasympathetic nervous system, and improvements of cardiovascular risk factors, such as blood lipids and body composition, can further aid in the reduction of blood pressure.

Demonstration Case Study 4.2

Exercise Responses

Cabrilla is an exercise physiologist working for a hospital's chronic disease management program. Part of Cabrilla's responsibilities is to supervise patients with hypertension as they exercise. Currently, Cabrilla is monitoring Liam, a 52-year-old male being medicated for stage II hypertension. In addition to having hypertension, Liam has a history of being sedentary and as such likes to skip out on the cooldown session. Cabrilla confronts Liam, in a very professional manner, and tells Liam that exercise causes his blood vessels to dilate and abruptly stopping exercise takes away the muscle pump, which returns blood to the heart. Therefore, Cabrilla correctly claims that abruptly stopping exercise may lead to postexercise hypotension, especially in an individual being medically managed for hypertension.

Demonstration Case Study 4.3

Exercise Responses

Cabrilla is an exercise physiologist working for a hospital's chronic disease management program. Part of Cabrilla's responsibilities is to supervise patients with hypertension as they exercise. Recently, Cabrilla worked with a patient named Charlotte. Charlotte is a 62-year-old female with stage I hypertension. During an exercise session, Charlotte appeared unusually fatigued, although she did not complain of fatigue. Cabrilla assessed Charlotte's blood pressure and discovered that Charlotte's systolic blood pressure had decreased by 20 mmHg from her pre-exercise value. Cabrilla correctly stopped the exercise session and consulted a physician at the hospital. Cabrilla told the physician she stopped Charlotte's exercise session because of an abnormal systolic blood pressure response as she feared Charlotte may experience myocardial ischemia.

EXERCISE TESTING FOR CLIENTS WITH HYPERTENSION

Exercise testing should be considered for clients with hypertension to collect baseline data for individualized exercise prescriptions and to assess physiological responses to exercise. Exercise test selection, test termination criteria, and test interpretation for clients with hypertension are similar to those for healthy adults. Thus exercise professionals should feel encouraged to select and conduct any appropriate health-related fitness test. Ideally, a test should be chosen to assess each component of health-related physical fitness in accordance with client goals, exercise history, and health status.

The contraindications and test termination criteria for exercise testing are the same for clients with hypertension as healthy populations. A complete list of exercise testing contraindications can be found and reviewed in the ACSM's *Guidelines for Exercise Testing and Prescription*.[38] In addition to these contraindications, clients with hypertension may present with medical scenarios that would require physician consultation for exercise testing and programming. Any client presenting with uncontrolled hypertension (i.e., not medically managed and/or medically managed with a resting systolic blood pressure ≥140 mmHg and/or a diastolic blood pressure ≥90 mmHg), stage II hypertension (resting systolic blood pressure ≥160 mmHg and/or a diastolic blood pressure ≥100 mmHg), or target organ disease (i.e., left ventricular hypertrophy, kidney failure, or retinopathy) should be evaluated by a physician prior to exercise testing and exercise participation and have a medically supervised exercise test.[39]

Further, exercise professionals must be knowledgeable of the mechanisms of action for common antihypertensive drugs and consider how exercise may interact with these mechanisms to influence the interpretation and safety of exercise testing. For instance, beta-blockers can blunt the heart rate response to exercise, resulting in diminished exercise capacity, while diuretics can cause hypokalemia, resulting in cardiac arrythmias and electrocardiographic changes. In addition, antihypertensive drugs that target peripheral resistance (i.e., angiotensin-converting enzyme (ACE) inhibitors and angiotensin receptor blockers) may compound vasodilatory effects of exercise and thus extended cooldowns should be implemented.

Demonstration Case Study 4.4

Exercise Testing and Hypertension

Tara is an exercise physiologist working for a local hospital. She is responsible for overseeing the risk reduction exercise program. Tara's facility is well equipped with various exercise modalities, but it is somewhat limited for body composition assessment capabilities—her facility has skinfold calipers, bioelectrical impedance, and anthropomorphic measuring tape. Her newest client is a sedentary 65-year-old male named Nathaniel. Nathaniel has controlled stage I hypertension with a resting blood pressure of 130/86 mmHg. He weighs 221 pounds with a BMI of 33.7 kg/m² and has no previous history with exercise. Nathaniel wants to undergo an exercise program to better manage his blood pressure and stave off cardiovascular disease so that he can be a productive part of his grandchildren's lives. Nathaniel takes one antihypertension drug, enalapril, an ACE inhibitor. Occasionally, Nathaniel complains of mild coughing episodes—a common side effect of ACE inhibitors. Nathaniel tells Tara that he is open to all kinds of exercise but vehemently opposes uphill walking and running, as he does not like how this form of exercise hurts his knees. Nathaniel's physician has cleared him to participate in exercise testing and an exercise program.

Given Nathaniel's physician clearance, Tara moves to exercise testing. Tara wants to prescribe a comprehensive exercise program consisting of cardiorespiratory, resistance, and flexibility. Further, Tara knows that obesity contributes to hypertension, so she wants to address Nathaniel's body composition. Tara's first exercise test selection is the Astrand-Rhyming cycle test. She chose this test because of Nathaniel's unwillingness to walk and run uphill. In addition, the Astrand-Rhyming cycle test is appropriate for previously sedentary individuals. Tara notes that Nathaniel is taking an ACE inhibitor and suggests a prolonged cooldown to avoid postexercise hypotension. With Nathaniel's exercise history, Tara doesn't wish to pursue maximal strength testing and instead opts for muscular endurance testing using Nathaniel's body weight as the resistance. Thus Tara selects the modified push-up test and the body squat test. For body composition, Tara keeps things simple by assessing girth measurements, which is appropriate considering Nathaniel is classified as obese, which can limit the accuracy of skinfold testing. To wrap up testing, Tara choose the simple sit-and-reach test to assess Nathaniel's flexibility. Following testing, Tara notes no abnormal responses to exercise and proceeds to exercise prescription.

Demonstration Case Study 4.5

Exercise Testing and Hypertension

Justine is an exercise physiologist working for a local hospital. She is responsible for overseeing the risk reduction exercise program. Justine spends most of her time working with clients with hypertension. Justine's facility is "state of the art" and contains all possible exercise equipment, physiological monitoring capabilities, and air displacement plethysmography for body composition assessment. Her newest client is a sedentary 42-year-old male named Gerald. Gerald reported to the facility with stage II hypertension but was cleared to exercise by his cardiologist just two weeks prior. Gerald's resting blood pressure was 156/92 mmHg at the beginning of his first visit. Gerald is class II obese with a BMI of 36.2 kg/m^2. Gerald has not been physically active since he threw the shot put in college. Gerald wants to undergo a comprehensive exercise program to get his health under control so that he can be a reliable father and husband. Gerald takes a plethora of antihypertensive drugs, including a beta-blocker, an ACE inhibitor, and a loop diuretic (strongest diuretic). Gerald reports no side effects from his medications. Gerald tells Justine that he is open to any and all forms of exercise.

Given Gerald's stage II hypertension, sedentary lifestyle, and numerous medications, Justine wants to be thorough, yet cautious, with her exercise test selections and protocols. Justine starts with cardiorespiratory fitness testing with medical supervision. Here she selects the modified Bruce protocol because of Gerald's current health status and sedentary lifestyle and because a treadmill modality can increase the accuracy of cardiorespiratory exercise test results. Justine is concerned about the numerous medications Gerald has been prescribed. Therefore, Justine options to assess continuous electrocardiography to keep a "watchful eye" for cardiac arrythmias. For resistance testing, Justine selects machine-based modalities and targets muscular endurance because of the lengthy delay in Gerald's physical activity. For body composition, Justine doesn't deem it necessary to place Gerald through the stress of air displacement plethysmography and thus selects girth measurements. For flexibility, Justine selects the sit-and-reach test. Following testing, Justine notes no abnormal responses to exercise and proceeds to exercise prescription.

Demonstration Case Study 4.6

Exercise Testing and Hypertension

David is an exercise physiologist working for a hospital's chronic disease management program. David specializes in exercise as a means of managing hypertension. To add to David's responsibilities, he is currently supervising an intern and wants to be thorough in his training. David's most recent client is Gwendolyn. Gwendolyn is a 51-year-old female with a BMI of 32.9 kg/m². David notices that Gwendolyn has not been officially cleared to exercise by a licensed physician. David realizes this doesn't immediately delay exercise testing, but he is cautious nevertheless. David continues reviewing Gwendolyn's medical records and finds a diagnosis of stage II hypertension. David assesses Gwendolyn's blood pressure and notes a resting blood pressure of 168/102 mmHg. Given that Gwendolyn has not been medically cleared, has stage II hypertension as a diagnosis, and present with a blood pressure revealing probable stage II hypertension, David correctly refers Gwendolyn for medical clearance. David then explains to his intern that patients with hypertension need to be referred for medical clearance and have a medically supervised exercise test if they present with no medical clearance and have stage II hypertension, uncontrolled hypertension, or target organ disease.

Demonstration Case Study 4.7

Exercise Testing and Hypertension

Gene is an exercise physiologist working for a local hospital. He specializes in exercise as a means of managing hypertension. Gene's facility is well equipped and contains all possible exercise equipment, physiological monitoring capabilities, and air displacement plethysmography for body composition assessment. His newest client is a highly active 38-year-old female named Felicia. Felicia has a family history of hypertension and despite her best efforts to beat the "family curse" through regular exercise training, she was recently diagnosed with stage I hypertension. Felicia reported to the facility with a resting blood pressure of 134/82 mmHg and a list of one medication—a diuretic. Felicia is otherwise very healthy and has no other cardiovascular disease risk factors. Felicia's main goal is to get a more science-based and supervised exercise program. Felicia is an avid cycler and enjoys weight lifting. Felecia was recently medically cleared to exercise and even participate in vigorous-intensity exercise.

   Given Felecia's exercise history, Gene feels he can really challenge her by prescribing more vigorous exercises. To test Felecia, Gene selects all maximum-effort tests. He chooses a maximal cycle test to evaluate Felecia's cardiorespiratory endurance using open-circuit spirometry, 1RM tests for the bench press, leg press, seated row, seated crunch, overhead press, air displacement plethysmography for body composition, and a sit-and-reach test for flexibility. Gene only has one concern and that is the influence of Felecia's diuretic. To put Gene's mind at ease, he chooses to assess continuous electrocardiography throughout the maximal cycle test. When asked by Felecia why he felt vigorous exercise was safe, Gene correctly stated that vigorous-intensity exercise can be safe for controlled patients with hypertension with a lifestyle consisting of regular exercise.

EXERCISE PRESCRIPTION FOR CLIENTS WITH HYPERTENSION

Regular exercise is beneficial in the management and or prevention of hypertension. With regular exercise overall blood pressure can be reduced by 5–7 mmHg[40] and improve many factors that contribute to hypertension, such as dyslipidemia, obesity, and an inactive lifestyle.[41] From a physiological perspective, the increased rate of blood flow that occurs with exercise causes vascular sheer stress, which leads to the release of vasodilators, such as nitric oxide and prostacyclin.[42,43] This vasodilatory effect can last up to 24 hours postexercise, and with repeated bouts of exercise throughout the week, blood pressure can remain reduced.[44] In the long-term, blood pressure can be reduced via several purposed mechanisms, including renal, cardiovascular, and parasympathetic nervous system adaptations.[45,46,47] Clients with hypertension benefit from both cardiorespiratory and resistance exercise.[48] Exercise professionals must continuously monitor clients' blood pressure, changes in medication status, and new diagnoses, such as target organ disease, as well as adjust exercise and/or make recommendations for medical examinations accordingly. Further, exercise professionals must always consider fitness level, exercise history, health status, goals, and physician orders when modifying the FITT-VP for clients with hypertension. This section explains these modifications for cardiorespiratory, muscular fitness, and flexibility exercises for clients with hypertension.

Cardiorespiratory Exercise Prescription

The general exercise recommendations discussed in Chapter 2 apply to clients with hypertension with some modifications. However, with the 24-hour postexercise temporary vasodilatory effect of an exercise bout, the ACSM recommends that an initial cardiorespiratory exercise prescription for clients with hypertension consist of greater exercise frequency. Instead of three to five days per week, clients with hypertension should be encouraged to perform cardiorespiratory exercise five to seven days per week.[49] In total, cardiorespiratory exercise time should be between 150 and 210 minutes per week (30 minutes per day).[50] Should clients be deconditioned, or long-term sedentary, ten-minute bouts can be used to accumulate 30 minutes of cardiorespiratory exercise daily. Like healthy populations, exercise time and frequency should be adjusted with changes in exercise intensity.

Exercise intensity plays a role in a hypertensive client's adaptations to cardiorespiratory exercise.[51] If a client has controlled hypertension and has been regularly participating in moderate-intensity cardiorespiratory exercise, vigorous exercise intensity can provide additional benefit and a greater reduction in long-term blood pressure. Previously sedentary clients or clients with multiple comorbidities, uncontrolled hypertension, stage II hypertension, or target organ disease should not be initially prescribed vigorous-intensity cardiorespiratory exercise. Further, inappropriately prescribed exercise intensity can result in early dropout of clients with hypertension and exaggerated blood pressure responses to exercise. In general, it is a reasonable philosophy to start low and progress slow.

Depending on medication status, heart rate may not be a reliable method of quantifying exercise intensity—especially if beta-blockers are prescribed. Therefore, RPE and $\dot{V}O_2R$ are the most reliable methods of quantifying cardiorespiratory exercise intensity. The starting cardiorespiratory endurance intensity for clients with hypertension should be 40 to 60 percent $\dot{V}O_2R$/HRR or an RPE of 12 to 13. Vigorous intensity, if warranted, can be prescribed at 60 to 89 percent of $\dot{V}O_2R$/HRR or an RPE of 14 to 17. For optimal adaptations, exercise professionals should make use of the metabolic equations in Chapter 2.

The type of cardiorespiratory endurance exercise that should be prescribed for clients with hypertension is the same for improving health in apparently healthy adults and other special populations. Modalities that stress larger muscle groups are optimal, as this can aid in addressing many of the factors that contribute to hypertension. However, such modalities are not necessary to elicit favorable adaptations for the client with hypertension. Ultimately, exercise professionals should select exercise modalities based on a client's goals, personal preferences, and safety.

Exercise professionals can modify exercise frequency, intensity, and time to accomplish adequate progress for clients with hypertension. A biweekly increase in exercise volume of 5 to 10 percent is a reasonable progression scheme for clients with hypertension. Like with other clients, exercise frequency and time should be increased before intensity.

Demonstration Case Study 4.8

Cardiorespiratory Exercise Prescription and Hypertension

Karen is an exercise physiologist who specializes in serving clients with hypertension. Her most recent client is Margus, and his profile is as follows: 52-year-old male, stage I controlled hypertension, 235 pounds, BMI 34.2 kg/m², 11 years of sedentary behavior.

Margus takes lisinopril and hydrochlorothiazide to control his blood pressure. Margus has physician approval to undergo exercise testing and an exercise program. A Bruce protocol test was completed without symptoms. The client's resting heart rate was 67 beats per minute, resting blood pressure was 136/82 mmHg, and estimated $\dot{V}O_{2max}$ was 35.5 mL/kg · min. The client is open to any exercise.

After analyzing Margus's profile, Karen, begins to write a cardiorespiratory exercise prescription. Karen first selects an exercise frequency. Karen wants to have Margus exercise five or more days per week to take advantage of the 24-hour vasodilatory effect of exercise. Next, Karen selects an exercise time of 30 minutes per exercise session, broken into ten-minute bouts because of his sedentary behavior. After that, Karen calculates the appropriate exercise intensity. She wants to be precise and specific, so she uses the $\dot{V}O_2R$ method to quantify the intensity and select corresponding workloads on several modalities. Karen chooses a narrow intensity range equal to 40 to 45 percent of $\dot{V}O_2R$, the lower end of a moderate-intensity range because of Margus's sedentary lifestyle. Karen's calculations are shown next.

$\dot{V}O_2R = \dot{V}O_{2max} - 3.5$ mL/kg · min

$\dot{V}O_2R = 35$ mL/kg · min $- 3.5$ mL/kg · min

$\dot{V}O_2R = 31.5$ mL/kg · min

40 percent of $\dot{V}O_2R = (31.5$ mL/kg · min x .4) $+ 3.5$ mL/kg · min

40 percent of $\dot{V}O_2R = 16.1$ mL/kg · min

45 percent of $\dot{V}O_2R = (31.5$ mL/kg · min x .45) $+ 3.5$ mL/kg · min

45 percent of $\dot{V}O_2R = 17.7$ mL/kg · min

$\dot{V}O_2R$ range $= 16.1 - 17.7$ mL/kg · min

Karen choses to have Margus perform walking and leg cycling at specific workloads. Karen's calculations (for the lower end of the intensity range), using metabolic equations, are provided next.

Walking Calculations:

Karen feels that Margus can walk comfortably at 2.5 mph. Therefore, she solves for incline using the walking equation that would elicit 40 percent of Margus's $\dot{V}O_2R$.

16.1 mL/kg · min $= (0.1 \times 2.5 \times 26.8) + (1.8 \times 2.5 \times 26.8 \times$ incline$) + 3.5$

Incline $= 4.9$ %

Leg Cycling Calculations:

Because of Margus's sedentary behavior, Karen feels that Margus should cycle at 60 revolutions per minute when leg cycling. Using the cycling equation, Karen calculates the resistance that should be placed on the flywheel of a Monark cycle to elicit 40 percent of Margus's $\dot{V}O_2R$.

16.1 mL/kg · min $= (1.8 \times 60 \times$ resistance $\times 6/106.8$ kg$) + 7$

Resistance $= 1.49$ kp

Karen then designs an exercise progression plan that involves a slow increase in exercise dose each week. First, Karen will suggest daily exercise intervals of 15 minutes after the first two weeks. From here, Karen will add five total minutes to the daily exercise time until Margus can sustain 60 minutes of continuous cardiorespiratory endurance exercise per daily session. At this point, Karen will increase exercise intensity as tolerated while slightly decreasing exercise time. The long-term exercise plan calls for eventual vigorous-intensity exercise, but only once Margus can achieve 60 minutes of cardiorespiratory endurance exercise per day at an intensity of 60 percent of his $\dot{V}O_2R$.

Demonstration Case Study 4.9

Cardiorespiratory Exercise Prescription and Hypertension

Charles is an exercise physiologist who specializes in serving clients with hypertension. His most recent client is Gianna. Gianna's profile is provided as follows: 39-year-old female, controlled stage I hypertension, 115 pounds, hikes or runs daily.

Gianna, unfortunately, is the exception to the rule when it comes to hypertension. Despite her physical activity level, she falls in line with many of her family members and battles high blood pressure. Gianna wants to undergo a supervised exercise program to improve her fitness as much as possible to hopefully offset her cardiovascular disease risk factor of hypertension. Gianna's primary care physician cleared her for full participation in moderate to vigorous-intensity exercise. Stephen optioned to conduct a maximal treadmill test, which was completed with no complications and a $\dot{V}O_{2max}$ of 40 mL/kg · min. Gianna's resting heart rate was 59 beats per minute and resting blood pressure was 134/86 mmHg.

Impressed by Gianna's exercise history, fitness status, goals, and full physician clearance, Charles begins to put together an aggressive exercise prescription to further improve Gianna's cardiorespiratory fitness. Charles wants Gianna to perform vigorous-intensity exercise, so he starts with an exercise frequency of four days per week and an exercise time of 45 minutes per day—further suggesting light recreational activities on exercise off days. After that, Charles calculates the appropriate exercise intensity. To be precise and specific, he uses the $\dot{V}O_2R$ method to quantify the intensity and select workloads on two challenging modalities. Charles chooses a narrow-intensity range equal to 70–75 percent of $\dot{V}O_2R$. Charles's calculations are shown next.

$\dot{V}O_2R = \dot{V}O_{2max} - 3.5$ mL/kg · min

$\dot{V}O_2R = 40$ mL/kg · min $- 3.5$ mL/kg · min

$\dot{V}O_2R = 36.5$ mL/kg · min

70 percent of $\dot{V}O_2R = (36.5$ mL/kg · min x .70) $+ 3.5$ mL/kg · min

70 percent of $\dot{V}O_2R = 26.05$ mL/kg · min

75 percent of $\dot{V}O_2R = (36.5$ mL/kg · min x .75) $+ 3.5$ mL/kg · min

75 percent of $\dot{V}O_2R = 30.87$ mL/kg · min

$\dot{V}O_2R$ range $= 26.05 - 30.87$ mL/kg · min

Running Calculations:

Given Gianna's history of hiking and running, Charles feels that Gianna can run up a 2 percent incline. Charles solves for speed using the running equation to elicit 70 percent of Gianna's $\dot{V}O_2R$.

26.05 mL/kg · min $= (0.2$ x speed) $+ (0.9$ x speed x 0.02) $+ 3.5$

Speed $= 111.74$ meters · min

Speed $= 4.17$ mph

<u>Stepping Calculations:</u>

To further challenge Gianna, Charles selects a stepping exercise to be performed on a 30-centimeter step. Charles then solves for stepping rate to elicit 70 percent of Gianna's $\dot{V}O_2R$.

$$26.05 \text{ mL/kg} \cdot \text{min} = (0.2 \times \text{stepping rate}) + (1.33 \times 1.8 \times 0.30 \times \text{stepping rate}) + 3.5$$

$$\text{Stepping rate} = 24.55 \text{ steps per minute}$$

The last issue Charles addresses is exercise progression. Charles plans to progress Gianna by adding five minutes per exercise session every two weeks. Once Gianna reaches 60 minutes per day, four days per week, Charles plans to add an extra exercise session per week. When Gianna reaches five days per week, 60 minutes per day, Charles will increase intensity as tolerated with the goal of incorporating ventilatory threshold and high-intensity interval training.

Muscular Fitness Exercise Prescription

Unlike with diabetes, resistance training doesn't appear to offer a strong direct physiological mechanism for lowering blood pressure in the long term. However, some reports do suggest that resistance exercise alone can lower blood pressure in clients with hypertension.[52] Currently, the ACSM emphasizes cardiorespiratory exercise for clients with hypertension with resistance training offered as a supplement.[53] Accordingly, the current muscular fitness exercise recommendations for clients with hypertension are the same as the general healthy adult population (see Chapter 2). Modifications to the FITT-VP are made based on health status, fitness level, exercise history, patient goals, and physician orders.

Demonstration Case Study 4.10

Muscular Fitness Exercise Prescription and Hypertension

Andrew is an exercise physiologist specializing in working with clients with hypertension. His newest is a 56-year-old male with stage I hypertension named Franklin. Franklin is slightly overweight but not obese, with a BMI of 28.1 kg/m². Franklin has a physically demanding job as a construction worker but does not regularly exercise—although he does have some experience with resistance exercises. Franklin is concurrently completing cardiorespiratory exercise with Andrew and as such was previously cleared to participate in all forms of exercise by his primary care physician.

Because of Franklin's previous experience with resistance exercise and the physical nature of his occupation, Andrew decided to conduct a series of maximal strength tests on six different exercise machines: (1) leg press 1RM = 300 lbs, (2) chest press 1RM = 250 lbs, (3) seated row 1RM = 200 lbs, (4) leg curls 1RM = 100 lbs, (5) leg extensions 1RM = 150 lbs, and (6) seated crunches = 100 lbs. From this information, Andrew put together a muscular fitness exercise prescription, which is provided next.

<u>Frequency:</u>
Andrew suggested that Franklin perform resistance exercises two days per week because of no recent history with resistance exercise.

<u>Intensity:</u>
Andrew suggested that Franklin complete each prescribed exercise at an intensity of 60 percent of 1RM. Andrew feels this is an appropriate starting point because of the physicality of Franklin's occupation coupled with his exercise history.

<u>Time:</u>
Andrew chose to have Franklin perform two sets of eight repetitions per each prescribed exercise. Andrew chose this starting point because of Franklin's time gap with resistance training.

<u>Type:</u>
Andrew chose to have Franklin initially complete machine-based resistance training to ensure safety with the long-term goal of progressing to free weights.

<u>Progression:</u>
Andrew correctly chose to progress Franklin slowly. The rationale for this was to enhance exercise adherence, especially to cardiorespiratory exercise. Therefore, Andrew did not want to injure Franklin or make him feel excessively uncomfortable. Andrew's overall progression scheme consisted of increases in repetitions, then sets, and, lastly, intensity. Once the upper end of the muscular fitness recommendations is satisfied, Andrew will introduce a broader variety of exercises, including free-weight training.

Flexibility Exercise Prescription

Flexibility exercises are recommended as a part of any general exercise program, including exercise programs for clients with hypertension.[54] The flexibility prescription for clients with hypertension is the same as general healthy adults.[55] A variety of flexibility exercises are suitable for clients with hypertension, and the accumulation of exercises should target each major musculotendon group. It is usually recommended to avoid ballistic stretches in nonathletic populations to avoid injury. Flexibility exercises can be performed prior to or after an exercise session, although flexibility exercises may be more effective after an exercise session, as the muscles will be more pliable. General recommendations for progression apply to clients with hypertension, so long as the flexibility program adheres to medical orders.

Exercise Safety Considerations

Most exercises are safe for clients with hypertension. However, there are certain safety recommendations for exercise professionals to consider. First, exercise professionals should record all antihypertension medications prescribed, monitor any changes in medication status, and be familiar with the mechanisms of action for the common antihypertensive drugs. The rationale for this is to be able to consider changes to the FITT-VP to avoid exercise reductions in postexercise blood pressure. Clients prescribed calcium channel blockers, alpha-blockers, and fast-acting vasodilators should be carefully monitored to avoid serious reductions in postexercise blood pressure. It is useful to have clients with hypertension perform extended cooldowns until the heart rate and blood pressure return to resting values. Such a measure is to avoid significant reductions in peripheral resistance postexercise. Further, exercise professionals should be able to monitor any side effects of common medications and not hesitate to communicate these side effects to the client's prescribing physician.

Clients with hypertension often do not present with isolated hypertension, essential or nonessential. Usually, hypertension is accompanied by other comorbidities or cardiovascular disease risk factors. Exercise professionals should be able to think critically and adjust the FITT-VP to target as many comorbidities and cardiovascular disease risk factors as possible. In addition, exercise professionals must pay close attention to client's medical records to look for key diagnoses, such as target organ disease. If target organ disease is present, exercise professionals should recommend medical clearance prior to exercise testing or training.

Exercise adaptations are highly tied to the intensity at which exercise is prescribed. However, vigorous exercise should be medically supervised if a client with hypertension is at risk of cardiovascular complications (i.e., arrhythmias, myocardial ischemia or infarction, and left ventricular dysfunction).[56] During exercise sessions, exercise professionals should continuously monitor blood pressure, record blood pressure responses, avoid large "spikes" in blood pressure, and keep systolic blood pressure at or below 220 mmHg and diastolic blood pressure at or below 105 mmHg.[57] To avoid these changes, the FITT-VP should be modified, and the Valsalva maneuver avoided. Further, exercise professionals must recognize that blunted heart rate and therefore systolic blood pressure responses may occur in clients prescribed beta-blocker medications.

Overall, exercise professionals must carefully monitor all clients with hypertension and use sound judgment in the design and execution of a comprehensive exercise program. Whenever questionable responses occur, exercise professionals should err on the side of safety and caution. Key takeaways are that exercise professionals must keep the safety of their clients at the forefront and all medical orders are followed.

Student Case Study 4.1

Exercise Test Selection for Clients with Hypertension

Consider an exercise physiologist at a health-fitness facility performing several exercise tests per day. The newest client has hypertension. The client's profile is provided next.

Demographics: (1) female and (2) 60 years old

Biometrics: (1) resting heart rate = 81 beats per minute; (2) resting blood pressure = 138/88 mmHg; (3) LDL-c = 122 mg/dL, HDL-c = 40 mg/dL, total cholesterol = 193 mg/dL; (4) blood glucose = 121 mg/dL; (5) weight = 220 lbs; and (6) BMI = 33.9 kg/m^2

Medical Diagnoses: (1) stage I hypertension (controlled)

Medications: (1) losartan and (2) hydrochlorothiazide

Symptoms: (1) none

Exercise History: (1) occasional light-paced walk along the lake—weather permitting—and (2) no resistance exercise experience

Exercise Goals and Needs: (1) manage blood pressure and (2) reduce medication requirements

1. Assuming the client has been medically cleared to exercise, would it be safe to conduct exercise testing on this client? In two to three sentences, provide a defense for the answer.
2. Assuming it is safe to test this client, should one conduct a maximal or submaximal cardiorespiratory fitness test? In four to five sentences, provide a defense for the decision based on the client's profile.
3. Assuming it is safe to test this client, which cardiorespiratory fitness test should be conducted? In four to five sentences, provide a defense for the decision based on the client's profile.
4. Specific to this case, which body composition test should one prefer to conduct? In four to five sentences, provide a defense for the decision based on the client's profile.
5. Assuming it is safe to test this client, to assess muscular fitness, should one conduct muscular endurance assessments or muscular strength assessments, or both? In four to five sentences, provide a defense for the decision based on the client's profile.
6. Assuming it is safe to test this client, provide a list of four specific muscular fitness tests one could conduct on the client. Then provide a four- to five-sentence defense supporting the selections.
7. List any special considerations that should be considered when choosing exercise tests for this client.

Student Case Study 4.2

Exercise Test Selection for Clients with Hypertension

Consider an exercise physiologist at a health-fitness facility performing several exercise tests per day. The newest client has hypertension. The client hasn't been cleared to exercise within the past two years. The client's profile is provided next.

Demographics: (1) male and (2) 50 years old

Biometrics: (1) resting heart rate = 96 beats per minute; (2) resting blood pressure = 166/108 mmHg; (3) LDL-c = 129 mg/dL, HDL-c = 40 mg/dL, total cholesterol = 199 mg/dL; (4) blood glucose = 125 mg/dL; (5) weight = 265 lbs; and (6) BMI = 38.9 kg/m²

Medical Diagnoses: (1) stage II hypertension, (2) left ventricular hypertrophy

Medications: (1) amlodipine and (2) lisinopril

Symptoms: (1) none

Exercise History: (1) none

Exercise Goals and Needs: (1) manage blood pressure and (2) improve overall health

1. Assuming the client has been medically cleared to exercise, would it be safe to conduct exercise testing on this client? In two to three sentences, provide a defense for the answer.
2. Assuming it is safe to test this client, should a maximal or submaximal cardiorespiratory fitness test be conducted? In four to five sentences, provide a defense for the decision based on the client's profile.
3. Assuming it is safe to test this client, which cardiorespiratory fitness test should be conducted? In four to five sentences, provide a defense for the decision based on the client's profile.
4. Specific to this case, which body composition test should be conducted? In four to five sentences, provide a defense for the decision based on the client's profile.
5. Assuming it is safe to test this client, to assess muscular fitness, should one conduct muscular endurance assessments or muscular strength assessments, or both? In four to five sentences, provide a defense for the decision based on the client's profile.
6. Assuming it is safe to test this client, provide a list of four specific muscular fitness tests one could conduct on the client. Then provide a four- to five-sentence defense supporting the selections.
7. List any special considerations when choosing exercise tests for this client.

Student Case Study 4.3

Exercise Test Selection for Clients with Hypertension

Consider an exercise physiologist at a health-fitness facility performing several exercise tests per day. The newest client has hypertension. The client's profile is provided next.

Demographics: (1) female and (2) 42 years old

Biometrics: (1) resting heart rate = 62 beats per minute; (2) resting blood pressure = 136/82 mmHg; (3) LDL-c = 105 mg/dL, HDL-c = 48 mg/dL, total cholesterol = 187 mg/dL; (4) blood glucose = 100 mg/dL; (5) weight = 125 lbs; and (6) BMI = 24.2 kg/m²

Medical Diagnoses: (1) stage I hypertension (controlled)

Medications: (1) hydrochlorothiazide

Symptoms: (1) none

Exercise History: (1) jogging, five days per week, two miles per day, (2) muscular endurance exercises two days per week, and (3) likes new challenges

Exercise Goals and Needs: (1) manage blood pressure and (2) further improve fitness

1. Assuming the client has been medically cleared to exercise, would it be safe to conduct exercise testing on this client? In two to three sentences, provide a defense for the answer.

2. Assuming it is safe to test this client, should a maximal or submaximal cardiorespiratory fitness test be conducted? In four to five sentences, provide a defense for the decision based on the client's profile.

3. Assuming it is safe to test this client, which cardiorespiratory fitness test should one conduct? In four to five sentences, provide a defense for the decision based on the client's profile.

4. Specific to this case, which body composition test would be preferred? In four to five sentences, provide a defense for the decision based on the client's profile.

5. Assuming it is safe to test this client, to assess muscular fitness, should one conduct muscular endurance assessments or muscular strength assessments, or both? In four to five sentences, provide a defense for the decision based on the client's profile.

6. Assuming it is safe to test this client, provide a list of four specific muscular fitness test to conduct on the client. Then provide a four- to five-sentence defense supporting the selections.

7. List any special considerations one should consider when choosing exercise tests for this client.

Student Case Study 4.4

Exercise Test Interpretation: YMCA Cycle Test

An exercise physiologist specializes in serving clients with hypertension. He just completed a YMCA cycle test on a 55-year-old male client with stage I hypertension (controlled) weighing 200 pounds. The results of the test are provided in Figure 4.1. After reading the results, use the graph and leg cycling equation to interpret the results and answer the questions.

1. Using graph paper (Figure 4.2), estimate maximal work rate (kpm/min). Then insert the estimated maximal work rate into the following equation to estimate $\dot{V}O_{2max}$:

   $\dot{V}O_2$ max mL/kg · min = (1.8 x estimated maximal work rate/kg body weight) + 7.

2. Assuming this client is taking a calcium channel blocker, how would an exercise physiologist ensure the safety of the client?
3. Assuming this client is taking a beta-blocker medication, could the accuracy of this test be limited? Why?
4. What could an exercise physiologist do to further assure the safety of this client during testing?

Figure 4.1 This table depicts hypothetical data from a YMCA cycle test

Stage	Kpm/min	Heart Rate	Blood Pressure	RPE	ECG	Symptoms/ Comments
Resting	0	80	134/88	NA	Sinus	No symptoms
I	150	104	152/88	11	Sinus	No symptoms
II	300	119	170/86	13	Sinus	No symptoms
III	450	139	192/86	15	Sinus	No symptoms
Immediate	0	139	190/88	NA	Sinus	No symptoms
Recovery 1 min	0	125	170/84	NA	Sinus	No symptoms
Recovery 5 min	0	90	142/82	NA	Sinus	No symptoms

Figure 4.2 Students may use these gridlines to graph data from the YMCA cycle test

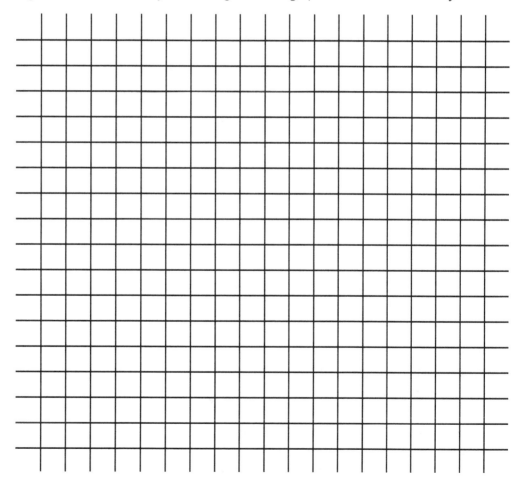

Exercise Test Interpretation: Astrand-Rhyming Cycle Test

An exercise physiologist specializes in serving clients with hypertension. She just completed an Astrand-Rhyming cycle test on a 61-year-old previously sedentary female client with stage I hypertension who weighs 230 pounds. The results of the test are provided in Figure 4.3. After reading the results, use the modified Astrand-Rhyming nomogram to interpret the results and answer the questions.

Figure 4.3 This table depicts hypothetical data from an Astrand-Rhyming cycle test

Stage/Minute	Kpm/m	Heart Rate	Blood Pressure	RPE	ECG	Symptoms
Resting		85	138/88	NA	Sinus	No symptoms
I	300	140	172/88	12	Sinus	No symptoms
II	300	142	180/86	13	Sinus	No symptoms
III	300	143	182/86	15	Sinus	No symptoms
IV	300	143	184/84	15	Sinus	No symptoms
V	300	144	186/84	15	Sinus	No symptoms
VI	300	144	186/86	16	Sinus	No symptoms
Immediate	150	143	190/86	NA	Sinus	No symptoms
Recovery 1 min	150	121	172/84	NA	Sinus	No symptoms
Recovery 5 min	75	90	142/82	NA	Sinus	No symptoms

1. Using the Astrand-Rhyming nomogram, estimate $\dot{V}O_{2max}$ in L · min. Be sure to multiply by a correction factor. Then convert $\dot{V}O_{2max}$ to mL/kg · min.

   Find estimated $\dot{V}O_{2max}$ in L · min

   Find estimated $\dot{V}O_{2max}$ in mL/kg · min

2. If this client reported to a clinic with uncontrolled stage I hypertension and a blood pressure of 156/92 mmHg, would the exercise physiologist have conducted this test? Why or why not? What if the client's blood pressure was controlled and had physician clearance?

3. Under which circumstances would the exercise physiologist have to terminate a submaximal cardiorespiratory fitness test being conducted on a client with hypertension?

Exercise Test Interpretation: Submaximal Treadmill Test

An exercise physiologist specializes in serving clients with hypertension. She just completed a submaximal treadmill test on a 63-year-old male, mildly physically active, with medically managed stage II hypertension and weighs 205 pounds. The client is medicated with a calcium channel blocker and an ACE inhibitor. The test was terminated at a heart rate equal to 70 percent of the client's heart rate reserve. The results of the test are provided in Figure 4.4. After reading the results, use the walking or running equation and a proportion equation to interpret the results and answer the questions.

Figure 4.4 This table depicts hypothetical data from a submaximal treadmill test

Stage	Speed (mph)	Grade %	Heart Rate	Blood Pressure	RPE	ECG	Symptoms
Resting	0	0	93	144/92	NA	Sinus	No symptoms
I	1.7	10.0	111	178/92	9	Sinus	No symptoms
II	2.5	12.0	129	192/90	12	Sinus	No symptoms
III	3.4	14.0	138	204/90	16	Sinus	No symptoms
Immediate	1.5	0	137	200/90	NA	Sinus	No symptoms
Recovery 1 min	1.5	0	122	180/90	NA	Sinus	No symptoms
Recovery 5 min	1	0	100	162/88	NA	Sinus	No symptoms

1. Using one of the following two equations, estimate $\dot{V}O_2$ for the last completed stage:

   Walking: $\dot{V}O_2$ = (0.1 x speed in m/min) + (1.8 x speed in m/min x grade) + 3.5

   Running: $\dot{V}O_2$ = (0.2 x speed in m/min) + (0.9 x speed in m/min x grade) + 3.5

   Find $\dot{V}O_2$ in last stage in mL/kg · min

   Find estimated $\dot{V}O_{2max}$ in mL/kg · min

2. Given the client's medical status, should the exercise physiologist have optioned for a medically supervised exercise test? Why or why not?

Student Case Study 4.7

Muscular Strength Testing for Clients with Hypertension

An exercise physiologist specializes in serving clients with hypertension. The newest client is a 48-year-old female with controlled stage I hypertension who weighs 175 pounds. The exercise physiologist wants to prescribe this client a resistance training program to help supplement her cardiorespiratory exercise program and to add additional benefit for blood pressure control. Therefore, the exercise physiologist conducts a series of muscular strength tests. The following data were collected (Figure 4.5).

Figure 4.5 This table depicts hypothetical data from a 3–5RM test

Leg Press Strength Test

Trial 1	5	repetitions
	125	weight
Trial 2	3	repetitions
	135	weight
Trial 3	3	repetitions
	140	weight
Best Trial	3	repetitions
	140	weight

Chest Press Strength Test

Trial 1	5	repetitions
	135	weight
Trial 2	3	repetitions
	145	weight
Trial 3	3	repetitions
	150	weight
Best Trial	3	repetitions
	150	weight

1. Use the Lander equation to predict the client's maximal leg press strength.
2. Calculate a weight pushed to body weight ratio and compare the client's results to normative data.
3. Use the Lander equation to predict the client's maximal chest press strength.
4. Calculate a weight pushed to body weight ratio and compare the client's results to normative data.
5. What steps can the exercise physiologist take to ensure safety during these strength tests?

Student Case Study 4.8

Body Composition Test Interpretation: Skinfolds

An exercise specialist is responsible for interpreting body composition assessments conducted on clients with hypertension. She was recently presented with the following skinfold and anthropomorphic data from a 191 pound, 54-year-old female client with hypertension. Analyze the results (Figure 4.6) to interpret body composition and answer the questions.

Figure 4.6 This table depicts hypothetical data from a seven-site skinfold assessment

Site	Trial 1	Trial 2	Trial 3	Average
Triceps	28	28	27	mm
Subscapular	31	33	32	mm
Chest	22	24	24	mm
Abdominal	34	36	36	mm
Suprailiac	38	40	41	mm
Midaxillary	27	28	29	mm
Thigh	30	31	31.5	mm
Waist Circumference	39 inches			

1. Using the seven-site skinfold body density equation for women, calculate body density.
2. Using the Siri equation, estimate the client's body fat percentage.
3. Calculate the client's fat and nonfat weight in pounds.
4. Compare the results to normative data.
5. Using the three-site skinfold body density equation for women, calculate body density.
6. Using the Siri equation, estimate the client's body fat percentage.
7. Calculate the client's fat and nonfat weight in pounds.
8. Was there a difference between the seven- and three-site skinfold calculations for body density and body fat? If there was a difference, why would the difference exist?
9. Classify the client's waist circumference according to disease risk.
10. Should a different body composition assessment be used for this client? If so, which assessment(s)? Would these tests be more accurate for this client?
11. Would this client benefit from fat loss? If so, in what way(s)?

Student Case Study 4.9

Exercise Prescription for Clients with Hypertension: Cardiorespiratory Endurance

An exercise professional specializes in serving clients with hypertension. The newest client is a 60-year-female with medically managed stage I hypertension. The client's resting blood pressure is 138/88 mmHg, weight is 173 pounds and BMI is 29.9 kg/m². The exercise professional just conducted an Astrand-Rhyming cycle test, completed without complications, and the client achieved an estimated $\dot{V}O_{2max}$ of 29.5 mL/kg · min. Prior to the test, the client's resting heart rate was 86 beats per minute. The client is prescribed an alpha-blocker medication to control pressure. The client is open to any form of exercise.

1. Calculate a heart rate range based on the heart rate reserve that the client should maintain during aerobic exercise. Should an exercise professional use this heart rate range during exercise training or consider other methods of quantifying exercise intensity? Why or why not?

2. Calculate a $\dot{V}O_2$ range based on the $\dot{V}O_2$ reserve that the client should maintain during aerobic exercise.

3. Provide an exercise type (be specific), frequency, and time at the $\dot{V}O_2$ range found in question 2 for the client to improve her cardiorespiratory fitness and better manage her blood pressure.

4. Suggest four possible aerobic exercises that would be appropriate for this client. Then explain the rationale for each selection.

5. Use the walking equation to calculate a walking speed (in mph) for the client that elicits the lower end of the $\dot{V}O_2$ reserve range found in question 2. The percent grade of the treadmill is 3.5 percent.

6. Use the stepping equation to calculate a stepping rate for the client that elicits the upper end of the $\dot{V}O_2$ reserve range found in question 2. The height of the step is 23 centimeters.

7. Use the arm cycle equation to calculate a resistance to be placed on the flywheel for the client that elicits the lower end of the $\dot{V}O_2$ reserve range found in question 2. The client turns the arm crank at 70 rpm.

8. Suggest a progression scheme to advance the client toward a goal of improving her blood pressure. Should vigorous-intensity exercise eventually be considered? Why or why not?

9. Provide three training considerations to help this client improve her blood pressure through cardiorespiratory exercise safely. One consideration must address medication status.

10. Provide the upper limit systolic and diastolic blood pressures during an exercise session. Should one of these pressures go above the upper limit, use critical thinking and good judgment to explain the actions you would take.

Student Case Study 4.10

Exercise Prescription for Clients with Hypertension: Cardiorespiratory Endurance

An exercise specialist is responsible for designing exercise prescriptions for clients with hypertension. The most recent client is a 205-pound, 57-year-old male with medically managed stage II hypertension. The client has a history of exaggerated blood pressure responses to physical activity as evidenced during his medically supervised submaximal cycle exercise test. The client's estimated a $\dot{V}O_{2\,max}$ was 25 mL/kg · min. Prior to the test, the exercise specialist recorded a resting heart rate of 66 beats per minute and resting blood pressure was 152/82 mmHg. The client was medically cleared to participate in a moderate-intensity exercise program with orders to keep systolic blood pressure below 190 mmHg. The client takes a beta-blocker and an ACE inhibitor.

1. Calculate a heart rate range based on the heart rate reserve that the client should maintain during aerobic exercise. Should the exercise specialist use this heart rate range during exercise training or consider other methods of quantifying exercise intensity? Why or why not?

2. Calculate a $\dot{V}O_2$ range based on the $\dot{V}O_2$ reserve that the client should maintain during aerobic exercise.

3. Provide an exercise type (be specific), frequency, and time at the $\dot{V}O_2$ range found in question 2 for the client to improve his cardiorespiratory fitness and better manage his blood pressure.

4. Suggest four possible aerobic exercises that would be appropriate for this client. Then explain the rationale for each selection.

5. Use the walking equation to calculate an appropriate walking speed (in mph) and incline for the client that elicits the lower end of the $\dot{V}O_2$ reserve range found in question 2.

6. Use the leg cycling equation to calculate an appropriate peddling frequency and resistance to elicit the upper end of the $\dot{V}O_2$ reserve range found in question 2.

7. Use the arm cycle equation to calculate an appropriate peddle frequency and resistance to be placed on the flywheel for the client that elicits the lower end of the $\dot{V}O_2$ reserve range found in question 2.

8. Suggest a progression scheme to advance the client toward a goal of improving his blood pressure.

9. Would progressing to high-intensity interval training be appropriate for this client? If so, what cautions should be considered? If not, explain why.

10. Provide three training considerations to help this client improve his blood pressure through cardiorespiratory exercise safely. One consideration must address the client's exaggerated blood pressure responses to exercise.

Student Case Study 4.11

Exercise Prescription for Clients with Hypertension: Muscular Fitness

An exercise physiologist specializes in training clients with hypertension. The exercise physiologist was recently presented with the following client data: (1) 50-year-old male, (2) controlled stage I hypertension, (3) resistance training in his 20s and 30s, (4) goals to improve blood pressure and improve muscular strength, (5) medicated with hydrochlorothiazide, (6) chest press 1RM = 195 pounds, (7) leg press 1RM = 240 pounds, and (8) open to any resistance exercise program.

1. Provide a range for the weight that the client should chest press.
2. Provide a range for the weight that the client should leg press.
3. Provide a resistance exercise prescription for frequency, number of exercises, sets, and repetitions to improve muscular strength.
4. Suggest at least four specific resistance training exercises that are appropriate for this client.

5. Suggest a progression scheme to advance the client toward the goal of improving muscular strength.

6. How would the resistance training program be different if the client expressed interest in specifically targeting muscular endurance?

7. Explain how to design the resistance training program to maximize client adherence.

8. Provide three training considerations to help this client improve his muscular strength through resistance exercise safely. One of the considerations must address a breathing technique during the completion of repetitions.

Student Case Study 4.12

Exercise Testing and Prescription: Comprehensive Case Study

An exercise physiologist works for a chronic disease risk reduction program. He thoroughly collected the following data from his most recent client:

Demographics: (1) female and (2) 48 years old

Family History: (1) father had stage II hypertension and suffered a myocardial infarction at the age of 54 and (2) mother has had stage I hypertension since the age of 40

Biometrics: (1) resting heart rate = 63 beats per minute; (2) resting blood pressure = 132/84 mmHg; (3) LDL-c = 108 mg/dL, HDL-c = 60 mg/dL, total cholesterol = 188 mg/dL; (4) glycosylated hemoglobin = 6.3 percent and blood glucose = 103 mg/dL; and (5) weight = 140 lbs., BMI = 23.1 kg/m²

Medical Diagnoses: (1) medically managed and controlled stage I hypertension

Medications: (1) hydrochlorothiazide

Symptoms: (1) none

Exercise History: (1) jogging, (2) cycling, and (3) resistance exercise

Exercise Goals and Needs: (1) maximize fitness to offset hypertension and (2) maintain control of hypertension

1. Should the exercise physiologist conduct a maximal or submaximal cardio-respiratory fitness test? In four to five sentences, provide a defense for the decision based on the client's profile.

2. Which cardiorespiratory fitness test should be conducted? In four to five sentences, provide a defense for the decision based on the client's profile.

3. Given limitless resources, which body composition test should the exercise physiologist conduct? In four to five sentences, provide a defense for the decision based on the client's profile.

4. Given minimal resources with a small budget, which body composition test should be conducted? In four to five sentences, provide a defense for the decision based on the client's profile.

5. Specific to this case, which body composition test would be preferred? In four to five sentences, provide a defense for the decision based on the client's profile.
6. To assess muscular fitness, should muscular endurance assessments or muscular strength assessments be conducted, or both? In four to five sentences, provide a defense for the decision based on the client's profile.
7. Provide a list of four specific muscular fitness tests to be conducted on the client. Then provide a four- to five-sentence defense supporting the selections.
8. Based on the answer for questions 1 and 2, calculate the client's $\dot{V}O_{2max}$ from the most appropriate of the following cardiorespiratory fitness tests (Figures 4.7–4.11).

Figure 4.7 This table depicts hypothetical data from a YMCA cycle test

YMCA Cycle Test

Stage	Kpm/min	Heart Rate	Blood Pressure	RPE	ECG	Symptoms/ Comments
Resting	0	63	132/84	NA	Sinus	No symptoms
I	150	110	158/82	11	Sinus	No symptoms
II	300	115	170/80	12	Sinus	No symptoms
Immediate	100	114	166/80	NA	Sinus	No symptoms
Recovery 1 min	50	90	150/80	NA	Sinus	No symptoms
Recovery 5 min	25	64	130/80	NA	Sinus	No symptoms

Figure 4.8 Students may use these gridlines to graph data from the YMCA cycle test

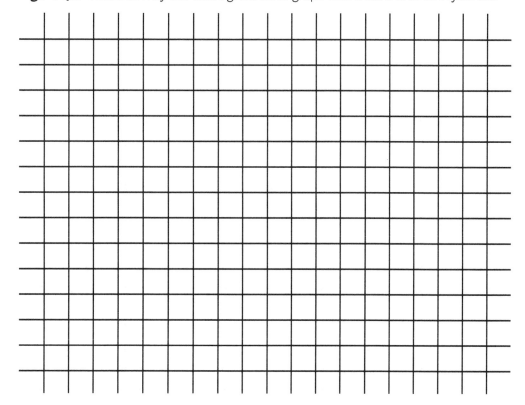

Figure 4.9 This table depicts hypothetical data from an Astrand-Rhyming cycle test

Astrand-Rhyming Cycle Test

Stage/Minute	Kpm/m	Heart Rate	Blood Pressure	RPE	ECG	Symptoms
Resting		63	132/84	NA	Sinus	No symptoms
I	300	125	152/82	10	Sinus	No symptoms
II	300	126	152/82	11	Sinus	No symptoms
III	300	126	152/80	11	Sinus	No symptoms
IV	300	126	154/80	11	Sinus	No symptoms
V	300	127	154/80	11	Sinus	No symptoms
VI	300	127	156/80	11	Sinus	No symptoms
Immediate	150	130	154/80	NA	Sinus	No symptoms
Recovery 1 min	75	117	140/80	NA	Sinus	No symptoms
Recovery 5 min	50	107	130/78	NA	Sinus	No symptoms

Figure 4.10 This table depicts hypothetical data from a maximal cycle test

Maximal Cycle Test

Stage	Time	Kpm /min	Heart Rate	Blood Pressure	RPE	$\dot{V}O_2$ (mL/kg · min.)	RER	Blood Lactate (mmol)	ECG
Resting		0	63	132/84	NA	3.9	0.75	NA	Sinus
I	2:00	600	94	146/82	11	13.5	0.90	1.0	Sinus
II	4:00	900	140	176/82	14	22.9	1.01	4.0	Sinus
III	6:00	1200	160	192/80	16	31.7	1.09	5.9	Sinus
IV	8:00	1500	170	204/80	18	36.3	1.17	9.0	Sinus
Immediate	NA	300	160	200/80	NA	28.4	1.14	NA	Sinus
Recovery 1 min	NA	150	130	152/80	NA	20.2	1.02	NA	Sinus
Recovery 5 min	NA	75	70	134/78	NA	18.6	0.97	NA	Sinus

Comments: Test terminated because of volitional fatigue

Figure 4.11 This table depicts hypothetical data from a maximal treadmill test

Maximal Treadmill Test

Stage	Time	Speed (mph)	Grade %	Blood Pressure	$\dot{V}O_2$ (mL/kg · min)	Blood Lactate (mmol)	RPE	Heart Rate	RER
Resting	NA	0	0	132/84	4.1	NA	NA	63	0.71
I	2:00	3.5	2	144/80	16.0	1.9	11	125	0.89
II	4:00	4.5	4	172/80	21.7	3.0	13	157	0.99
III	6:00	5.5	6	188/80	29.9	5.7	15	166	1.09
IV	8:00	6.5	8	202/80	38.9	8.8	19	173	1.16
Immediate	NA	1.5	0	200/80	38.6	NA	NA	170	1.15

(Continued)

Figure 4.11 This table depicts hypothetical data from a maximal treadmill test (Continued)

Maximal Treadmill Test

Stage	Time	Speed (mph)	Grade %	Blood Pressure	$\dot{V}O_2$ (mL/kg · min)	Blood Lactate (mmol)	RPE	Heart Rate	RER
Recovery 1 min	NA	1.5	0	172/80	17.3	NA	NA	141	1.03
Recovery 5 min	NA	1	0	136/78	6.7	NA	NA	71	0.91

Comments: Test terminated because of volitional fatigue

9. For the cardiorespiratory fitness test chosen to interpret question 8, should the test have been terminated prior to completion? Explain why or why not.
10. Assuming the skinfold assessment for body composition test was selected, calculate body fat percentage from the following seven-site skinfold data (Figure 4.12).

Figure 4.12 This table depicts hypothetical data from a seven-site skinfold assessment

Site	Trial 1	Trial 2	Trial 3	Average
Triceps	13	14	14	mm
Subscapular	18	18	20	mm
Chest	17	19	17	mm
Abdominal	14	13	12.5	mm
Suprailiac	22	22.5	22.75	mm
Midaxillary	20	20.75	21	mm
Thigh	23	21	23	mm

11. If the client's waist circumference were 36 inches, what would be her risk classification?
12. Assuming muscular strength was selected, interpret and classify the client's leg and chest press strength from the following data (Figure 4.13).

Figure 4.13 This table depicts hypothetical data from a 3–5RM test

Leg Press Strength Test

Trial 1	_____5_____ repetitions _____170_____ weight
Trial 2	_____3_____ repetitions _____190_____ weight
Trial 3	_____3_____ repetitions _____195_____ weight
Best Trial	_____3_____ repetitions _____195_____ weight

(Continued)

Chest Press Strength Test

Trial 1	5	repetitions
	140	weight
Trial 2	3	repetitions
	155	weight
Trial 3	3	repetitions
	165	weight
Best Trial	3	repetitions
	165	weight

13. Calculate a heart rate range based on the heart rate reserve that the client should maintain during aerobic exercise. Is this the most reliable method for quantifying cardiorespiratory endurance exercise? Why or why not?

14. Calculate a $\dot{V}O_2$ range based on the $\dot{V}O_2$ reserve that the client should maintain during aerobic exercise.

15. Provide an exercise type (be specific), frequency, and time at the $\dot{V}O_2$ range found in question 14 for the client to improve her cardiorespiratory fitness and manage her blood pressure.

16. Suggest four possible aerobic exercises that would be appropriate for this client.

17. Provide a walking speed and grade for the client to maintain on the treadmill to elicit the lower end of the $\dot{V}O_2$ range listed in question 14.

18. Provide a resistance and peddle frequency for leg cycling to elicit the lower end of the $\dot{V}O_2$ range listed in question 14.

19. Provide a resistance and peddle frequency for arm cycling to elicit the lower end of the $\dot{V}O_2$ range listed in question 14.

20. Suggest a progression scheme for improving cardiorespiratory fitness. Would vigorous-intensity or high-intensity interval training be warranted? Why or why not?

21. Provide a range for the weight that the client should chest press.

22. Provide a range for the weight that the client should leg press.

23. Provide a resistance exercise prescription for frequency, number of exercises, sets, and repetitions to improve muscular fitness.

24. Suggest at least four specific resistance training exercises that are appropriate for this client.

25. Suggest a progression scheme to help the client improve overall muscular fitness.

26. Provide a frequency, intensity, number of stretches, sets, and amount of time each stretch should be held to help improve the client's flexibility.

27. Provide a list consisting of all safety considerations that should be considered when supervising this client's exercise program.

REFERENCES

1. B. M. Egan, Y. Zhao, and R. N. Axon, "U.S. Trends in Prevalence, Awareness, Treatment, and Control of Hypertension, 1998–2008," *JAMA* 303, no. 20 (2010): 2043–50.

2. American College of Sports Medicine, *ACSM's Guidelines for Exercise Testing and Prescription*, 11th ed. (Philadelphia: Wolters Kluwer Health, 2022).

3. A. V. Chobanian, G. L. Bakris, H. R. Black, et al., "The Seventh Report of The Joint National Committee on Prevention, Detection, Evaluation, and Treatment of High Blood Pressure: the JNC7 Report," *JAMA* 289, no. 19 (2003): 2560–72.

4. American College of Sports Medicine, *ACSM's Guidelines*.

5. A. Briasoulis, V. Agarwal, and F. H. Messerli, "Alcohol Consumption and the Risk of Hypertension in Men and Women: A Systematic Review and Meta-Analysis," *Journal of Clinical Hypertension* 14, no. 11 (2012): 792–98.

6. Y. E. Bogaert, and S. Linas, "The Role of Obesity in the Pathogenesis of Hypertension," *Nature Review Nephrology* 5, no. 2 (2009): 101–11.

7. T. M. Spruill, "Chronic Psychosocial Stress and Hypertension," *Current Hypertension Reports* 12, no. 1 (2010): 10–16.

8. American College of Sports Medicine, *ACSM's Guidelines*.

9. L. S. Lilly, *Pathophysiology of Heart Disease: A Collaborative Project of Medical Students and Faculty*, 4th ed. (Philadelphia: Wolters Kluwer Health, 2007).

10. American College of Sports Medicine, *ACSM's Guidelines*.

11. O. A. Carrentero and S. Oparil, "Essential Hypertension, Part I: Definition and Etiology," *Circulation* 101 (2000): 329–35.

12. E. Mannarino and M. Pino, "Molecular Biology of Atherosclerosis," *Clinical Cases in Mineral and Bone Metabolism* 5, no. 1 (2008): 57–62.

13. D. H. Endemann and E. L. Schiffrin, "Endothelial Dysfunction," *Journal of the American Society of Nephrology* 15 (2004): 1983–1992.

14. Lilly, *Pathophysiology*.

15. ibid.

16. W. Johnson, M. L. Nguyen, and R. Patel. "Hypertension Crisis in the Emergency Department," *Cardiology Clinics* 30, no. 4 (2012): 533–43.

17. American College of Sports Medicine, *ACSM's Guidelines*.

18. T. Hayashi, K. Tsumura, C. Suematsu, et al., "Walking to Work and the Risk for Hypertension in Men: The Osaka Health Survey," *Annals of Internal Medicine* 131, no. 1 (1999): 21–6.

19. J. P. Wallace, "Exercise in Hypertension: A Clinical Review," Sports Medicine 33, no. 8 (2003): 585–98.

20. K. M. Diaz and D. Shimbo, "Physical Activity and the Prevention of Hypertension," *Current Hypertension Reports* 15, no. 6 (2012): 659–68.

21. P. Kokkinos, "Cardiorespiratory Fitness, Exercise, and Blood Pressure," *Hypertension* 64 (2014): 1160–64.

22. L. S. Pesatello, H. V. MacDonald, L. Lamberti, and B. T. Johnson, "Exercise for Hypertension: A Prescription Update Integrating Existing Recommendations with Emerging Research," *Current Hypertension Reports* 17, no. 11 (2015): 87.

23. ibid.

24. Hayashi et al., "Walking to Work."

25. American College of Sports Medicine, *ACSM's Guidelines*.

26. ibid.

27. ibid.

28. G. F. Fletcher, P. A. Ades, P. Kligfield, et al., "Exercise Standards for Testing and Training: A Scientific Statement for the American Heart Association," *Circulation* 128, no. 8 (2013): 873–934.

29. M. D. Delp and M. H. Laughlin, "Regulation of Skeletal Muscle Perfusion during Exercise," *Acta Physiologica Scandinavia* 162 (1998): 411–19.

30. ibid.

31. G. A. Brooks, T. D. Fahey, and K. M. Baldwin, *Exercise Physiology: Human Bioenergetics and its Applications*, 4th ed. (New York: McGraw-Hill Higher Education, 2005).

32. D. R. Bassett and E. T. Howley, "Limiting Factors for Maximum Oxygen Uptake and Determinants of Endurance Performance," *Medicine and Science in Sports and Exercise* 32, no. 1 (200): 70–84.

33. Brooks et al., *Exercise Physiology*.

34. L. S. Pescatello, M. A. Guidry, B. E. Blanchard, et al., "Exercise Intensity Alters Postexercise Hypotension. *Journal of Hypertension* 22 (2004): 1881–88.

35. K. Goessler, M. Polito, and V. A. Cornelissen, "Effect of Exercise Training on the Renin-Angiotensin-Aldosterone System in Healthy Individuals: A Systematic Review and Meta-Analysis," *Hypertension Research* 39 (2016): 119–26.

36. V. A. Cornelissen and R. H. Fagardm, "Effects of Endurance Training on Blood Pressure, Blood Pressure-Regulating Mechanisms and Cardiovascular Risk Factors," *Hypertension* 46 (2005): 667–75.

37. J. B. Carter, E. W. Banister, and A. P. Blaber, "Effect of Endurance Exercise on Autonomic Control of Heart Rate. *Sports Medicine* 33, no. 1 (2003): 33–46.

38. American College of Sports Medicine, *ACSM's Guidelines*.

39. ibid.

40. Pescatello et al., "Exercise Intensity."

41. C. E. Garber, B. Blissmer, M. R. Deschenes, et al., "Quantity and Quality of Exercise for Developing and Maintaining Cardiorespiratory, Musculoskeletal, and Neuromotor Fitness in Apparently Healthy Adults: Guidance for Prescribing Exercise. *Medicine and Science in Sports and Exercise* 43, no. 7 (2011): 1334–59.

42. Delp and Laughlin, "Regulation of Skeletal."

43. Brooks et al., *Exercise Physiology*.

44. Pescatello et al., "Exercise Intensity."

45. Goessler et al., "Effect of Exercise."

46. Cornelissen et al., "Effect of Exercise Training."

47. Carter et al., "Effect of Endurance."

48. Pescatello et al., "Exercise Intensity."

49. American College of Sports Medicine, *ACSM's Guidelines*.

50. ibid.

51. Pescatello et al., "Exercise Intensity."

52. M. R. Moras, R. F. P. Bacurau, D. E. Casarini, et al., "Chronic Conventional Resistance Exercise Reduced Blood Pressure in Stage I Hypertensive Men," *Journal of Strength and Conditioning Research* 26, no. 4 (2012): 1122–29.

53. American College of Sports Medicine, *ACSM's Guidelines*.

54. ibid.

55. ibid.

56. ibid.

57. ibid.

CHAPTER 5

Exercise Testing and Prescription for Overweight and Obese Clients

INTRODUCTION

OBESITY IS DEFINED as having a BMI ≥30 kg/m², while overweight is defined as having a BMI ≤30 kg/m2 but ≥25 kg/m².[1] Although BMI does not necessarily reflect body composition, which is the relative amount of fat and nonfat mass, BMI does predict body composition and long-term health consequences. Recent data suggest that obesity rates are rising with approximately 39.8% of US adults classified as obese.[2] When combined with the percentage of adults who are classified as overweight, over two-thirds of US adults are, at a minimum, overweight and would benefit from a weight-loss program.[3, 4]

There are numerous long-term health consequences associated with obesity and overweightness. These consequences include type 2 diabetes, cardiovascular diseases, hepatic disease, sleep apnea, certain cancers, orthopedic ailments, and poor mortality and morbidity.[5,6,7] Further, obesity at younger ages and even during childhood is highly predictive of negative health outcomes later in life. From the standpoint of cardiometabolic diseases, obesity, as brought on by a sedentary lifestyle, fuels the atherosclerotic cascade and can even result in the development of lipolytic-induced diabetes mellitus. Moreover, being obese or overweight at a younger age is highly predictive of negative health outcomes later in life.[8,9,10,11] Accordingly, exercise professionals must be knowledgeable of the challenges associated with exercise programs and lifestyle modifications intended to aid in modest and or significant long-term weight loss and maintenance.

Exercise is a commonly recommended treatment strategy for managing and preventing obesity or overweightness and offers numerous health-related benefits. Some of these benefits include improved cardiometabolic health, decreased central adiposity and body fat, increased fat-free body mass, decreased cancer risk, and an overall reduction in mortality risk.[12,13,14] Sustained reductions in as little as 3 percent of body weight offers improvement in many cardiovascular disease risk factors in obese individuals.[15,16] Furthermore, the benefits also apply to nonobese or overweight individuals.

The reduction of body weight and body fat among overweight or obese individuals involves creating an energy deficit. That is, expending more calories than consumed. Although simple in theory, this practice presents challenges for exercise professionals. Weight and fat loss through exercise alone is very difficult and only results in modest weight and fat reduction.[17] Instead, exercise needs to be married to alterations in dietary habits. Further, metabolic complications, deconditioning, the presence of other cardiovascular disease risk factors, and orthopedic limitations associated with obesity present additional challenges for clients and exercise professionals. Exercise professionals must be able to use sound judgment to ensure safety, select appropriate exercise tests, modify the FITT-VP of an exercise prescription, and make lifestyle modification recommendations to help overweight or obese clients achieve their goals.

The purpose of this chapter is to teach students how to apply their knowledge of exercise as a means of modifying body composition, exercise testing, and exercise prescription. On completion of the case studies within this chapter, students will be able to achieve the following:

1. Explain to and educate clients on the concepts of energy expenditure and energy deficit and how cardiorespiratory and muscular fitness exercise influences each

2. Recognize obesity-related limitations when selecting and interpreting exercise tests

3. Apply the cardiorespiratory, muscular fitness, and flexibility FITT-VP recommendations and modifications to overweight or obese clients

4. Identify and understand safety considerations for training overweight or obese clients

THE ROLE OF EXERCISE ON ENERGY EXPENDITURE AND ENERGY DEFICIT

Whether the objective of a weight-loss program is to reduce total body weight or body fat, both are achieved by inducing an energy deficit. Simply, an energy deficit reflects the negative difference between the number of kilocalories (kcals) consumed through diet and the number of kcals expended through metabolism.[18] Thus preventing weight regain requires the equalization of kcal consumption and kcal expenditure. Reductions in body weight or body fat through exercise training occur because of repeated elevations in resting metabolic rate, which occurs following exercise bouts.[19] As such, greater exercise volume is necessary to elicit the energy deficit necessary for weight or fat loss. Exercise professionals should educate overweight or obese clients to make minor reductions in daily kcal intake while increasing kcal expenditure through exercise.

Exercise increases energy expenditure through numerous mechanisms. A notable mechanism is the phenomenon of excess postexercise oxygen consumption (EPOC). EPOC represents the elevation of oxygen consumption up to 48 hours after exercise.[20] The elevation of oxygen consumption after exercise occurs for several reasons, including elevated body temperature, increased circulation of catecholamines, the replenishment of phosphocreatine stores, and the removal of blood lactate, all of which increase kcal expenditure.[21,22] For fat loss, the elevations of catecholamine hormones are particularly importance, as they enhance the rate of lipolysis.[23] The influence of postexercise oxygen consumption on kcal expenditure highlights the need for increasing exercise frequency. Further, excess postexercise consumption is greater with higher exercise intensities. Therefore, if clients are capable, vigorous-intensity training can aid in reducing body weight or body fat.

Another notable influence of exercise on energy expenditure is muscle mass. Skeletal muscle accounts for approximately 40 percent of body mass and 30 percent of resting energy expenditure.[24] Therefore, when designing exercise programs aimed at managing or preventing obesity, exercise professionals should consider muscular fitness exercises to maintain or increase muscle mass and thereby increase resting kcal expenditure.

Although the concept of increasing kcal expenditure while simultaneously decreasing kcal consumption is simple, eliciting large kcal deficits can negatively influence weight loss and result in weight regain. First, any energy deficit must be attainable and sustainable. Thus a slight kcal deficit is recommended. Second, from a metabolic standpoint, excessive kcal deficits can result in the downregulation of resting kcal expenditure, leading to a stall in weight loss and regain of weight if positive dietary behaviors lapse.[25]

Demonstration Case Study 5.1

Exercise and Energy Expenditure

Derek is an exercise physiologist working at a weight-loss clinic. He routinely councils overweight and obese clients on weight-loss strategies. His most recent client was a college professor who likes detailed explanations prior to engaging in new activities. The client asks Derek "how exercise causes weight loss, how often should exercise be performed, how hard exercise must be completed, and how many calories need to be reduced per day?" Derek offered his client the following response:

> *Exercise's main influence on weight loss is increasing the number of daily calories expended by the body to maintain function. With each exercise bout, the body needs to consume more oxygen and therefore expend more calories to return the body to its normal resting state. This increase in caloric expenditure lasts 24–48 hours after each exercise session, which is why exercise really should be performed five or more days per week. All kinds of exercises can increase caloric expenditure, but cardiorespiratory exercise elicits a greater caloric expenditure. Further, oxygen consumption and therefore caloric expenditure at rest is enhanced with higher exercise intensities. Resistance exercise should be included at least two days per week. The reason for this is to maintain or increase muscle mass, as the more muscle people have, the more calories they expend at rest. All in total, this is how exercise influences weight loss. As for diet, the total calories consumed should only be modestly reduced. Significantly reducing the calories consumed in addition to exercise can actually slow down metabolism and even result in weight gain if diet adherence falters.*

EXERCISE TESTING FOR OVERWEIGHT OR OBESE CLIENTS

Depending on the overweight or obese client, exercise testing may not necessarily be warranted. This is particularly true when training clients who are only intent on completing low-intensity exercise. However, to increase the efficacy of exercise programs, exercise professionals should consider exercise testing to collect data useful for exercise prescription and tracking goals throughout an exercise program. When exercise tests are conducted on obese or overweight clients, tests should be conducted in a similar manner as with healthy adults with the same contraindications and test termination criteria.

Exercise professionals do have to keep in mind special testing considerations for obese or overweight clients. To ensure exercise tests are completed safely, comfortably, and accurately, exercise professionals should focus on an overweight or obese client's physical/fitness capacity and medication status. Client's with orthopedic limitations should undergo non-weight-bearing tests, such as arm or leg cycling. In addition, obesity or overweightness may make cycling uncomfortable and, ultimately, interfere with the test's reliability. Tests with low starting workloads and small 0.5–1 MET increases per stage should be selected for deconditioned clients. Further, certain body composition assessments, such as skinfold assessments, may not be accurate on obese clients. Like other special populations, overweight and obese clients may be prescribed medications that can interfere with the results of exercise tests.

Demonstration Case Study 5.2

Exercise Testing for Overweight or Obese Clients

Luke is an exercise physiologist working for a weight-loss clinic. His job is to conduct exercise tests on the facility's clients and recommend exercise plans accordingly. His most recent client is Douglass. Douglass is a 43-year-old male with a BMI of 38 kg/m². Douglass is completely sedentary and has not been physically active since he was in high school. Douglass came to Luke's clinic to begin a low-intensity exercise program just to get eased into exercise. Douglass was recently medically cleared to exercise by his endocrinologist.

After having read Douglass's medical records and his goals, Luke chooses not to have Douglass complete any exercise tests. Luke's rationale is that Douglass will only be completing low-intensity exercise to get back into the behavior of regular exercise. Luke decides that he will get more specific with his exercise plan once Douglass has been exercising regularly for several weeks. Early on, Luke wants Douglass to focus on increasing total physical activity and weekly exercise time.

Demonstration Case Study 5.3

Exercise Testing for Overweight or Obese Clients

Glenda is an exercise physiologist working for a weight-loss clinic. She primarily oversees exercise testing at the clinic. Her most recent client is Pauline. Pauline is a 45-year-old female with a BMI of 37.7 kg/m². Pauline has been participating in low-intensity walking exercise at the clinic for three months and is now ready to progress to moderate-intensity exercise. Pauline does not feel comfortable on leg cycle ergometers, as they cause upper leg pain. Pauline was cleared by her primary care physician to undergo exercise testing and participate in a comprehensive exercise program.

Glenda feels that a submaximal modified Naughton treadmill test is most appropriate to assess Pauline's cardiorespiratory fitness. She reaches this conclusion because the submaximal modified Naughton treadmill test is most appropriate since it consists of small MET increases from one stage to the next, only moderate-intensity exercise is to be completed after the test, and it avoids conducting a cycling protocol.

Glenda wants to reassess Pauline's body composition. Because of class II obesity, Glenda correctly assumes that skinfold assessment will likely not be accurate and thus decides to assess girth measurements. Glenda knows that changes in anthropomorphic measurements can encourage Pauline to continue with exercise. As for resistance exercise, Glenda options for body weight muscular endurance tests, such as sit to stand and modified push-ups. Lastly, Glenda decides it is appropriate to assess lumbo-pelvic-hip flexibility via the sit-and-reach test.

EXERCISE PRESCRIPTION FOR OVERWEIGHT AND OBESE CLIENTS

Regular exercise plays a significant role in reducing body weight and body fat in overweight and obese individuals, as it contributes to kcal expenditure during and after exercise. It is important for exercise professionals to communicate to their clients that exercise is only a portion of an effective weight-loss program and that dietary modifications are necessary. A key point concerning exercise for body weight management is the dose-response relationship between exercise and exercise-induced benefits—more exercise time is necessary for optimal results. The long-term goal of a weight-loss exercise program is to maximize kcal expenditure. For exercise to be minimally effective at reducing body weight, weekly exercise time should be, at a minimum, 150 minutes.[26,27] For continued and more modest weight loss, weekly exercise time should be more than 150 minutes with the most optimal results occurring with more than 225 minutes per week.[28,29] To accumulate the weekly exercise time necessary to elicit meaningful weight loss, exercise professionals should recommend exercise at least five days per week.

Both cardiorespiratory and muscle fitness exercises should be part of an exercise program intended for weight loss. Cardiorespiratory exercise results in the greatest kcal expenditure during exercise and contributes to postexercise kcal expenditure at rest. Increasing cardiorespiratory exercise intensity results amplified kcal expenditure postexercise, even at rest. However, exercise professionals should emphasize increasing exercise time and frequency prior to intensity. Resistance training offers the benefit of muscular hypertrophy, which can add to kcal expenditure at rest.

Exercise professionals should always encourage overweight or obese clients to adhere to exercise as a part of broader lifestyle modification. The reason such encouragement is necessary is because of the slow nature of weight loss. Further, weight loss may be challenging for clients who have been obese for a long period of time and for those with unhealthy behaviors, such as tobacco use. Exercise professionals should continuously monitor clients' responses and progress throughout an exercise program and modify the FITT-VP accordingly. This section explains these modifications for cardiorespiratory, muscular fitness, and flexibility exercise for overweight or obese clients.

Cardiorespiratory Exercise Prescription

Many of the cardiorespiratory exercise prescription recommendations for overweight or obese clients remains the same as for healthy adults. However, the main emphasis of cardiorespiratory exercise for weight loss is accumulating exercise time. Therefore, it is recommended that overweight or obese clients accumulate at least 150 minutes of cardiorespiratory exercise per week.[30] Such an exercise volume is not likely attainable for deconditioned or previously sedentary clients. In these cases, exercise professionals can prescribe daily ten-minute bouts with the goals of progressing to 30 minutes of exercise daily. Once 150 minutes of cardiorespiratory exercise is routinely achieved, exercise professionals should continue to progress clients weekly exercise time to eventually reach 300 minutes.[31] Once a weight-loss goal is achieved, at least 250 minutes of cardiorespiratory exercise should be prescribed to avoid weight regain.

Starting cardiorespiratory exercise intensities can range from low- to moderate-intensity, depending on exercise and health history/status. In general, it is recommended that overweight or obese clients start with moderate-intensity exercise (40–60 percent of $\dot{V}O_2R$/HRR), five to seven days per week.[32] Exercise professionals can consider progressing to vigorous-intensity exercise as the lipolysis and kcal expenditure are enhanced with higher intensities. However, the first progression should always be accumulating exercise time. Exercise intensity can be quantified by the $\dot{V}O_2R$ or HRR method, depending on medication status. An excellent method for quantifying exercise for clients wanting to lose weight is by kcal expenditure. Use of such equations can help determine the total time necessary for reaching a weight-loss goal. It is recommended that weekly energy deficits elicit one to two pounds of weight loss per week, and once a weight-loss goal is reached, 2,000 kcal expenditure through exercise per week is recommended.[33] The equations for quantifying kcal expenditure are provided next.

Energy Expenditure Equations:

> 1 pound of body fat = 3,500 kcals
>
> 1 liter of oxygen consumption per minute (L · min) = 5 kcals expended per minute (kcal/min)
>
> *Use net $\dot{V}O_2$ (target $\dot{V}O_2$ – 3.5 mL/kg · min) if target kcal expenditure is being used where target VO_2 is the oxygen consumed at the target kcal expenditure.*

Overweight and obese clients should be encouraged to perform a variety of cardiorespiratory exercises. Exercise professionals should seek to find modalities that are enjoyable, safe, and comfortable to increase client adherence. If clients are willing and capable of modalities that use more muscle masses, such as rowing, elliptical training, or cross-country skiing, such modalities can be prescribed to enhance kcal expenditure.

Exercise professionals can modify exercise frequency, intensity, and time to adequately progress overweight or obese clients. A biweekly increase in exercise volume of 5 to 10 percent is a reasonable progression scheme. A target goal for sustained weight loss should be 300 minutes of cardiorespiratory exercise per week. Exercise frequency and time should be increased before intensity.

Demonstration Case Study 5.4

Cardiorespiratory Exercise Prescription for Overweight or Obese Clients

Reagan is an exercise physiologist specializing in weight loss. Her most recent client is Kimberly. Kimberly is a 50-year-old female, 270 pounds, BMI = 44 kg/m², and mostly sedentary. Kimberly was medically cleared to exercise and previously completed a modified Naughton treadmill test with an estimated $\dot{V}O_{2max}$ of 19.4 mL/kg · min.

After analyzing Kimberly's profile, Reagan begins to write a cardiorespiratory exercise prescription. Reagan first recommends that Kimberly exercise five days per week, ten minutes per day. The reason Reagan chose this starting point is because Kimberly is classified as class III obese and is sedentary. Further, Reagan believes this will help Kimberly change her lifestyle to include regular exercise. To initially quantify exercise intensity, Reagan chooses to use the $\dot{V}O_2R$ method and sets an initial intensity range equal to 40 to 45 percent of $\dot{V}O_2R$. Reagan's calculations are shown next.

$\dot{V}O_2R = \dot{V}O_{2max} - 3.5$ mL/kg · min

$\dot{V}O_2R = 19.4$ mL/kg · min – 3.5 mL/kg · min

$\dot{V}O_2R = 15.9$ mL/kg · min

40 percent of $\dot{V}O_2R$ = (15.9 mL/kg · min x .4) + 3.5 mL/kg · min

40 percent of $\dot{V}O_2R$ = 9.86 mL/kg · min

45 percent of $\dot{V}O_2R$ = (15.9 mL/kg · min x .45) + 3.5 mL/kg · min

45 percent of $\dot{V}O_2R$ = 10.65 mL/kg · min

$\dot{V}O_2R$ range = 9.86 – 10.65 mL/kg · min

Because of Kimberly's previously sedentary lifestyle and class III obesity, Reagan chooses walking and arm cycling as exercise modalities. Reagan's calculations (for the lower end of the intensity range), using metabolic equations, are provided next.

Walking Calculations:

Reagan feels that Kimberly can sustain walking at 2 mph for ten minutes. She, therefore, solves for incline using the walking equation to elicit 40 percent of Kimberly's $\dot{V}O_2R$.

9.86 mL/kg · min = (0.1 x 2.0 x 26.8) + (1.8 x 2.0 x 26.8 x incline) + 3.5

Incline = ~1 %

<u>Arm Cycling Calculations:</u>

Because of Kimberly's excessive weight, Reagan feels arm cycling would be a more comfortable modality. She believes Kimberly can arm cycle at 65 revolutions per minute for ten-minute bouts. Reagan calculates the resistance that should be placed on the flywheel of a Monark arm cycle to elicit 40 percent of Kimberly's' $\dot{V}O_2R$.

9.86 mL/kg · min = (3 x 65 x resistance x 2.4/122.7 kg) + 3.5

Resistance = 1.66 kp

Reagan chooses a progression scheme that emphasizes accumulating exercise time so as to maximize kcal expenditure. Reagan decides to increase daily exercise time by 5 percent each week until 60 minutes per day is achieved. At that point, Reagan will increase exercise intensity as tolerated.

Demonstration Case Study 5.5

Cardiorespiratory Exercise Prescription for Overweight or Obese Clients

Allen is an exercise physiologist specializing in weight loss at local weight-loss clinic. His most recent client is Zoe. Zoe is a 42-year-old female, 210 pounds, BMI = 33 kg/m^2, and she has been performing stepping exercises 30 minutes daily for the past three months. Zoe was medically cleared to exercise and previously completed a Bruce treadmill test with an estimated $\dot{V}O_{2max}$ of 34.9 mL/kg · min. Zoe wants to lose a total of 50 pounds and is open to any form of cardiorespiratory exercise.

After analyzing Zoe's profile, Allen realizes he can be more aggressive with Zoe's exercise program because she is only classified as class I obese and is physically active. Therefore, Allen starts Zoe's exercise frequency at five days per week and daily exercise time at 60 minutes per day. Given Zoe's specific weight-loss goal, Allen wants to quantify exercise by kcal expenditure. He wants Zoe to initially lose one pound per week through exercise. To accomplish this, Allen uses algebra and the energy expenditure equations. Allen determines that if Zoe exercises at an intensity that elicits a net $\dot{V}O_2$ of 20.95 mL/kg · min, the equivalent of 55 percent of $\dot{V}O_2R$, Zoe will lose one pound per week through exercise alone. Using the stepping equation, this would mean at a stepping rate of 20 steps per minute. Zoe would need to use a 28-centimeter-high step. His work is shown next.

3,500 kcals = 1 pound of body fat

300 minutes of exercise per week = 11.7 kcals expended per minute

11.7 kcal per minute ÷ 5 kcals per minute per liter of oxygen consumed = $\dot{V}O_2$ of 2.33 L · min

($\dot{V}O_2$ of 2.33 L · min x 1,000 mL) ÷ 95.45 kg body weight = 24.45 mL/kg · min

24.45 mL/kg · min – 3.5 mL/kg · min = 20.95 net $\dot{V}O_2$

20.95 mL/kg · min = (0.2 x 20 steps per minute) + (1.33 x 1.8 x step height x 20 steps per minute) + 3.5

Step height = 0.28 meters, which = 28 centimeters

For a progression scheme, Allen chooses to add an additional day per week of exercise every other week until Zoe is exercising seven days per week. At that point, Allen plans to have Zoe perform vigorous-intensity exercise.

Muscular Fitness and Flexibility Exercise Prescription

Although cardiorespiratory exercise is emphasized for overweight or obese clients, resistance training can offer additional benefits, such as the improvement of other cardiovascular disease risk factors.[34] Further, resistance exercise can lead to muscular hypertrophy, which would increase kcal expenditure at rest. As clients progress through a weight-loss program, muscular fitness exercise can be prescribed using the same guidelines as for healthy adults.[35] Like the muscular fitness recommendations, the flexibility recommendations for obese or overweight clients is the same as for healthy adults. Any modifications to the FITT-VP are made based on health status, fitness level, exercise history, patient goals, and physician orders.

Exercise Safety Considerations

Exercise is generally safe for overweight or obese clients. A main safety consideration for excessively obese clients is to ensure that the weight specifications for exercise equipment are not exceeded. Another potential hazard for obese clients is extreme caloric restrictions. Exercise professionals should only recommend a weekly caloric reduction of 500–1,000 kcals.[36] Further reductions should occur under either medical or dietician supervision. Next, exercise professionals must be aware of any existing comorbidity and other cardiovascular risk factors. By knowing existing comorbidities, exercise professionals can monitor for specific signs and symptoms, such as hypoglycemia among clients with diabetes. Lastly, exercise professionals need to record all patient medications, research those medications mechanisms of action, and determine how exercise interacts with those medications and modify the FITT-VP accordingly.

Student Case Study 5.1

Exercise Test Selection for Overweight or Obese Clients

Consider an exercise physiologist at a weight-loss clinic performing several exercise tests per day. The newest client is obese, and the client's profile is provided next.

Demographics: (1) male and (2) 54 years old

Biometrics: (1) resting heart rate = 85 beats per minute; (2) resting blood pressure = 128/84 mmHg; (3) LDL-c = 129 mg/dL, HDL-c = 42 mg/dL, total cholesterol = 199 mg/dL; (4) blood glucose = 125 mg/dL; (5) weight = 277 lbs; and (6) BMI = 41.2 kg/m²

<u>Medical Diagnoses:</u> (1) class III obesity

<u>Medications:</u> (1) none

<u>Symptoms:</u> (1) none

<u>Exercise History:</u> (1) weight lifting in high school (2) manual labor

<u>Exercise Goals and Needs:</u> (1) weight loss and (2) fat loss

1. Assuming the client has been medically cleared to exercise, would it be safe to conduct exercise testing on this client? In two to three sentences, provide a defense for the answer.
2. Assuming it is safe to test this client, should one conduct a maximal or sub-maximal cardiorespiratory fitness test? In four to five sentences, provide a defense for the decision based on the client's profile.
3. Assuming it is safe to test this client, which cardiorespiratory fitness test should be conducted? In four to five sentences, provide a defense for the decision based on the client's profile.
4. Specific to this case, which body composition test should one prefer to conduct? In four to five sentences, provide a defense for the decision based on the client's profile.
5. Assuming it is safe to test this client, to assess muscular fitness, should one conduct muscular endurance assessments or muscular strength assessments, or both? In four to five sentences, provide a defense for the decision based on the client's profile.
6. Assuming it is safe to test this client, provide a list of four specific muscular fitness tests one could conduct on the client. Then provide a four to five-sentence defense supporting the selections.
7. List any special considerations that should be taken into account when choosing exercise tests for this client.

Student Case Study 5.2

Exercise Test Selection for Overweight or Obese Clients

Consider an exercise physiologist at a weight-loss clinic performing several exercise tests per day. The newest client is obese, and the client's profile is provided next.

<u>Demographics:</u> (1) female and (2) 49 years old

<u>Biometrics:</u> (1) resting heart rate = 80 beats per minute; (2) resting blood pressure = 124/80 mmHg; (3) LDL-c = 125 mg/dL, HDL-c = 43 mg/dL, total cholesterol = 191 mg/dL; (4) blood glucose = 119 mg/dL; (5) weight = 247 lbs; and (6) BMI = 34 kg/m²

<u>Medical Diagnoses:</u> (1) class I obesity

<u>Medications:</u> (1) atenolol (beta-blocker)

<u>Symptoms:</u> (1) none

<u>Exercise History:</u> (1) 20 minutes of moderate-intensity cycling, previous three months, (2) does not like walking up hills or stairs

<u>Exercise Goals and Needs:</u> (1) weight loss and (2) fat loss

1. Assuming the client has been medically cleared to exercise, would it be safe to conduct exercise testing on this client? In two to three sentences, provide a defense for the answer.
2. Assuming it is safe to test this client, should a maximal or submaximal cardiorespiratory fitness test be conducted? In four to five sentences, provide a defense for the decision based on the client's profile.
3. Assuming it is safe to test this client, which cardiorespiratory fitness test should be conducted? In four to five sentences, provide a defense for the decision based on the client's profile.
4. Specific to this case, which body composition test should be conducted? In four to five sentences, provide a defense for the decision based on the client's profile.
5. Assuming it is safe to test this client, to assess muscular fitness, should one conduct muscular endurance assessments or muscular strength assessments, or both? In four to five sentences, provide a defense for the decision based on the client's profile.
6. Assuming it is safe to test this client, provide a list of four specific muscular fitness tests one could conduct on the client. Then provide a four- to five-sentence defense supporting the selections.
7. List any special considerations when choosing exercise tests for this client.

Student Case Study 5.3

Exercise Test Selection for Overweight or Obese Clients

Consider an exercise physiologist at a weight-loss clinic performing several exercise tests per day. The newest client is obese, and the client's profile is provided next.

<u>Demographics:</u> (1) female and (2) 38 years old

<u>Biometrics:</u> (1) resting heart rate = 71 beats per minute; (2) resting blood pressure = 118/80 mmHg; (3) LDL-c = 112 mg/dL, HDL-c = 53 mg/dL, total cholesterol = 190 mg/dL; (4) blood glucose = 111 mg/dL; (5) weight = 180 lbs; and (6) BMI = 30.7 kg/m^2

<u>Medical Diagnoses:</u> (1) class I obesity

<u>Medications:</u> (1) none

<u>Symptoms:</u> (1) none

Exercise History: (1) moderate-intensity cycling, five days per week, previous three months, (2) muscular endurance exercises two days per week, and (3) wants a supervised exercise program

Exercise Goals and Needs: (1) continued weight loss and (2) fat loss

1. Assuming the client has been medically cleared to exercise, would it be safe to conduct exercise testing on this client? In two to three sentences, provide a defense for the answer.
2. Assuming it is safe to test this client, should a maximal or submaximal cardiorespiratory fitness test be conducted? In four to five sentences, provide a defense for the decision based on the client's profile.
3. Assuming it is safe to test this client, which cardiorespiratory fitness test should one conduct? In four to five sentences, provide a defense for the decision based on the client's profile.
4. Specific to this case, which body composition test would be preferred? In four to five sentences, provide a defense for the decision based on the client's profile.
5. Assuming it is safe to test this client, to assess muscular fitness, should one conduct muscular endurance assessments or muscular strength assessments, or both? In four to five sentences, provide a defense for the decision based on the client's profile.
6. Assuming it is safe to test this client, provide a list of four specific muscular fitness tests to conduct on the client. Then provide a four- to five-sentence defense supporting the selections.
7. List any special considerations that should be taken into account when choosing exercise tests for this client.

Student Case Study 5.4

Exercise Test Interpretation: YMCA Cycle Test

An exercise physiologist specializes in serving obese clients. She just completed a YMCA cycle test on a 51-year-old male client weighing 260 pounds with a BMI of 33.3 kg/m². The results of the test are provided in Figure 5.1. After reading the results, use the graph and leg cycling equation to interpret the results and answer the questions.

Figure 5.1 This table depicts hypothetical data from a YMCA cycle test

Stage	Kpm/min	Heart Rate	Blood Pressure	RPE	ECG	Symptoms/Comments
Resting	0	75	120/80	NA	Sinus	No symptoms
I	150	125	134/80	12	Sinus	No symptoms
II	300	140	158/78	13	Sinus	No symptoms
Immediate	0	138	156/78	NA	Sinus	No symptoms

(Continued)

Figure 5.1 This table depicts hypothetical data from a YMCA cycle test (Continued)

Stage	Kpm/min	Heart Rate	Blood Pressure	RPE	ECG	Symptoms/Comments
Recovery 1 min	0	120	134/78	NA	Sinus	No symptoms
Recovery 5 min	0	80	122/76	NA	Sinus	No symptoms

1. Using graph paper (Figure 5.2), estimate maximal work rate (kpm/min). Then insert the estimated maximal work rate into the following equation to estimate $\dot{V}O_{2\,max}$:
2. $\dot{V}O_2$ max mL/kg · min = (1.8 x estimated maximal work rate/kg body weight) + 7.
3. What could an exercise physiologist do to further assure the safety and comfort of this client during testing?

Figure 5.2 Students may use these gridlines to graph data from the YMCA cycle test

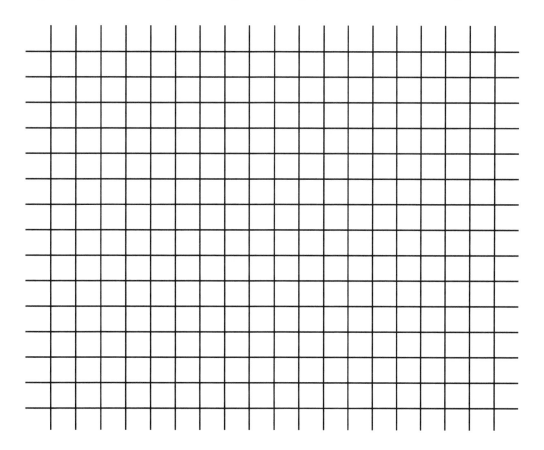

Student Case Study 5.5

Exercise Test Interpretation: Submaximal Treadmill Test

An exercise physiologist specializes in serving obese clients. He just completed a submaximal treadmill test using the modified Naughton protocol on a 48-year-old female who is sedentary, with a BMI of 40 kg/m² and weighs 218 pounds. The test was terminated at a heart rate equal to 70 percent of the client's heart rate reserve. The results of the test are provided in Figure 5.3. After reading the results, use the walking or running equation and a proportion equation to interpret the results and answer the questions.

Figure 5.3 This table depicts hypothetical data from a submaximal treadmill test

Stage	Speed (mph)	Grade %	Heart Rate	Blood Pressure	RPE	ECG	Symptoms
Resting	0	0	70	138/86	NA	Sinus	No symptoms
1	1.0	0	108	158/86	10	Sinus	No symptoms
2	1.5	0	129	170/84	13	Sinus	No symptoms
3	2.0	3.5	141	188/86	16	Sinus	No symptoms
Immediate	1.5	0	140	190/86	NA	Sinus	No symptoms
Recovery 1 min	1.5	0	130	168/84	NA	Sinus	No symptoms
Recovery 5 min	1	0	80	140/84	NA	Sinus	No symptoms

1. Using one of the following two equations, estimate $\dot{V}O_2$ for the last completed stage:

    Walking: $\dot{V}O_2 = (0.1 \times \text{speed in m/min}) + (1.8 \times \text{speed in m/min} \times \text{grade}) + 3.5$

    Running: $\dot{V}O_2 = (0.2 \times \text{speed in m/min}) + (0.9 \times \text{speed in m/min} \times \text{grade}) + 3.5$

    Find $\dot{V}O_2$ in last stage in mL/kg · min

    Find estimated $\dot{V}O_{2max}$ in mL/kg · min

2. Given the client's BMI, should the exercise physiologist have optioned for a different protocol? Defend the answer in two to three sentences. Then design a submaximal cardiorespiratory test—at least three stages—that could be used instead of the modified Naughton or other tests covered in this casebook.

Student Case Study 5.6

Muscular Strength Testing for Overweight or Obese Clients

An exercise physiologist specializes in serving obese clients. The newest client is a 50-year-old male with a BMI of 36.7 kg/m² who weighs 255 pounds. The exercise physiologist wants to prescribe this client a resistance training program to help maximize caloric expenditure. Therefore, the exercise physiologist conducts a series of muscular strength tests. The following data were collected (Figure 5.4).

Figure 5.4 This table depicts hypothetical data from a 3–5RM test

Leg Press Strength Test

Trial 1	5	repetitions
	300	weight
Trial 2	3	repetitions
	320	weight
Trial 3	3	repetitions
	330	weight
Best Trial	3	repetitions
	330	weight

Chest Press Strength Test

Trial 1	5	repetitions
	220	weight
Trial 2	4	repetitions
	235	weight
Trial 3	3	repetitions
	250	weight
Best Trial	3	repetitions
	250	weight

1. Use the Lander equation to predict the client's maximal leg press strength.
2. Calculate a weight pushed to body weight ratio and compare the client's results to normative data.
3. Use the Lander equation to predict the client's maximal chest press strength.
4. Calculate a weight pushed to body weight ratio and compare the client's results to normative data.
5. What steps can the exercise physiologist take to ensure safety during these strength tests?

Student Case Study 5.7

Exercise Prescription for Overweight or Obese Clients: Cardiorespiratory Endurance

An exercise professional specializes in serving obese clients. The newest client is a 51-year-female with a BMI of 37.5 kg/m² weighing 231 pounds. The exercise professional just conducted an arm cycle submaximal exercise test, completed without complications, and the client achieved an estimated $\dot{V}O_{2max}$ of 23.5 mL/kg · min. Prior to the test, the client's resting heart rate was 78 beats per minute. The client is open to any form of exercise.

1. Calculate a heart rate range based on the heart rate reserve that the client should maintain during aerobic exercise. Should an exercise professional use this heart rate range during exercise training or consider other methods of quantifying exercise intensity? Why or why not?
2. Calculate a $\dot{V}O_2$ range based on $\dot{V}O_2$ reserve that the client should maintain during aerobic exercise.
3. Provide an exercise type (be specific), frequency, and time at the $\dot{V}O_2$ range found in question 2 for the client to improve her cardiorespiratory fitness and better manage her body composition.
4. Suggest four possible aerobic exercises that would be appropriate for this client. Then explain the rationale for each selection.
5. Use the walking equation to calculate a walking speed (in mph) for the client that elicits the lower end of the $\dot{V}O_2$ reserve range found in question 2. The percent grade of the treadmill is 3.5 percent.
6. Use the stepping equation to calculate a stepping rate for the client that elicits the upper end of the $\dot{V}O_2$ reserve range found in question 2. The height of the step is 23 centimeters.
7. Use the arm cycle equation to calculate a resistance to be placed on the flywheel for the client that elicits the lower end of the $\dot{V}O_2$ reserve range found in question 2. The client turns the arm crank at 70 rpm.
8. Suggest a progression scheme to advance the client toward a goal of improving her body composition. Should vigorous-intensity exercise eventually be considered? Why or why not?
9. Using the lower end of the $\dot{V}O_2$ reserve range found in question 2 and exercise time and frequency from question 3, how many weeks will it take for the client to lose 20 pounds through exercise alone?
10. Provide three training considerations to help this client improve her body composition through cardiorespiratory exercise safely.

Student Case Study 5.8

Exercise Prescription for Overweight or Obese Clients: Cardiorespiratory Endurance

An exercise professional specializes in serving obese clients. The newest client is a 44-year-male with a BMI of 31.5 kg/m² weighing 245 pounds. The exercise professional just conducted a submaximal Bruce protocol test, completed without complications, and the client achieved an estimated $\dot{V}O_{2max}$ of 28.1 mL/kg · min. Prior to the test, the client's resting heart rate was 70 beats per minute. The client is open to any form of exercise.

1. Calculate a heart rate range based on the heart rate reserve that the client should maintain during aerobic exercise. Should the exercise professional use this heart rate range during exercise training or consider other methods of quantifying exercise intensity? Why or why not?
2. Calculate a $\dot{V}O_2$ range based on $\dot{V}O_2$ reserve that the client should maintain during aerobic exercise.
3. Provide an exercise type (be specific), frequency, and time at the $\dot{V}O_2$ range found in question 2 for the client to improve his cardiorespiratory fitness and better manage their body composition.
4. Suggest four possible aerobic exercises that would be appropriate for this client. Then explain the rationale for each selection.
5. Use the walking equation to calculate an appropriate walking speed (in mph) and incline for the client that elicits the lower end of the $\dot{V}O_2$ reserve range found in question 2.
6. Use the leg cycling equation to calculate an appropriate peddling frequency and resistance to elicit the upper end of the $\dot{V}O_2$ reserve range found in question 2.
7. Use the arm cycle equation to calculate an appropriate peddle frequency and resistance to be placed on the flywheel for the client that elicits the lower end of the $\dot{V}O_2$ reserve range found in question 2.
8. Using the upper end of the $\dot{V}O_2$ reserve range found in question 2 and exercise time and frequency from question 3, how many weeks will it take for the client to lose 30 pounds through exercise alone?
9. Suggest a progression scheme to advance the client toward a goal of improving his body composition.
10. Would progressing to high-intensity interval training be appropriate for this client? If so, what cautions should be considered? If not, explain why.
11. Provide three training considerations to help this client improve his body composition through cardiorespiratory exercise safely.

Student Case Study 5.9

Exercise Prescription for Overweight and Obese Clients: Muscular Fitness

An exercise physiologist specializes in training obese clients. The exercise physiologist was recently presented with the following client data: (1) 47-year-old female, (2) class II obesity, (3) goals to maximize caloric expenditure and improve muscular strength, (4) chest press 1RM = 105 pounds, (5) leg press 1RM = 155 pounds, and (6) open to any resistance exercise program.

1. Provide a range for weight that the client should chest press.
2. Provide a range for weight that the client should leg press.
3. Provide a resistance exercise prescription for frequency and number of exercises, sets, and repetitions to improve muscular strength.

4. Suggest at least four specific resistance training exercises that are appropriate for this client.
5. Suggest a progression scheme to advance the client toward the goal of improving muscular strength.
6. How would the resistance training program be different if the client expressed interest in specifically targeting muscular endurance?
7. Explain how one might design the resistance training program to maximize client adherence.
8. Explain in four to five sentences how adherence to this resistance training program will help improve the overall health of the client in addition to amplifying her caloric expenditure.

Student Case Study 5.10

Exercise Testing and Prescription: Comprehensive Case Study

An exercise physiologist works for a weight-loss clinic. He thoroughly collected the following data from his most recent client:

Demographics: (1) male and (2) 53 years old

Family History: (1) father had an ischemic stroke at the age of 53 and (2) mother was diagnosed with type II diabetes mellitus at the age of 40

Biometrics: (1) resting heart rate = 82 beats per minute; (2) resting blood pressure = 136/74 mmHg; (4) LDL-c = 128 mg/dL, HDL-c = 42 mg/dL, total cholesterol = 199 mg/dL; (5) glycosylated hemoglobin = 6.45 percent and blood glucose = 124.5 mg/dL; and (6) weight = 300 lbs, BMI = 44.3 kg/m²

Medical Diagnoses: (1) class III obesity

Medications: (1) lisinopril, (2) carvedilol

Symptoms: (1) none

Exercise History: (1) no recent exercise history, (2) does not like walking up hill

Exercise Goals and Needs: (1) maximize fitness to offset hypertension and (2) maintain control of hypertension

1. Should the exercise physiologist conduct a maximal or submaximal cardiorespiratory fitness test? In four to five sentences, provide a defense for the decision based on the client's profile.
2. Which cardiorespiratory fitness test should be conducted? In four to five sentences, provide a defense for the decision based on the client's profile.
3. Given limitless resources, which body composition test should the exercise physiologist conduct? In four to five sentences, provide a defense for the decision based on the client's profile.

4. Given minimal resources with a small budget, which body composition test should be conducted? In four to five sentences, provide a defense for the decision based on the client's profile.

5. Specific to this case, which body composition test would be preferred? In four to five sentences, provide a defense for the decision based on the client's profile.

6. To assess muscular fitness, should muscular endurance assessments or muscular strength assessments be conducted, or both? In four to five sentences, provide a defense for the decision based on the client's profile.

7. Provide a list of four specific muscular fitness tests to be conducted on the client. Then provide a four- to five-sentence defense supporting the selections.

8. Based on the answers for questions 1 and 2, calculate the client's $\dot{V}O_{2\,max}$ from the most appropriate of the following cardiorespiratory fitness tests (Figures 5.5–5.9).

Figure 5.5 This table depicts hypothetical data from a YMCA cycle test

Stage	**Kpm/ min**	**Heart Rate**	**Blood Pressure**	**RPE**	**ECG**	**Symptoms/ Comments**
Resting	0	82	136/74	NA	Sinus	No symptoms
I	150	124	148/76	13	Sinus	No symptoms
II	300	142	166/76	14	Sinus	No symptoms
Immediate	100	140	160/76	NA	Sinus	No symptoms
Recovery 1 min	50	121	152/74	NA	Sinus	No symptoms
Recovery 5 min	25	93	140/72	NA	Sinus	No symptoms

YMCA Cycle Test

Figure 5.6 Students may use these gridlines to graph data from the YMCA cycle test

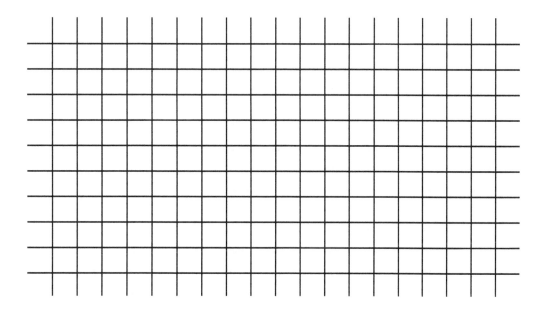

Figure 5.7 This table depicts hypothetical data from an Astrand-Rhyming cycle test

Astrand-Rhyming Cycle Test

Stage/Minute	Kpm/m	Heart Rate	Blood Pressure	RPE	ECG	Symptoms
Resting		82	136/74	NA	Sinus	No symptoms
I	300	136	160/76	12	Sinus	No symptoms
II	300	140	162/76	13	Sinus	No symptoms
III	300	141	164/78	13	Sinus	No symptoms
IV	300	141	168/74	13	Sinus	No symptoms
V	300	142	168/74	15	Sinus	No symptoms
VI	300	142	170/76	15	Sinus	No symptoms
Immediate	150	130	168/76	NA	Sinus	No symptoms
Recovery 1 min	75	117	150/74	NA	Sinus	No symptoms
Recovery 5 min	50	107	142/72	NA	Sinus	No symptoms

Figure 5.8 This table depicts hypothetical data from a maximal cycle test

Maximal Cycle Test

Stage	Time	Kpm/min	Heart Rate	Blood Pressure	RPE	$\dot{V}O_2$ (mL/kg · min)	RER	Blood Lactate (mmol)	ECG
Resting		0	82	136/74	NA	4.0	0.85	NA	Sinus
I	2:00	600	117	148/74	11	11.2	0.74	1.1	Sinus
II	4:00	900	133	158/74	15	18.7	0.99	4.4	Sinus
III	6:00	1200	149	170/76	16	21.4	1.02	6.7	Sinus
IV	8:00	1500	164	184/76	18	27.9	1.14	8.4	Sinus
Immediate	NA	300	160	182/74	NA	26.2	1.12	NA	Sinus
Recovery 1 min	NA	150	120	162/70	NA	18.2	1.00	NA	Sinus
Recovery 5 min	NA	75	90	140/70	NA	11.3	0.96	NA	Sinus

Comments: Test terminated because of volitional fatigue

Figure 5.9 This table depicts hypothetical data from a maximal treadmill test

Maximal Treadmill Test

Stage	Time	Speed (mph)	Grade %	Blood Pressure	$\dot{V}O_2$ (mL/ kg · min)	Blood Lactate (mmol)	RPE	Heart Rate	RER
Resting	NA	0	0	136/74	4.3	NA	NA	82	0.80
I	2:00	3.5	2	144/76	10.6	1.4	13	125	0.92
II	4:00	4.5	4	158/76	14.9	4.0	14	157	1.06
III	6:00	5.5	6	172/76	21.7	5.3	17	166	1.09
IV	8:00	6.5	8	182/76	29.3	8.9	18	167	1.15
Immediate	NA	1.5	0	180/74	27.6	NA	NA	164	1.14
Recovery 1 min	NA	1.5	0	164/74	20.1	NA	NA	133	1.01
Recovery 5 min	NA	1	0	146/72	8.8	NA	NA	90	0.97

Comments: Test terminated because of volitional fatigue

9. For the cardiorespiratory fitness test chosen to interpret the answer for question 8, should the test have been terminated prior to completion? Explain why or why not.

10. What is the minimal threshold for this client's waist circumference to warrant a high-risk classification?

Assuming muscular strength was selected, interpret and classify the client's leg and chest press strength from the following data (Figure 5.10).

Figure 5.10 This table depicts hypothetical data from a 3–5RM test

Leg Press Strength Test

Trial 1	5 repetitions
	110 weight
Trial 2	4 repetitions
	120 weight
Trial 3	3 repetitions
	125 weight
Best Trial	3 repetitions
	125 weight

(Continued)

Chest Press Strength Test

Trial 1	5	repetitions
	80	weight
Trial 2	4	repetitions
	100	weight
Trial 3	4	repetitions
	110	weight
Best Trial	4	repetitions
	110	weight

11. Calculate a heart rate range based on the heart rate reserve that the client should maintain during aerobic exercise. Is this the most reliable method for quantifying cardiorespiratory endurance exercise? Why or why not?

12. Calculate a $\dot{V}O_2$ range based on $\dot{V}O_2$ reserve that the client should maintain during aerobic exercise.

13. Provide an exercise type (be specific), frequency, and time at the $\dot{V}O_2$ range found in question 12 for the client to improve his cardiorespiratory fitness and manage his body composition.

14. Suggest four possible aerobic exercises that would be appropriate for this client.

15. Provide a walking speed and grade for the client to maintain on the treadmill to elicit the lower end of the $\dot{V}O_2$ range listed in question 12.

16. Provide a resistance and peddle frequency for leg cycling to elicit the lower end of the $\dot{V}O_2$ range listed in question 12.

17. Provide a resistance and peddle frequency for arm cycling to elicit the lower end of the $\dot{V}O_2$ range listed in question 12.

18. Suggest a progression scheme for improving cardiorespiratory fitness. Would vigorous-intensity or high-intensity interval training be warranted? Why or why not?

19. Based on the lower end of the intensity range in question 12 and exercise frequency and time found in question 13 how many weeks will it take for the client to lose 45 pounds through exercise alone?

20. Provide a range for weight that the client should chest press.

21. Provide a range for weight that the client should leg press.

22. Provide a resistance exercise prescription for frequency and number of exercises, sets, and repetitions to improve muscular fitness.

23. Suggest at least four specific resistance training exercises that are appropriate for this client.

24. Suggest a progression scheme to help the client improve overall muscular fitness.

25. Provide the frequency, intensity, number of stretches, sets, and amount of time each stretch should be to help improve the client's flexibility.

26. Provide a list consisting of all safety considerations that should be taken into account when supervising this client's exercise program.

REFERENCES

1. American College of Sports Medicine, *ACSM's Guidelines for Exercise Testing and Prescription*, 11th ed. (Philadelphia: Wolters Kluwer Health, 2022).

2. C. M. Hales, M. D. Carroll, C. D. Fryar, and C. L. Ogden, *Prevalence of Obesity Among Adults and Youth: United States, 2015–2016, NCHS Data Brief, no 219.* (Hyattsville, MD: National Center for Health Statistics, 2017).

3. American College of Sports Medicine, *ACSM's Guidelines.*

4. K. M. Flegal, B. K. Kit, H. Orpana, and B. I. Graubard, "Association of All-Cause Mortality with Overweight and Obesity Using Standard Body Mass Index Categories: A Systematic Review and Meta-Analysis," *JAMA* 309, no. 1 (2013): 71–82.

5. Flegal et al., "Association of All-Cause."

6. L. F. Drager, S. M. Togeiro, V. Y. Polotsky, and G. Lorenzi-Filho, "Obstructive Sleep Apnea: A Cardiometabolic Risk in Obesity and the Metabolic Syndrome," *Journal of the American College of Cardiology* 62, no. 7 (2013): 569–76.

7. A. Must, J. Spadano, E. H. Coakley, A. E. Field, et al., "The Disease Burden Associated with Overweight and Obesity, *JAMA* 282, no. 16 (1999): 1523–29.

8. H. L. Cheng, S. Medlow, and K. Steinbeck, "The Health Consequences of Obesity in Young Adulthood," *Current Obesity Reports* 5, no. 1 (2016): 30–7.

9. M. M. Kelsey, A. Zaepfel, P. Bjornstad, and K. J. Nadeau, "Age-Related Consequences of Childhood Obesity. *Gerontology* 60, no. 3 (2014): 222–28.

10. J. J. Reilly and J. Kelly, "Long-Term Impact of Overweight and Obesity in Childhood and Adolescence on Morbidity and Premature Mortality in Adulthood: Systematic Review," *International Journal of Obesity* 35, no. 7 (2011): 891–98.

11. P. E. Zebekakis, T. Nawrot, L. Thijs, E. J. Balkestein, et al., "Obesity Is Associated with Increased Arterial Stiffness from Adolescence Until Old Age," *Journal of Hypertension* 23, no. 10 (2005): 1839–46.

12. V. W. Barry, M. Baruth, M. W. Beets, J. L. Durstine, et al., "Fitness vs. Fatness on All-Cause Mortality: A Meta-Analysis," *Progress in Cardiovascular Diseases* 56, no. 4 (2014): 382–90.

13. C. Dalzill, A. Nigam, M. Juneau, et al., "Intensive Lifestyle Intervention Improves Cardiometabolic and Exercise Parameters in Metabolically Healthy Obese and Metabolically Unhealthy Obese Individuals," *Canadian Journal of Cardiology* 30, no. 4 (2014): 434–40.

14. S. P. Messier, S. L. Mihalko, C. Legault, et al., "Effects of Intensive Diet and Exercise on Knee Joint Loads, Inflammation, and Clinical Outcomes among Overweight and Obese Adults with Knee Osteoarthritis: The IDEA Randomized Clinical Trial," *JAMA* 310, no. 12 (2013): 1263–73.

15. J. E. Donnelly, S. N. Blair, J. M. Jakicic, et al., "American College of Sports Medicine Position Stand: Appropriate Physical Activity Intervention Strategies for Weight Loss and Prevention of Weight Regain for Adults," *Medicine and Science in Sports and Exercise* 41, no. 2 (2009): 459–71.

16. American College of Sports Medicine, *ACSM's Guidelines.*

17. ibid.

18.	D. M. Thomas, C. Bouchard, T. Church, et al., "Why Do Individuals Not Lose More Weight from an Exercise Intervention at a Defined Dose? An Energy Balance Analysis," *Obesity Reviews* 13, no. 10 (2012): 835–47.

19.	M. Rosenkilde, P. Auerbach, M. H. Reichkendler, et al., "Body Fat Loss and Compensatory Mechanisms in Response to Different Doses of Aerobic Exercise—A Randomized Controlled Trial in Overweight Sedentary Males. *American Journal of Physiology-Regulatory, Integrative and Comparative Physiology* 303, no. 6 (2012): 571–79.

20.	S. Maehlum, M. Grandmontagne, E. A. Newsholme, and O. M. Sejersted, "Magnitude and Duration of Excess Postexercise Oxygen Consumption in Healthy Young Subjects," *Metabolism* 35, no. 5 (1986): 425–29.

21.	R. G. McMurray and A. C. Hackney, "Interactions of Metabolic Hormones, Adipose Tissue and Exercise," *Sports Medicine* 35, no. 5 (2005): 393–412.

22.	D. A. Sedlock, M. G. Lee, M. G. Flynn, et al., "Excess Postexercise Oxygen Consumption after Aerobic Exercise Training. *International Journal of Sports Nutrition* 20, no. 4 (2010): 336–49.

23.	M. Lafontan and D. Langin, "Lipolysis and Lipid Mobilization in Human Adipose Tissue," *Progress in Lipid Research* 48, no. 5 (2009): 275–97.

24.	F. Zurlo, K. Larson, C. Bogardus, and E. Ravussin, "Skeletal Muscle Metabolism Is A Major Determinant of Resting Energy Expenditure, *Journal of Clinical Investigation* 86, no. 5 (1990): 1423–27.

25.	M. Hopkins, C. Gibbons, P. Caudwell, et al., "The Adaptive Metabolic Response to Exercise-Induced Weight Loss Influences Both Energy Expenditure and Energy Intake," *European Journal of Clinical Nutrition* 68 (2014): 581–86.

26.	Donnelly et al., "American College of Sports."

27.	American College of Sports Medicine, *ACSM's Guidelines.*

28.	Donnelly et al., "American College of Sports."

29.	American College of Sports Medicine, *ACSM's Guidelines.*

30.	ibid.

31.	ibid.

32.	ibid.

33.	ibid.

34.	Ibid.

35.	ibid.

36.	ibid.

Exercise Testing and Prescription for Clients with Dyslipidemia

INTRODUCTION

DYSLIPIDEMIA IS AN umbrella term that references an abnormal concentration of blood lipids. Recent research suggests that approximately 105 million US adults, nearly 30 percent of the US population, have dyslipidemia.[1,2] Dyslipidemia is a well-known contributor in the development of chronic diseases—specifically atherosclerotic diseases, such as coronary,[3] cerebral,[4] and peripheral artery diseases.[5] In addition, dyslipidemia contributes to the development of lipolytic-induced type II diabetes mellitus[6] and other cardiometabolic abnormalities, which further augments the development of atherosclerotic diseases.

Three types of lipids are targeted during dyslipidemia therapy. The first type is LDL-c. LDL-c is the primary target of dyslipidemia treatment because of the role it plays in accelerating atherosclerosis and inflammation. In excess amounts, LDL-c can penetrate damaged areas of the endothelium of both coronary and peripheral arteries contributing to the formation of atherosclerotic plaque and increasing the risk for coronary,[7] cerebral,[8] and peripheral artery disease.[9] Accordingly, the optimal concentration of LDL-c in the blood should be less than 130 mg/dL.[10] The second lipid addressed is HDL-c. HDL-c works in reverse lipid transport by sequestering blood lipids back to the liver. As such, HDL-c is seen as cardioprotective, and health professionals aim to implement strategies to increase HDL-c to at least 40 mg/dL in men and 50 mg/dL in women[11] secondary to lowering LDL-c. The third type of lipid addressed is the triglyceride. Triglycerides can be seen in the blood and within adipose and muscle cells. There is an association between high blood triglyceride levels and cardiovascular disease and type II diabetes, although LDL-c is the primary concern. Triglyceride levels should be less than 150 mg/dL.[12]

There are many causes of dyslipidemia, with the main cause being lifestyle. Diet is arguably the most potent contributor to dyslipidemia. Diets high in saturated fat introduce exogenous cholesterol into the body and can elevate LDL-c.[13] High-fat diets, in general, lead to chronically elevated triglyceride levels.[14] Other lifestyle decisions, such as cigarette smoking, lower HDL-c levels while physical inactivity contributes to obesity, insulin resistance, and, ultimately, dyslipidemia.[15,16] Given the potency of lifestyle factors to the development of dyslipidemia, lifestyle modification will be prescribed in addition to antilipemic medications as a part of dyslipidemia therapy.

With the prevalence of dyslipidemia and lifestyle modification as the first-line treatment or prevention strategy for individuals with dyslipidemia, exercise professionals will be increasingly tasked with serving this population. It is crucial that exercise professionals know the various strategies for optimizing LDL-c, HDL-c, and triglycerides. This includes dietary advice and the complex role that exercise plays in cholesterol and lipid metabolism and optimization. Further, exercise professionals will need to be aware of antilipemic side effects and target lipid levels as recommended by the ACSM[17] or the prescribing physician. Therefore, the purpose of this chapter is to teach students how to apply their knowledge of exercise as a means of modifying lipid profile, exercise testing, and exercise prescription. On completion of the case studies within this chapter, students will be able to achieve the following:

1. Explain to and educate clients on the role of lipids in the body, basic lipid metabolism, and health-related consequences of abnormal blood lipid levels
2. Explain to and educate clients on how dietary choices and exercise influence blood lipid levels
3. Select and interpret appropriate exercise tests and apply the cardiorespiratory, muscular fitness, and flexibility FITT-VP recommendations and modifications to clients with dyslipidemia
4. Identify and understand safety considerations for training clients with dyslipidemia

LIPIDS' ROLE IN THE BODY

Lipids are organic compounds that are insoluble in water. Although the definition of lipids is simple, there are several categories of lipids. Each category of lipid plays an important role in the structure and function of the human body, including bioenergetics, cellular structure, thermoregulation, insulation, and hormone biosynthesis. So as not to confuse clients, the categories of lipids discussed for client education should be limited and simplified. Fatty acids, triglycerides, lipoproteins, and cholesterol are important lipid categories that can be discussed in a comprehensible manner and can be used to offer an explanation on the importance of lipids in the body, their dangers in abnormal concentrations, and how diet and exercise influence levels.

Lipids are an important storage form of energy used by the body's cells to perform work. Lipids are energy-dense and primarily stored within adipose and hepatic cells but are also stored within cardiac and muscle cells. Within these cells, fatty acids are stored as triglycerides—three fatty acids and a glycerol backbone. To meet energy needs at rest, in the fasted state, during low-intensity exercise, or when carbohydrate stores are scarce, triglycerides are broken down into three fatty acids and their glycerol backbone through a process called lipolysis. The fatty acids are then used via oxidative phosphorylation to produce adenosine triphosphate molecules to be used as energy to carry out cellular work. From an educational standpoint, it is useful to discuss with clients that lipids are easily stored and in excess can cause metabolic problems, such as insulin resistance.[18] Sufficient exercise elicits adaptions, which facilitate adequate lipolysis and the mitochondrial density necessary for oxidation of free fatty acids, thereby reducing excess fat and lipid storage in the body.[19,20]

Aside from meeting the energy needs of cells, lipids also play important roles in cellular structure. Cholesterol is a component of the outer layer of the body's cells. Without adequate cholesterol production and/or consumption, cells would lose their fluidity and possibly rupture and spill their contents in the blood, which can harm the kidneys. When such damage occurs to muscle cells, myoglobin can enter the blood and eventually cause kidney injury. This condition is called rhabdomyolyses and is a possible side effect of antilipemic therapy with statin drugs or under extreme exercise conditions.

Cholesterol plays an additional role as a metabolic intermediate in the production of steroid hormones, such as testosterone and estrogen. Both testosterone and estrogen are critical for reproductive health, growth, and development. Testosterone promotes anabolic processes, such as protein synthesis and the development of muscle mass and strength. Estrogen is a cardioprotective hormone, as it can limit the accumulation of atherosclerotic plaque.[21]

Because of the hydrophobic nature of lipids, they are packaged and transported in the blood as components of lipoproteins. Lipoproteins contain cholesterol, triglycerides, and protein. Lipoproteins are categorized according to the density of their content, with lower density lipoproteins being the most detrimental to health in high concentrations, and higher density lipoproteins being more cardioprotective. Lower density lipoproteins work in forward lipid transport and carry triglycerides and cholesterol throughout circulation from the liver and intestines to fat and muscle cells. High-density lipoproteins work in reverse lipid transport and act as scavengers to transport cholesterol back to the liver, which theoretically reduces the number of circulating cholesterols that can penetrate the endothelium of blood vessels and form atherosclerotic plaque.

Demonstration Case Study 6.1

Role of Lipids in the Body

Denise is an exercise professional working for an employee wellness program at a large company. She oversees client education where she focuses on offering lifestyle modification recommendations and providing teaching seminars about lowering chronic disease risk. Most recently, Denise had a walk-in client who wanted to discuss his recent diagnosis of dyslipidemia. The client's physician told him he needed to lower his "bad" cholesterol, and he wanted clarification on the purpose of cholesterol and other fats in the body and why they could be bad for his health. Denise offered the following explanation:

> *In and of themselves, fats and cholesterols are not harmful to your health, as they are necessary for everyday functions. Fats and cholesterols are both forms of what are called lipids. Fats are packaged in the body as triglycerides, which are*

either stored or broken down for energy. Right now, you and I are both relaxed and sitting down, but our body still needs to function—our hearts need to beat, our diaphragms need to contract so we can breathe, and our bodies need energy to maintain body temperature. At low intensities, fats are our primary source for this energy, and we all have substantial fat stores in the body, enough to keep our bodies functioning for days.

As for cholesterol, our cells have an outer layer that keeps its contents within the cell and keeps unwanted fluids out. Cholesterol is needed to form this layer, and without enough cholesterol, our cells might rupture. Also, cholesterol is used to make testosterone, which allows you to maintain and build muscle mass.

When fats and cholesterols become problematic for your health is when there are either too many or not enough. In your case, you were told to lower your bad cholesterol, which is called LDL-c. LDL-c carries triglycerides and cholesterol to other cells, which is a necessary process. But when LDL-c levels are too high, they can get inside the walls of your blood vessels, and this is how plaque forms. This plaque can eventually block the flow of blood causing a heart attack or stroke. To lower your LDL-c you will want to decrease the amount of animal products you consume because they are high in cholesterol, get more exercise, and if you are prescribed a cholesterol medication, take that medication as ordered by your doctor.

Demonstration Case Study 6.2

Role of Lipids in the Body

Tyree is an exercise professional working for an employee health program at a large accounting firm. Tyree focuses on developing educational programs for assisting employees in chronic disease risk reduction. A client recently visited Tyree and asked questions because he was confused about cholesterol. The client was told by his nurse practitioner that he was borderline for dyslipidemia. The nurse practitioner told Tyree's client that he needed to increase his good cholesterol and lower his bad cholesterol. The client was confused by this because he thought all cholesterol was bad. Thus the client wanted clarification. Tyree offered the following explanation:

> *First off, let's dispel the notion that cholesterol as a molecule is bad. Cholesterol is actually needed in the body because it forms the outer layers of our cells and is necessary for constructing hormones, such as testosterone and estrogen. Cholesterol needs to be transported in the blood by what are called lipoproteins because it is not soluble in water. There are five types of lipoproteins, but to keep things simple, let's focus on two: LDL-c and HDL-c.*
>
> *LDL-c carries fats and cholesterol throughout the blood to cells that need them, which is a necessary process. In high amounts, LDL-c can get into the walls of blood vessels and form atherosclerosis. This is why your nurse practitioner refers*

to these cholesterols as bad. To lower the amounts of LDL-c in the blood, you should avoid consuming too many animal products, as they contain cholesterol. HDL-c works in reverse of LDL-c. HDL-c picks up cholesterol in the blood and transports it back to the liver, which decreases the opportunity for cholesterol to get into your blood vessel walls. This is why your nurse practitioner refers to these cholesterols as good. To increase your HDL-c, you should get plenty of exercise and avoid tobacco products.

BASIC LIPID METABOLISM AND THE INFLUENCE OF DIET AND EXERCISE

The overall process of lipid metabolism is very complex and involves numerous enzymatic reactions. Much of these metabolic processes are beyond the scope of this text. Instead, the aim of this section is to provide a framework from which to design safe and effective exercise programs for clients with dyslipidemia and to educate clients about the interplay of diet and exercise for managing blood lipids.

Most lipids enter the body through the diet in the form of dietary triglycerides. Dietary triglycerides are first digested in the small intestine where they are emulsified by the action of bile salts. Bile salts are synthesized in the liver from cholesterol and are stored in the gallbladder. Exercise and health professionals often recommend diets high in fiber for clients with dyslipidemia because soluble fiber, found in whole grains, fruits, and vegetables, binds to bile salts, forcing the hepatic production of new bile salts from cholesterol, which can lower circulating cholesterol levels.

Once triglycerides are emulsified by bile salts, they are hydrolyzed to free fatty acids and its glycerol backbone. The bile salts continue acting on the free fatty acids, forming small particles called micelles. Micelles then diffuse across the intestine wall where they are repacked into triglycerides. The repacked triglycerides are combined with cholesterol and encapsulated by a protein shell forming a large lipoprotein called a chylomicron.

Once formed, chylomicrons enter the lymphatic system, eventually ending up in the blood. In the blood, chylomicrons circulate to various tissues, including skeletal, fat, and cardiac and the liver. At these sites, the chylomicrons' triglycerides are broken down into free fatty acids by the enzyme lipoprotein lipase, which is found along capillary walls of target tissues. Free fatty acids then enter target cells for storage as intracellular triglycerides, which are eventually broken down for energy via the enzyme hormone-sensitive lipase. Each time lipoprotein lipase acts on lipoproteins, they get smaller, thus going from the large chylomicron to, eventually, the LDL-c.

HDL-c is primarily synthesized in the liver. HDL-c is a relatively smaller lipoprotein than chylomicrons and other LDL-cs. HDL-c operates in reverse lipid transport. That is, HDL-c is a scavenger and as it circulates, it picks up cholesterol and transports it to the liver for repackaging as a LDL-c. In addition, HDL-c can exchange cholesterol for triglycerides, form very low-density lipoproteins, and transport those triglycerides to the liver. The remaining very low-density lipoprotein is degraded to LDL-c. HDL-c is thought to be cardioprotective by eliminating excess cholesterol in circulation and thereby reducing the accumulation of atherosclerotic plaque.

Cholesterol can be consumed via the diet and can also be produced in the liver via the mevalonate pathway. All of the cholesterol required for normal bodily functions can be produced in the liver. Exogenous cholesterol consumed through the diet can add to the cholesterol already being produced in the liver and increase the amount of LDL-c in circulation. The rate-limiting enzyme in the mevalonate pathway is the target of antilipemic drugs called statins. By inhibiting the rate-limiting enzyme HMG CoA reductase, hepatic production of cholesterol is reduced.

Although exercise professionals are often not licensed as dieticians, they can offer basic dietary advice. Given the metabolism of lipids, the takeaway message can be that consuming exogenous cholesterol and large quantities of dietary triglycerides can elevate blood lipid levels over time. Although fat is an important part of daily dietary intake, most of the fat consumed should be in the form of polyunsaturated fats—found mainly in plant-based foods. Further, it is useful to recommend that dyslipidemia clients limit consumption of animal-based products, as they are high in exogenous cholesterol. Further, a reasonable dietary recommendation would be to increase consumption of soluble fiber to reduce circulating cholesterol. Emerging research suggests that small-particle LDL-c is more dangerous for cardiovascular health and low carbohydrate diets are shown to slightly reduce the amount of small-particle LDL-c.[22,23]

Research results are mixed regarding the role regular exercise plays on blood lipid levels. Some research has shown both cardiorespiratory and resistance exercise training increases HDL-c, while others have shown no effect.[24,25,26,27] Research does appear to be more consistent in showing that both cardiorespiratory and resistance exercise lowers LDL-c and triglycerides.[28,29] The precise mechanisms behind the improvement in blood lipids, particularly lipoproteins, is somewhat unknown. Improvements in mitochondrial density, lipolytic enzyme activity, and lipoprotein clearance may account for favorable lipid profiles in response to exercise training.[30,31] Further, increased caloric expenditure and weight loss can increase the oxidation of lipids, making exercise time and frequency critical to lipid management. Exercise professionals should be prepared to prescribe both cardiorespiratory and resistance training to favorably influence lipid profiles in dyslipidemia clients.

Demonstration Case Study 6.3

Role of Diet and Exercise on Lipids

Ayasha is an exercise professional working for a government-funded health education and community action group. Ayasha conducts regular health education events and speaks with members of the community in groups and in person. At her most recent education event, Ayasha was approached by a community member who had a new diagnosis of dyslipidemia. The community member had a very curious mind and was seeking a comprehensive, yet understandable, answer as to how his lipids can be improved by diet and exercise and not just general recommendations. Ayasha offered the following response:

> *Diet, arguably, has the most profound influence on blood lipid levels. The reason for this is twofold. First, most of the lipids introduced into the body through the diet are triglycerides. These triglycerides, through several enzymatic reactions, get packaged with cholesterol to form lipoproteins. These lipoproteins circulate in the body, giving up their triglycerides for storage in fat, muscle, and cardiac cells. With high-fat diets, triglyceride storage and circulation in the blood increases and can negatively influence cardiac health. Second, most of the cholesterol in the body is produced in the liver, so in some cases, excess cholesterol can be attributed to eating too many cholesterol-rich foods, which are found in animal products. The excess cholesterol can then get inside artery walls to begin forming plaque, which can eventually lead to a heart attack or stroke.*
>
> *Exercise influences your lipid levels through a number of possible methods. The simplest of these methods is whenever you exercise, you increase the number of calories you burn to provide the cells with the energy they need to function. The cells get this energy, in part, from lipids—mainly fatty acids stored within triglycerides. These triglycerides come from within the muscle, fat cells, and even from the blood. So, by exercising regularly and consisting increasing the number of calories you burn, you can positively influence LDL-c or bad cholesterol circulating in the blood. Therefore, you should prioritize increasing the time you spend exercising each week.*

EXERCISE TESTING FOR CLIENTS WITH DYSLIPIDEMIA

Exercise testing is not necessarily recommended for asymptomatic clients with dyslipidemia prior to beginning a low- to moderate-intensity exercise program.[32] However, to make the effectiveness of exercise programs and designs more individualized and scientifically sound, exercise professionals should consider exercise testing. Exercise testing clients with dyslipidemia allows exercise professionals not only to establish baseline data for exercise prescription design but also affords exercise professionals and clients, alike, the ability to track exercise-induced improvements in fitness variables.

Exercise tests and procedures are selected in a similar manner to those conducted on healthy adults. There are some precautions that exercise professionals need to consider when testing clients with dyslipidemia. Given the relationship between dyslipidemia and cardiovascular disease, it is plausible that clients with dyslipidemia may have underlying and undetected cardiovascular disease. Therefore, exercise professionals need to closely monitor clients for cardiovascular symptoms during exercise testing. The presence of other comorbidities, such as obesity and deconditioning, may require exercise professionals to modify existing exercise testing protocols, as discussed in previous chapters. Clients with dyslipidemia may also have the presence of xanthomas (cholesterol deposits under the skin). These deposits do not exclude clients from exercise or exercise testing, but new developing xanthomas should be communicated with the client and his or her physician. The same contraindications and test termination criteria exist for clients with dyslipidemia as for healthy adults.

Demonstration Case Study 6.4

Exercise Testing for Clients with Dyslipidemia

Adam is an exercise physiologist working for a hospital's chronic disease risk reduction program. Adam's job is all-encompassing, as he is responsible for educational programs, exercise testing, exercise test interpretation, and exercise prescription. His newest client is Jensen. Jensen is a 51-year-old male with dyslipidemia. His lipid profile reveals LDL-c = 155 mg/dL, HDL-c = 37 mg/dL, and triglycerides = 200 mg/dL. Jensen is not obese, having a BMI of 29 kg/m². However, Jensen has been sedentary for 25 years and is extremely deconditioned. Jensen's primary care physician recommended that he visit Adam's program to begin an exercise regimen to positively influence his lipids. Jensen was medically cleared to participate in any exercise program.

After reading Jensen's medical records, exercise history, and goals, Adam decides not to initially conduct exercise tests, although he does conduct waist circumference and body fat measurements to track improvements in body composition. Adam believes that Jensen should focus on adhering to low- to moderate-intensity exercises that he enjoys for the first several weeks. Adam's primary focus at the beginning is simply to increase the calories Jensen expends and get him to adopt a new healthy lifestyle. Once Jensen has been exercising regularly for a few weeks, Adam will then complete a submaximal cardiorespiratory fitness test on a modality that Jensen enjoys, a series of muscular endurance tests, and a sit-and-reach test.

Demonstration Case Study 6.5

Exercise Testing for Clients with Dyslipidemia

Morgan is an exercise physiologist working for a cardiometabolic exercise management clinic. Morgan is primarily responsible for exercise testing, exercise test interpretation, and exercise prescription. Her most recent client is Carol. Carol is a 56-year-old female with dyslipidemia and a normal body weight and composition. Carol's lipid profile reveals LDL-c = 137 mg/dL, HDL-c = 39 mg/dL, and triglycerides = 174 mg/dL. Despite walking for 20 minutes daily and working in her garden, Carol still developed dyslipidemia. Recently, Carol's primary care physician started Carol on a statin and recommended she seek a supervised exercise program to receive and complete a more rigorous and scientifically sound exercise regimen. Carol was medically cleared to complete any exercise program as tolerated.

With Carol's history of walking for exercise, Morgan feels that Carol should complete a submaximal treadmill test prior to exercise prescription and is fully capable of completing the submaximal Bruce protocol. Also, given Carol's history of physical work in the garden, Morgan correctly believes it is acceptable to conduct 3–5 RM tests on machine-based resistance modalities to estimate Carol's muscular strength. For flexibility, Morgan selects a sit-and-reach test, and for body composition she opts for the convenient bioelectrical impedance test.

EXERCISE PRESCRIPTION FOR CLIENTS WITH DYSLIPIDEMIA

Regular exercise offers many benefits for clients with dyslipidemia. First, regular exercise can help modify abnormal lipid profiles.[33,34] Of the lipids most consistently modified in past research, regular exercise can lower LDL-c by up to 9 mg/dL.[35] Evidence also suggests that regular exercise can play a role in modestly increasing HDL-c.[36,37] Regular exercise also results in increased energy expenditure, which can increase the oxidation of intracellular and blood-based triglycerides. Second, given the propensity of individuals with dyslipidemia to develop cardiovascular disease and the numerous individuals with concurrent dyslipidemia and other cardiovascular disease risk factors (i.e., having metabolic syndrome), regular exercise helps prevent and/or manage cardiovascular disease by modifying other cardiovascular disease risk factors.

Both cardiorespiratory and resistance exercises can help clients manage and/or prevent dyslipidemia,[38] although the primary focus of exercise prescriptions for clients with dyslipidemia should be cardiorespiratory exercise.[39] The initial exercise prescription for clients with dyslipidemia is similar to the initial exercise prescription for healthy adults with one key exception: exercise should emphasize weight loss. Accordingly, clients with dyslipidemia will need to accumulate more exercise time, 350–420 minutes per week, to expend more calories[40] or 250–300 minutes to promote weight loss or maintain current weight.

Like addressing obesity, exercise professionals should encourage clients with dyslipidemia to adhere to exercise as a part of broader lifestyle modification. Regular exercise, proper diet, and medication compliance are essential for managing dyslipidemia and preventing further cardiometabolic abnormalities. Exercise professions should be mindful of other existing health conditions, such as obesity, hypertension, and diabetes mellitus, as dyslipidemia often does not occur in isolation. Therefore, exercise responses need to continuously be monitored throughout an exercise program, and the FITT-VP should be adjusted accordingly. This section explains these modifications for cardiorespiratory, muscular fitness, and flexibility exercise for clients with dyslipidemia.

Cardiorespiratory Exercise Prescription

Overall, the cardiorespiratory exercise prescription for clients with dyslipidemia is like the prescription for healthy adults. The major difference between the two prescriptions is the accumulation of exercise time, as the emphases of exercise for clients with dyslipidemia should be weight loss and weight-loss maintenance. Therefore, cardiorespiratory exercise should be completed five or more days per week for 30–60 minutes per day.[41] This equates to a target exercise volume of 250–300 minutes weekly. As with other populations, continuous 30–60 minutes of exercise per day may not be feasible because of health, disease, or fitness status. In such cases, intermittent bouts of ten-minute cardiorespiratory exercise can be used to accumulate daily exercise time recommendations.[42]

Clients with dyslipidemia should be prescribed an initial exercise intensity between 40 and 60 percent of $\dot{V}O_2R$/HRR, depending on health and fitness status.[43] Vigorous exercise intensity, up to 75 percent of $\dot{V}O_2R$/HRR, can be prescribed as a part of a progression scheme. As with other special populations, exercise intensity can be increased after exercise time and frequency have been increased to their upper limit recommendations. Exercise modalities are chosen based primarily on a client's preference and physical capabilities.

Demonstration Case Study 6.6

Cardiorespiratory Exercise Prescription for Clients with Dyslipidemia

Colbie is an exercise physiologist specializing in lipid management. Her most recent client is Lenny. Lenny is a 54-year-old male, 215 pounds, BMI = 28.7 kg/m², and technically sedentary, although he has a physically demanding occupation. Lenny's lipid profile reveals LDL-c = 150 mg/dL, HDL-c = 35 mg/dL and triglycerides = 180 mg/dL. Lenny takes atorvastatin to manage his cholesterol levels. Lenny was medically cleared to exercise and previously completed a modified submaximal Bruce treadmill test with an estimated $\dot{V}O_{2max}$ of 31.4 mL/kg · min.

After analyzing Lenny's profile, Colbie, begins to write a cardiorespiratory exercise prescription. To facilitate elevated and accumulated energy expenditure, Colbie recommends that Lenny exercise five days per week, 35 minutes per day—two 10-minute bouts and one 15-minute bout. To initially quantify exercise intensity, Colbie chooses to use $\dot{V}O_2R$ method. Because Lenny has a physically demanding occupation and would benefit from enhanced energy expenditure, Colbie sets an initial intensity range equal to 50 to 55 percent of $\dot{V}O_2R$. Colbie's calculations are shown next.

$\dot{V}O_2R = \dot{V}O_{2max} - 3.5$ mL/kg · min

$\dot{V}O_2R = 31.4$ mL/kg · min $- 3.5$ mL/kg · min

$\dot{V}O_2R = 27.9$ mL/kg · min

50 percent of $\dot{V}O_2R = (27.9$ mL/kg · min x .5$) + 3.5$ mL/kg · min

50 percent of $\dot{V}O_2R = 17.45$ mL/kg · min

55 percent of $\dot{V}O_2R = (27.9$ mL/kg · min x .55$) + 3.5$ mL/kg · min

55 percent of $\dot{V}O_2R = 18.84$ mL/kg · min

$\dot{V}O_2R$ range = 17.45 – 18.84 mL/kg · min

Because of Lenny's physically demanding occupation and to facilitate energy expenditure, Colbie chooses walking and stepping as exercise modalities. Colbie's calculations (for the lower end of the intensity range), using metabolic equations, are provided next.

Walking Calculations:

Colbie feels that Lenny can sustain walking for 15- and 10-minute bouts walking up a 3 percent incline. She, therefore, solves for speed using the walking equation to elicit 50 percent of Lenny's $\dot{V}O_2R$.

$$17.45 \text{ mL/kg} \cdot \text{min} = (0.1 \times \text{speed}) + (1.8 \times \text{speed} \times 0.03) + 3.5$$

$$\text{Speed} = 90.58 \text{ m} \cdot \text{min} = 3.38 \text{ mph}$$

Stepping Calculations:

Because of Lenny's occupation, Colbie believes that Lenny can successfully step at a rate of 25 steps per minute for 10- to 15-minute bouts. Colbie, therefore, calculates the step height needed to elicit 50 percent of Lenny's $\dot{V}O_2R$.

$$17.45 \text{ mL/kg} \cdot \text{min} = (0.2 \times 25) + (1.33 \times 1.8 \times \text{step height} \times 25) + 3.5$$

$$\text{Step height} = 0.1495 \text{ meters} = 14.95 \text{ cm}$$

Colbie chooses a progression scheme that emphasizes the accumulation of exercise time to maximize energy expenditure. Colbie decides to increase daily exercise time by 5 percent each week until 60 minutes per day is achieved. To accomplish this, she will have to modify the initial 10- to 15-minute bouts. Once 60 minutes of exercise per day is achieved, Colbie will increase exercise intensity as tolerated with the eventual goal of having Lenny complete vigorous-intensity exercise.

Muscular Fitness and Flexibility Exercise Prescription

Resistance training can be offered as a complement to cardiorespiratory exercise for clients with dyslipidemia. Although little research shows marked improvement of dyslipidemia in response to resistance training, resistance exercise can offer additional benefits to help manage cardiovascular and metabolic disease risk. Muscular fitness exercise can be prescribed to clients with dyslipidemia using the same guidelines as for healthy adults.[44] Flexibility exercise will not modify blood lipids but can be considered for functional health purposes. Flexibility exercise, like muscular fitness exercise, is prescribed the same for clients with dyslipidemia as for healthy adults.[45]

Exercise Safety Considerations

Overall, exercise is safe for individuals with dyslipidemia. Exercise professionals must be mindful of concurrent cardiovascular disease or unknown underlying cardiovascular disease in clients with dyslipidemia and always monitor for cardiovascular symptoms during exercise training. The most common medication prescribed for dyslipidemia is a statin. Statins inhibit HMG CoA reductase and thus limit hepatic cholesterol synthesis. Therefore, it is not unusual for clients with dyslipidemia to experience myalgia or muscle weakness during an exercise program. Such symptoms need to be monitored for worsening, and the FITT-VP should be adjusted accordingly. If muscle soreness worsens, medications may have dangerously lowered cholesterol production to the point of causing rhabdomyolysis. In the event of severe muscle soreness, clients should be referred to their prescribing physician's office immediately.

Student Case Study 6.1

Exercise Test Selection for Clients with Dyslipidemia

Consider an exercise physiologist at a health-fitness clinic performing several exercise tests per day. The newest client has dyslipidemia, and the client's profile is provided next.

Demographics: (1) female and (2) 47 years old

Biometrics: (1) resting heart rate = 71 beats per minute; (2) resting blood pressure = 124/80 mmHg; (3) LDL-c = 139 mg/dL, HDL-c = 32 mg/dL, triglycerides = 189 mg/dL; (4) blood glucose = 106 mg/dL; (5) weight = 170 lbs; and (6) BMI = 29.9 kg/m²

Medical Diagnoses: (1) dyslipidemia

Medications: (1) simvastatin

Symptoms: (1) none

Exercise History: (1) weight lifting and agility drills in college and (2) current college softball coach

Exercise Goals and Needs: (1) lower LDL-c, (2) lower triglycerides, (3) increase HDL-c, and (4) improve fitness

1. Assuming the client has been medically cleared to exercise, would it be safe to conduct exercise testing on this client? In two to three sentences, provide a defense for the answer.
2. Assuming it is safe to test this client, should one conduct a maximal or submaximal cardiorespiratory fitness test? In four to five sentences, provide a defense for the decision based on the client's profile.
3. Assuming it is safe to test this client, which cardiorespiratory fitness test should be conducted? In four to five sentences, provide a defense for the decision based on the client's profile.
4. Specific to this case, which body composition test should one prefer to conduct? In four to five sentences, provide a defense for the decision based on the client's profile.
5. Assuming it is safe to test this client, to assess muscular fitness, should one conduct muscular endurance assessments or muscular strength assessments, or both? In four to five sentences, provide a defense for the decision based on the client's profile.

6. Assuming it is safe to test this client, provide a list of four specific muscular fitness tests one could conduct on the client. Then provide a four- to five-sentence defense supporting the selections.

7. List any special considerations that should be taken into account when choosing exercise tests for this client.

Student Case Study 6.2

Exercise Test Selection for Clients with Dyslipidemia

Consider an exercise physiologist at a health-fitness clinic performing several exercise tests per day. The newest client has dyslipidemia, and the client's profile is provided next.

Demographics: (1) male and (2) 52 years old

Biometrics: (1) resting heart rate = 91 beats per minute; (2) resting blood pressure = 140/88 mmHg; (3) LDL-c = 148 mg/dL, HDL-c = 32 mg/dL, triglycerides = 201 mg/dL; (4) blood glucose = 123 mg/dL; (5) weight = 285 lbs; and (6) BMI = 36.7 kg/m²

Medical Diagnoses: (1) dyslipidemia and (2) class II obesity

Medications: (1) lovastatin and (2) Propranolol (beta-blocker)

Symptoms: (1) none

Exercise History: (1) none

Exercise Goals and Needs: (1) lower LDL-c (2) lower triglycerides (3) increase HDL-c (4) weight loss

1. Assuming the client has been medically cleared to exercise, would it be safe to conduct exercise testing on this client? In two to three sentences, provide a defense for the answer.

2. Assuming it is safe to test this client, should a maximal or submaximal cardiorespiratory fitness test be conducted? In four to five sentences, provide a defense for the decision based on the client's profile.

3. Assuming it is safe to test this client, which cardiorespiratory fitness test should be conducted? In four to five sentences, provide a defense for the decision based on the client's profile.

4. Specific to this case, which body composition test should be conducted? In four to five sentences, provide a defense for the decision based on the client's profile.

5. Assuming it is safe to test this client, to assess muscular fitness, should one conduct muscular endurance assessments or muscular strength assessments, or both? In four to five sentences, provide a defense for the decision based on the client's profile.

6. Assuming it is safe to test this client, provide a list of four specific muscular fitness tests one could conduct on the client. Then provide a four- to five-sentence defense supporting the selections.

7. List any special considerations when choosing exercise tests for this client.

Student Case Study 6.3

Exercise Test Interpretation: YMCA Cycle Test

An exercise physiologist specializes in serving clients with dyslipidemia. He just completed a YMCA cycle test on a 60-year-old client weighing 200 pounds with a BMI of 28.3 kg/m^2. The results of the test are provided in Figure 6.1. After reading the results, use the graph and leg cycling equation to interpret the results and answer the questions.

Figure 6.1 This table depicts hypothetical data from a YMCA cycle test

Stage	Kpm/ min	Heart Rate	Blood Pressure	RPE	ECG	Symptoms/ Comments
Resting	0	87	118/78	NA	Sinus	No symptoms
I	150	120	136/80	14	Sinus	No symptoms
II	300	136	160/80	15	Sinus	No symptoms
Immediate	0	135	162/80	NA	Sinus	No symptoms
Recovery 1 min	0	120	150/78	NA	Sinus	No symptoms
Recovery 5 min	0	90	120/78	NA	Sinus	No symptoms

1. Using graph paper (Figure 6.2), estimate the maximal work rate (kpm/min). Then insert the estimated maximal work rate into the following equation to estimate $\dot{V}O_{2\,max}$:

   $\dot{V}O_2$ max mL/kg · min = (1.8 x estimated maximal work rate/kg body weight) + 7.

2. What factors could influence the accuracy of this test?

3. What should an exercise physiologist consider to enhance safety during the completion of this test?

Figure 6.2 Students may use these gridlines to graph data from the YMCA cycle test

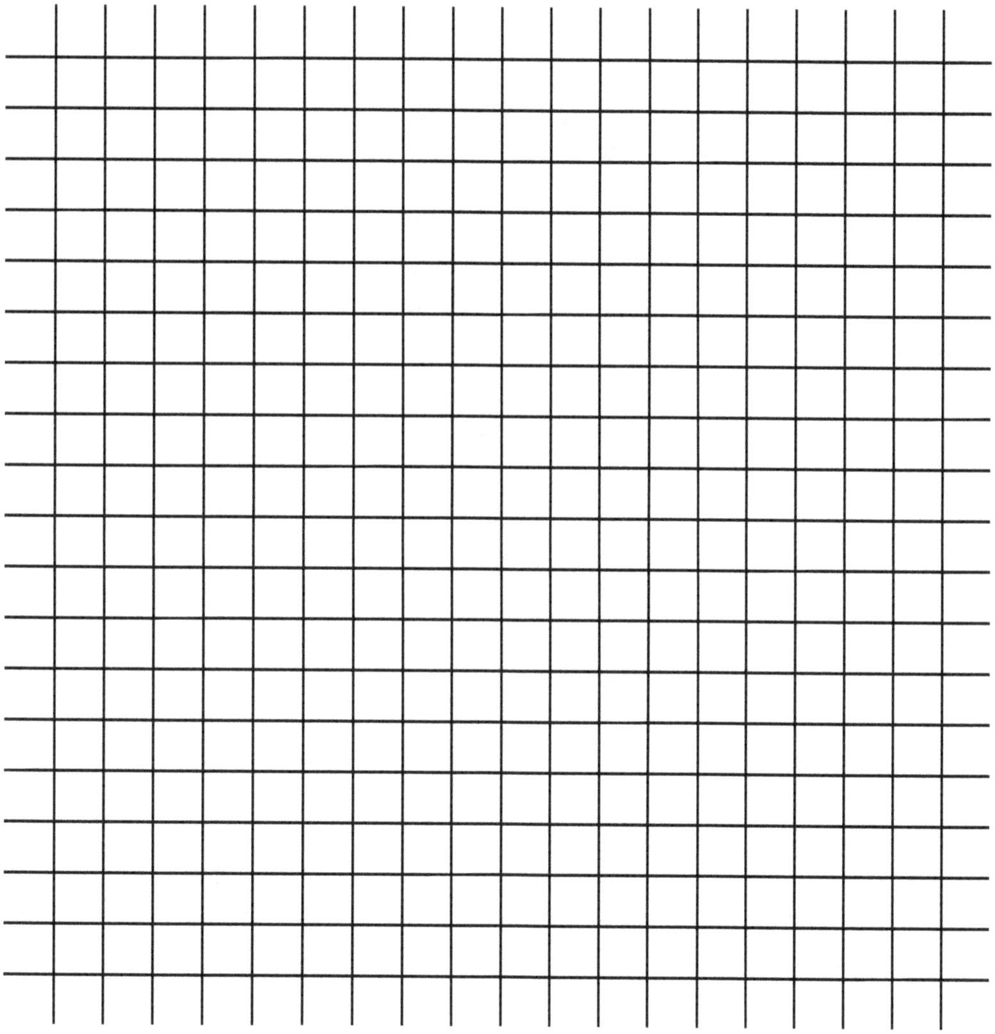

Student Case Study 6.4

Exercise Test Interpretation: Submaximal Treadmill Test

An exercise physiologist specializes in serving clients with dyslipidemia. She just completed a submaximal treadmill test using the modified Bruce protocol on a 50-year-old female who has dyslipidemia, is sedentary, weighs 130 pounds and is severely deconditioned. The test was terminated at a heart rate equal to 70 percent of the client's heart rate reserve. The results of the test are provided in Figure 6.3. After reading the results, use the walking or running equation and a proportion equation to interpret the results and answer the questions.

Figure 6.3 This table depicts hypothetical data from a submaximal treadmill test

Stage	Speed (mph)	Grade %	Heart Rate	Blood Pressure	RPE	ECG	Symptoms
Resting	0	0	80	136/88	NA	Sinus	No symptoms
I	1.7	0	107	160/88	10	Sinus	No symptoms
II	1.7	5	131	180/90	13	Sinus	No symptoms
III	1.7	10	143	198/88	16	Sinus	No symptoms
Immediate	1.5	0	144	200/88	NA	Sinus	No symptoms
Recovery 1 min	1.5	0	132	176/88	NA	Sinus	No symptoms
Recovery 5 min	1	0	100	154/86	NA	Sinus	No symptoms

1. Using one of the following two equations, estimate $\dot{V}O_2$ for the last completed stage:

   Walking: $\dot{V}O_2$ = (0.1 x speed in m/min) + (1.8 x speed in m/min x grade) + 3.5

   Running: $\dot{V}O_2$ = (0.2 x speed in m/min) + (0.9 x speed in m/min x grade) + 3.5

   Find $\dot{V}O_2$ in last stage in mL/kg · min

   Find estimated $\dot{V}O_{2max}$ in mL/kg · min

2. Given the client has dyslipidemia and is severely deconditioned, what steps should an exercise physiologist take to ensure safety during this test? Was this chosen protocol appropriate for the client? Defend the answer in two to three sentences. Then explain other potential health conditions that this client may have and be sure to defend the answer.

Student Case Study 6.5

Muscular Strength Testing for Clients with Dyslipidemia

An exercise physiologist specializes in serving clients with dyslipidemia. The newest client is a 57-year-old female with dyslipidemia and a BMI of 29.0 kg/m² who weighs 153 pounds. The exercise physiologist wants to prescribe this client a resistance training program as a complement to cardiorespiratory exercise to provide addition cardiovascular disease risk reduction benefits. Therefore, the exercise physiologist conducts a series of muscular strength tests. The following data were collected (Figure 6.4).

Figure 6.4 This table depicts hypothetical data from a 3–5RM test

Leg Press Strength Test

Trial 1	_____5_____ repetitions _____100_____ weight
Trial 2	_____4_____ repetitions _____110_____ weight
Trial 3	_____3_____ repetitions _____115_____ weight
Best Trial	_____3_____ repetitions _____115_____ weight

Chest Press Strength Test

Trial 1	_____4_____ repetitions _____70_____ weight
Trial 2	_____3_____ repetitions _____75_____ weight
Trial 3	_____3_____ repetitions _____75_____ weight
Best Trial	_____3_____ repetitions _____75_____ weight

1. Use the Lander equation to predict the client's maximal leg press strength.
2. Calculate a weight pushed to body weight ratio and compare the client's results to normative data.
3. Use the Lander equation to predict the client's maximal chest press strength.
4. Calculate a weight pushed to body weight ratio and compare the client's results to normative data.
5. What steps can the exercise physiologist take to ensure safety during these strength tests?

Student Case Study 6.6

Exercise Prescription for Clients with Dyslipidemia: Cardiorespiratory Endurance

An exercise professional specializes in serving clients with dyslipidemia. The newest client is a 46-year-male with dyslipidemia and a normal body weight of 175 pounds; he doesn't take any cardiac medications, is prescribed a low-dose statin, and has a history of moderate-intensity jogging twice per week. The exercise professional just conducted a maximal exercise test, completed without complications, and the client achieved a measured $\dot{V}O_{2max}$ of 35.7 mL/kg · min and a maximum heart rate of 172 bpm. Prior to the test, the client's resting heart rate was 66 beats per minute. The client is open to any form of exercise but prefers jogging and stepping.

1. Calculate a heart rate range based on the heart rate reserve that the client should maintain during aerobic exercise. Should an exercise professional use this heart rate range during exercise training or consider other methods of quantifying exercise intensity? Why or why not?
2. Calculate a $\dot{V}O_2$ range based on the $\dot{V}O_2$ reserve that the client should maintain during aerobic exercise.
3. Provide an exercise type (be specific), frequency, and time at the $\dot{V}O_2$ range found in question 2 for the client to improve his cardiorespiratory fitness and better manage his blood lipids.
4. Suggest four possible aerobic exercises that would be appropriate for this client. Then explain the rationale for each selection.
5. Use the walking or running equation to calculate a walking or running speed (in mph) for the client that elicits the upper end of the $\dot{V}O_2$ reserve range found in question 2. The percent grade of the treadmill is 2.0 percent.
6. Use the stepping equation to calculate a stepping rate for the client that elicits the lower end of the $\dot{V}O_2$ reserve range found in question 2. The height of the step is 25 centimeters.
7. Use the leg cycle equation to calculate a resistance to be placed on the Monark flywheel for the client that elicits the upper end of the $\dot{V}O_2$ reserve range found in question 2. The client peddles at 100 rpm.
8. Suggest a progression scheme to advance the client toward a goal of improving his blood lipids. Should vigorous-intensity exercise eventually be considered? Why or why not?
9. Provide three training considerations to help this client improve his blood lipids through cardiorespiratory exercise safely. One of the considerations must address potential issues with medication and exercise.

Student Case Study 6.7

Exercise Prescription for Clients with Dyslipidemia: Cardiorespiratory Endurance

An exercise professional specializes in serving clients with dyslipidemia. The newest client is a 59-year-female with dyslipidemia, taking a beta-blocker and a statin, with a BMI of 33.9 kg/m² weighing 209 pounds, and no history of exercise. The exercise professional just conducted an Astrand-Rhyming cycle test, completed without complications, and the client achieved an estimated $\dot{V}O_{2max}$ of 18.1 mL/kg · min. Prior to the test, the client's resting heart rate was 67 beats per minute. The client is open to any form of exercise.

1. Calculate a heart rate range based on the heart rate reserve that the client should maintain during aerobic exercise. Should the exercise professional use this heart rate range during exercise training or consider other methods of quantifying exercise intensity? Why or why not?

2. Calculate a $\dot{V}O_2$ range based on the $\dot{V}O_2$ reserve that the client should maintain during aerobic exercise.

3. Provide an exercise type (be specific), frequency, and time at the $\dot{V}O_2$ range found in question 2 for the client to improve her cardiorespiratory fitness and better manage her blood lipids.

4. Suggest four possible aerobic exercises that would be appropriate for this client. Then explain the rationale for each selection.

5. Use the walking equation to calculate an appropriate walking speed (in mph) and incline for the client that elicits the lower end of the $\dot{V}O_2$ reserve range found in question 2.

6. Use the leg cycling equation to calculate an appropriate peddling frequency and resistance on a BodyGuard ergometer to elicit the upper end of the $\dot{V}O_2$ reserve range found in question 2.

7. Use the arm cycle equation to calculate an appropriate peddle frequency and resistance to be placed on the flywheel for the client that elicits the lower end of the $\dot{V}O_2$ reserve range found in question 2.

8. Suggest a progression scheme to advance the client toward a goal of improving her blood lipids.

9. Would progressing to high-intensity interval training be appropriate for this client? If so, what cautions should be considered? If not, explain why.

10. Provide three training considerations to help this client improve her body lipids through cardiorespiratory exercise safely.

Student Case Study 6.8

Exercise Prescription for Clients with Dyslipidemia: Muscular Fitness

An exercise physiologist specializes in training clients with dyslipidemia. The exercise physiologist was recently presented with the following client data: (1) 55-year-old male, (2) dyslipidemia, (3) class I obesity weighing 222 pounds, (4) goals to improve muscular strength and further reduce cardiovascular disease risk, (5) chest press 1RM = 125 pounds, (6) leg press 1RM = 215 pounds, and (7) open to any resistance exercise program.

1. Provide a range for weight that the client should chest press.
2. Provide a range for weight that the client should leg press.
3. Provide a resistance exercise prescription for frequency and number of exercises, sets, and repetitions to improve muscular strength.

4. Suggest at least four specific resistance training exercises that are appropriate for this client.
5. Suggest a progression scheme to advance the client toward the goal of improving muscular strength.
6. How would the resistance training program be different if the client expressed interest in specifically targeting muscular endurance?
7. Explain how to design the resistance training program to maximize client adherence.
8. Explain, in four to five sentences, how adherence to this resistance training program will help improve the overall health of the client in addition to amplifying his caloric expenditure.

Student Case Study 6.9

Exercise Testing and Prescription: Comprehensive Case Study

An exercise physiologist works for a chronic disease risk reduction clinic. He thoroughly collected the following data from their most recent client:

Demographics: (1) female and (2) 60 years old

Family History: (1) father had a myocardial infarction at the age of 49, (2) mother had coronary revascularization at the age of 66.

Biometrics: (1) resting heart rate = 67 beats per minute; (2) resting blood pressure = 130/80 mmHg; (3) LDL-c = 136 mg/dL, HDL-c = 39 mg/dL, triglycerides = 187 mg/dL; (4) glycosylated hemoglobin = 6.0 percent and blood glucose = 119.7 mg/dL; and (5) weight = 247 lbs., BMI = 31.2 kg/m²

Medical Diagnoses: (1) dyslipidemia, (2) class I obesity

Medications: (1) atorvastatin

Symptoms: (1) none

Exercise History: (1) no recent exercise history, (2) does not like cycling

Exercise Goals and Needs: (1) optimize blood lipids, (2) weight loss

1. Should the exercise physiologist conduct a maximal or submaximal cardiorespiratory fitness test? In four to five sentences, provide a defense for the decision based on the client's profile.
2. Which cardiorespiratory fitness test should be conducted? In four to five sentences, provide a defense for the decision based on the client's profile.
3. Given limitless resources, which body composition test should the exercise physiologist conduct? In four to five sentences, provide a defense for the decision based on the client's profile.
4. Given minimal resources with a small budget, which body composition test should be conducted? In four to five sentences, provide a defense for the decision based on the client's profile.

5. Specific to this case, which body composition test would be preferred? In four to five sentences, provide a defense for the decision based on the client's profile.

6. To assess muscular fitness, should muscular endurance assessments or muscular strength assessments be conducted, or both? In four to five sentences, provide a defense for the decision based on the client's profile.

7. Provide a list of four specific muscular fitness tests to be conducted on the client. Then provide a four- to five- sentence defense supporting the selections.

8. Provide a list of four specific muscular fitness tests to be conducted on the client. Then provide a four- to five-sentence defense supporting the selections.

9. Based on the answers for questions 1 and 2, calculate the client's $\dot{V}O_{2max}$ from the most appropriate of the following cardiorespiratory fitness tests (Figures 6.5–6.9).

Figure 6.5 This table depicts hypothetical data from a YMCA cycle test

			YMCA Cycle Test			
Stage	**Kpm/ min**	**Heart Rate**	**Blood Pressure**	**RPE**	**ECG**	**Symptoms/ Comments**
Resting	0	67	130/80	NA	Sinus	No symptoms
I	150	92	136/82	11	Sinus	No symptoms
II	450	119	152/82	12	Sinus	No symptoms
III	600	132	168/82	13	Sinus	No symptoms
Immediate	100	133	166/80	NA	Sinus	No symptoms
Recovery 1 min	50	120	146/80	NA	Sinus	No symptoms
Recovery 5 min	25	73	132/78	NA	Sinus	No symptoms

Figure 6.6 Students may use these gridlines to graph data from the YMCA cycle test

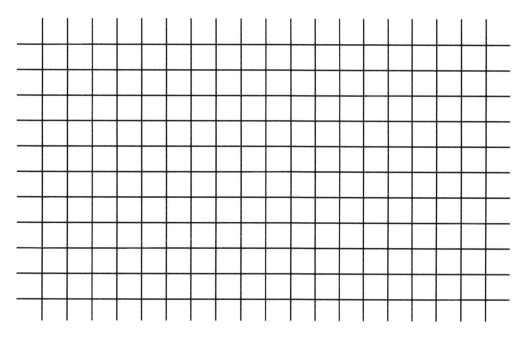

Figure 6.7 This table depicts hypothetical data from a submaximal treadmill test

Submaximal Bruce Protocol

Stage	Speed (mph)	Grade %	Heart Rate	Blood Pressure	RPE	ECG	Symptoms
Resting	0	0	67	130/80	NA	Sinus	No symptoms
I	1.7	10.0	88	142/80	10	Sinus	No symptoms
II	2.5	12.0	121	154/80	12	Sinus	No symptoms
III	3.4	14.0	132	174/80	15	Sinus	No symptoms
Immediate	1.5	0	132	176/80	NA	Sinus	No symptoms
Recovery 1 min	1.5	0	120	160/78	NA	Sinus	No symptoms
Recovery 5 min	1	0	71	138/78	NA	Sinus	No symptoms

Figure 6.8 This table depicts hypothetical data from a maximal treadmill test

Maximal Treadmill Test

Stage	Time	Speed (mph)	Grade %	Blood Pressure	$\dot{V}O_2$ (mL/ kg · min)	Blood Lactate (mmol)	RPE	Heart Rate	RER
Resting	NA	0	0	130/80	3.8	NA	NA	67	0.77
I	2:00	3.5	2	142/80	15.5	1.2	13	103	0.86
II	4:00	4.5	4	160/78	22.9	3.8	14	120	1.01
III	6:00	5.5	6	184/78	30.1	5.1	17	146	1.07
IV	8:00	6.5	8	198/80	33.7	8.7	18	160	1.16
Immediate	NA	1.5	0	200/82	27.6	NA	NA	161	1.15
Recovery 1 min	NA	1.5	0	176/80	20.1	NA	NA	140	1.02
Recovery 5 min	NA	1	0	140/76	8.8	NA	NA	81	0.99

Comments: Test terminated because of volitional fatigue

Figure 6.9 This table depicts hypothetical data from a maximal cycle test

Maximal Cycle Test

Stage	Time	Kpm /min	Heart Rate	Blood Pressure	RPE	$\dot{V}O_2$ (mL/ kg · min.)	RER	Blood Lactate (mmol)	ECG
Resting		0	67	130/80	NA	3.9	0.76	NA	Sinus
I	2:00	600	100	138/80	10	12.4	0.77	1.1	Sinus
II	4:00	900	115	158/80	15	22.9	0.97	4.4	Sinus
III	6:00	1200	130	170/82	16	28.7	1.00	6.1	Sinus
IV	8:00	1500	152	188/84	18	30.1	1.12	8.2	Sinus

(Continued)

Figure 6.9 This table depicts hypothetical data from a maximal cycle test (Continued)

Maximal Cycle Test

Stage	Time	Kpm /min	Heart Rate	Blood Pressure	RPE	$\dot{V}O_2$ (mL/ kg · min.)	RER	Blood Lactate (mmol)	ECG
Immediate	NA	300	154	186/84	NA	30.0	1.13	NA	Sinus
Recovery 1 min	NA	150	141	160/80	NA	20.1	1.01	NA	Sinus
Recovery 5 min	NA	75	80	142/78	NA	10.3	0.94	NA	Sinus

Comments: Test terminated because of volitional fatigue

10. For the cardiorespiratory fitness test chosen to interpret the answer for question 9, should the test have been terminated prior to completion? Explain why or why not.

11. Assuming the skinfold assessment for body composition test was selected, calculate body fat percentage from the following seven-site skinfold data (Figure 6.10).

Figure 6.10 This table depicts hypothetical data from a seven-site skinfold assessment

Site	Trial 1	Trial 2	Trial 3	Average
Triceps	15	17	16	mm
Subscapular	19	20	20.5	mm
Chest	20	22	21	mm
Abdominal	23	25	23.75	mm
Suprailiac	20	21	20.75	mm
Midaxillary	19	17.75	18.75	mm
Thigh	25	27	26.25	mm

12. Assuming muscular strength was selected, interpret and classify the client's leg and chest press strength from the following data (Figure 6.11; compare results with normative data).

Figure 6.11 This table depicts hypothetical data from a 3–5RM test

Leg Press Strength Test

Trial 1	_____5_____ repetitions
	_____180_____ weight
Trial 2	_____4_____ repetitions
	_____190_____ weight

(Continued)

Figure 6.11 This table depicts hypothetical data from a 3–5RM test (Continued)

Leg Press Strength Test

Trial 3	3	repetitions
	200	weight
Best Trial	3	repetitions
	200	weight

Chest Press Strength Test

Trial 1	5	repetitions
	105	weight
Trial 2	5	repetitions
	115	weight
Trial 3	5	repetitions
	120	weight
Best Trial	5	repetitions
	120	weight

13. Calculate a heart rate range based on the heart rate reserve that the client should maintain during aerobic exercise. Is this the most reliable method for quantifying cardiorespiratory endurance exercise? Why or why not?

14. Calculate a $\dot{V}O_2$ range based on the $\dot{V}O_2$ reserve that the client should maintain during aerobic exercise.

15. Provide an exercise type (be specific), frequency, and time at the $\dot{V}O_2$ range found in question 14 for the client to improve her cardiorespiratory fitness and manage her blood lipids.

16. Suggest four possible aerobic exercises that would be appropriate for this client.

17. Provide a walking speed and grade for the client to maintain on the treadmill to elicit the lower end of the $\dot{V}O_2$ range listed in question 14.

18. Provide a resistance and arm crank frequency for arm cycling to elicit the lower end of the $\dot{V}O_2$ range listed in question 14.

19. Provide a step height and stepping frequency to elicit the lower end of the $\dot{V}O_2$ range listed in question 14.

20. Suggest a progression scheme for improving cardiorespiratory fitness. Would vigorous-intensity or high-intensity interval training be warranted? Why or why not?

21. Based on the lower end of the intensity range in question 14 and exercise frequency and time found in question 15, how many weeks will it take for the client to lose 20 pounds through exercise alone?

22. Provide a range for weight that the client should chest press.

23. Provide a range for weight that the client should leg press.

24. Provide a resistance exercise prescription for frequency and number of exercises, sets, and repetitions to improve muscular fitness.

25. Suggest at least four specific resistance training exercises that are appropriate for this client.

26. Suggest a progression scheme to help the client improve overall muscular fitness.

27. Provide a frequency, intensity, number of stretches, sets, and the amount of time each stretch should be to help improve the client's flexibility.

28. Provide a list consisting of all safety considerations that should be considered when supervising this client's exercise program.

REFERENCES

1. P. P. Toth, D. Potter, and E. E. Ming, "Prevalence of Lipid Abnormalities in the United States: The National Health and Nutrition Examination Survey 2003–2006," *Journal of Clinical Lipidology* 6, no. 4 (2012): 325–30.

2. D. C. J. Goff, A. G. Bertoni, H. Kramer, et al., "Dyslipidemia Prevelance, Treatment, and Control in the Multi-Ethnic Study of Atherosclerosis: Gender, Ethnicity, and Coronary Artery Calcium," *Circulation* 113, no. 5 (2006): 647–56.

3. J. Stamler, M. L. Daviglus, D. B. Garside, et al., "Relationship of Baseline Serum Cholesterol Levels in 3 Large Cohorts of Younger Men to Long-Term Coronary, Cardiovascular, and All-Cause Mortality and to Longevity," *JAMA* 284, no. 3 (2000): 311–18.

4. R. M. Adibhatla and J. F. Hatcher, "Altered Lipid Metabolism in Brain Injury and Disorders," *Subcellular Biochemistry* 49 (2008): 241–68.

5. M. H. Criqui, "Peripheral Artery Disease—Epidemiological Aspects," *Vascular Medicine* 6, no. 1 (2001): 3–7.

6. D. Leroith, "Pathophysiology of the Metabolic Syndrome: Implications for the Cardiometabolic Risks Associated with Type 2 Diabetes," *American Journal of the Medical Sciences* 343, no. 1 (2012): 13–16.

7. Stamler et al., "Relationship of Baseline."

8. Adibhatla et al., "Altered Lipid Metabolism."

9. Criqui et al., "Peripheral Artery Disease."

10. American College of Sports Medicine, *ACSM's Guidelines for Exercise Testing and Prescription*, 11th ed. (Philadelphia: Wolters Kluwer Health, 2022).

11. ibid.

12. ibid.

13. A. Mente, L. de Koning, H. S. Shannon, and S. S. Anand, "A Systematic Review of the Evidence Supporting a Causal Link between Dietary Factors and Coronary Heart Disease," *Archives of Internal Medicine* 169, no. 7 (2009): 659–69.

14. ibid.

15. P. Jellinger, D. Smith, A. Mehta, et al., "American Association of Clinical Endocrinologists' Guidelines for Management of Dyslipidemia and Prevention of Atherosclerosis," *Endocrine Practice* 1(2012; 18 Suppl 1):1–78.

16. Leroith et al., "Pathophysiology of the Metabolic."

17. American College of Sports Medicine, *ACSM's Guidelines*.

18. Leroith et al., "Pathophysiology of the Metabolic".

19. G. A. Brooks, T. D. Fahey, and K. M. Baldwin, *Exercise Physiology: Human Bioenergetics and Its Applications, 4th edition* (New York: McGraw-Hill Higher Education, 2005).

20. D. A. Hood, "Mechanisms of Exercise-Induced Mitochondrial Biogenesis in Skeletal Muscle," *Applied Physiology, Nutrition, and Metabolism* 34, no. 3 (2009): 465–72.

21. H. N. Hodis, W. J. Mack, R. A. Lobo, et al., "Estrogen in the Prevention of Atherosclerosis: A Randomized, Double-Blind, Placebo-Controlled Trial," *Annals of Internal Medicine* 135, no. 11 (2001): 939–53.

22. A. C. St-Pierre, I. L. Ruel, B. Cantin, et al., "Comparison of Various Electrophoretic Characteristics of LDL Particles and Their Relationship to the Risk of Ischemic Heart Disease," *Circulation* 104 (2001): 2295–99.

23. K. Musunuru, "Atherogenic Dyslipidemia: Cardiovascular Risk and Dietary Intervention," *Lipids* 45, no. 10 (2010): 907–14.

24. S. Kodama, S. Tanaka, K. Saito, et al., "Effect of Aerobic Exercise Training on Serum Levels of High-Density Lipoprotein Cholesterol: A Meta-Analysis," *Archives of Internal Medicine* 167, no. 10 (2007): 999–1008.

25. M. A. Frey, B. M. Doerr, L. L. Laubach, et al., "Exercise Does Not Change High-Density Lipoprotein Cholesterol in Women after Ten Weeks of Training," *Metabolism* 31, no. 11 (1982): 1142–46.

26. K. J. Elliott, C. Sale, and N. T. Cable, "Effects of Resistance Training and Detraining on Muscle Strength and Blood Lipid Profiles in Postmenopausal Women," *BMJ* 36, no. 5 (2002): 340–44.

27. P. F. Kokkinos, B. F. Hurley, P. Vaccaro, et al., "Effects of Low- and High-Repetition Resistive Training on Lipoprotein-Lipid Profiles," *Medicine and Science in Sports and Exercise* 20, no. 1 (1988): 50–54.

28. S. Mann, C. Beedie, A. Jimenez, "Differential Effects of Aerobic Exercise, Resistance Training and Combined Exercise Modalities on Cholesterol and the Lipid Profile: Review, Synthesis and Recommendations," *Sports Medicine* 44, no. 2 (2014): 211–21.

29. American College of Sports Medicine, *ACSM's Guidelines.*

30. B. Egan and J. R. Zierath, "Exercise Metabolism and the Molecular Regulation of Skeletal Muscle Adaptation," Cell Metabolism 17, no. 2 (2013): 162–84.

31. C. Wei, M. Penumetcha, N. Santanam, et al., "Exercise Might Favor Reverse Cholesterol Transport and Lipoprotein Clearance: Potential Mechanism for Its Anti-atherosclerotic Effects," *BBA-General Subjects* 1723, no. 1 (2005): 124–27.

32. American College of Sports Medicine, *ACSM's Guidelines.*

33. Mann et al., "Differential Effects."

34. American College of Sports Medicine, *ACSM's Guidelines.*

35. ibid.

36. Kokkinos et al., "Effects of Low."

37. Kodama et al., "Effect of Aerobic Exercise."

38. Kodama et al., "Effect of Aerobic Exercise."

39. American College of Sports Medicine, *ACSM's Guidelines.*

40. ibid.

41. ibid.

42. ibid.

43. ibid.

44. ibid.

45. ibid.

Exercise Testing and Prescription for Clients with Arthritis, Fibromyalgia, and Osteoporosis

INTRODUCTION

Over half of the US adult population suffers from conditions such as arthritis, fibromyalgia, and osteoporosis.[1,2,3] These neuromusculoskeletal conditions can limit affected individuals' ability to carry out activities of daily living, physical activity, and regular exercise as they are often restricted by pain, fatigue, and joint stiffness.[4,5] Accordingly, it is not unusual for these populations to lose muscle mass and strength, store excess fat mass, acquire dyslipidemia and hypertension, and, ultimately, develop chronic diseases, such as cardiovascular disease, type II diabetes mellitus, and certain cancers—all because of a lack of regular movement.[6,7]

Exercise professionals are uniquely positioned to serve clients with neuromusculoskeletal ailments. Although exercise professionals cannot prescribe programs intended to rehabilitate these conditions, they can assist in modifying physical activities and exercises to bring about specific physiological and structural improvements, which in turn can reduce chronic disease risk and progression to disability. In addition, regular exercise can reduce pain and mitigate functional limitations, which act to improve overall quality of life among these populations.[8,9,10]

Each neuromusculoskeletal ailment presents with different pathologies, symptoms, and exercise-related challenges. Therefore, uniform recommendations for exercise testing and training that encompass these populations are not established. Thus the purpose of this chapter is to present the common neuromusculoskeletal conditions, teach students how to select appropriate fitness tests, and to modify the FITT-VP to bring about favorable adaptations for improving quality of life and reducing the risk of cardiometabolic diseases. On completion of the case studies within this chapter, students will be able to achieve the following:

1. Describe the causes and characteristics of arthritis (osteoarthritis and rheumatoid arthritis), fibromyalgia, and osteoporosis
2. Explain to and educate clients about how regular exercise can slow the progression of arthritis, fibromyalgia, and osteoporosis; improve quality of life; and prevent the onset of cardiometabolic diseases

3. Select and interpret appropriate exercise tests and apply the cardiorespiratory, muscular fitness, and flexibility FITT-VP recommendations and modifications to clients with arthritis, fibromyalgia, or osteoporosis
4. Identify and understand safety considerations for training clients with neuromusculoskeletal conditions

ARTHRITIS

Arthritis refers broadly to more than 100 different diseases that are characterized by the presence of persistent joint pain. In addition to joint pain, arthritis also leads to limitations in functional capacity, fatigue, muscle atrophy, and increased adiposity. Altogether, the physical limitation imposed from arthritis and other joint conditions account for the leading causes of disability in the United States.[11,12] Further, adverse changes in body composition and diminished movement capacity accelerate the development of cardiometabolic disease risk factors, such as dyslipidemia, elevated blood glucose, and hypertension. Therefore, finding methods to keep individuals with arthritis physically active is paramount in preventing the onset of disability and chronic diseases.

Of the more than 100 different types of arthritis, osteoarthritis and rheumatoid arthritis are the most common. Osteoarthritis occurs when cartilage within a given joint is degraded to the point that articulating bones come into contact and cause joint pain and inflammation. Osteoarthritis can occur in one or more joints and becomes a significant challenge for physical activity when it affects weight-bearing joints, such as the knees, intervertebral joints, and hips. Osteoarthritis is more common than rheumatoid arthritis and is caused by several factors, including obesity, previous injury, and age.

Rheumatoid arthritis is a chronic, systematic, and inflammatory autoimmune disease in which inflammation within joints leads to joint erosion. The inflammatory response of rheumatoid arthritis can also cause damage to internal organs, augment the development of atherosclerosis, and degrade skeletal muscle. Currently, the causes of rheumatoid arthritis are under debate. However, some evidence suggests that genetic predisposition and environmental factors, such as smoking and viral infections, can increase the risk of developing rheumatoid arthritis.[13]

Regular exercise offers important benefits for clients with arthritis. Aside from pain management, regular exercise can improve cardiorespiratory fitness and muscular strength, as well as promote the hypertrophy or maintenance of muscle mass. These adaptations are critical for avoiding progression to disability, cardiovascular disease, or type II diabetes. Further, regular exercise can reduce inflammation and pain, in addition to improving overall quality of life among clients with arthritis. The major challenge for exercise professionals is not necessarily exercise prescription design but promoting exercise adherence. Therefore, reassuring clients that exercise will not further worsen their condition and can help manage symptoms is a strategy that exercise professionals should adopt.

EXERCISE TESTING FOR CLIENTS WITH ARTHRITIS

Exercise testing should be considered when serving clients with arthritis. The results of exercise testing not only provide exercise professionals with the baseline data necessary for designing initial exercise prescriptions and tracking progression but also allows exercise professionals to know the extent to which clients with arthritis can tolerate exercise. The recommendations for exercise testing of clients with arthritis are the same as for healthy adults. However, there are additional considerations exercise professionals must take into account. First, maximal effort tests are contraindicated in the presence of systemic inflammation.[14] Systemic inflammation is characterized by warm, swollen, and painful joints. Second, exercise professionals should select exercise tests that are likely to be less painful. Third, pain should be recorded using a zero- to ten-point scale, and future exercise should be at intensities below pain thresholds.[15,16] Lastly, joint pain may impair muscular contractions and, therefore, maximal strength test results may not be completely reflective of true muscular strength—especially when muscles being targeted for testing traverse arthritic joints.[17]

Demonstration Case Study 7.1

Exercise Test Selection for Clients with Arthritis

Lani is an exercise professional who specializes in training clients with arthritis. She is supervising an exercise science intern from a nearby university when her newest client, Abigail, arrives for exercise testing. Abigail is a 50-year-old female with osteoarthritis in both knees. She takes nonsteroidal anti-inflammatory medications to manage her condition. Because of Abigail's osteoarthritis, she has not exercised in nearly ten years and as a result is deconditioned and slightly overweight. Abigail was recently medically cleared to participate in an exercise program.

Lani reviews Abigail's medical history with her intern and begins to explain her exercise test selections and rationale for each. First, Lani tells her intern that she will be conducting an Astrand-Rhyming cycle test to evaluate Abigail's cardiorespiratory fitness. She tells the intern that the Astrand-Rhyming cycle test is non-weight bearing and is appropriate for someone suffering from arthritis in weight-bearing joints. Further, Lani asserts that the Astrand-Rhyming cycle test is a single-stage test, which can help avoid struggles with pain and exertion. The second set of tests that Lani wants to conduct are muscular endurance tests. She tells the intern that she wants to assess Abigail's capacity for muscular fitness exercise and will do so by having Abigail complete simple body weight tests. For body composition, Lani tells the intern that she will conduct girth measurements and bioelectrical impedance. Lani explains that arthritis can lead to cardiovascular disease, and it is useful to track risk factors for this condition. Lani explains that these girth measurements and bioelectrical impedance, although not the most accurate tests, are appropriate for overweight individuals and can give good feedback on body composition improvements.

Prior to testing Abigail, Lani goes over safety considerations for exercise testing with her intern. Lani tells the intern that she will monitor pain throughout all tests. Lani explains that she wants to know the pain threshold so as to avoid inducing too much pain during exercise training, as it may discourage Abigail from continuing with her exercise program. Next, Lani tells the intern that she will suggest a warm-up prior to testing. The reason for this is to allow Abigail to get accustomed to the exercises she will be performing and to increase the temperature and pliability of skeletal muscles, which can help prevent pain during testing. Lastly, Lani explains that it is important to check for systemic inflammation, especially in clients with rheumatoid arthritis. Although Abigail does not have rheumatoid arthritis, this is still a worthwhile assessment. Lani explains to the intern that clients with systemic inflammation will have warm, swollen, and painful joints, and if systemic inflammation is present, exercise testing or exercise will need to be suspended until the inflammation subsides.

EXERCISE PRESCRIPTION FOR CLIENTS WITH ARTHRITIS

Exercise recommendations for clients with arthritis are like those for healthy adults. However, the FITT-VP principle must be modified to account for disease status, pain, fitness, physical capabilities, and exercise preferences. Clients with arthritis should perform cardiorespiratory exercises three to five days per week, at 40–60 percent of HRR/$\dot{V}O_2R$, and accumulate 150 minutes of exercise per week.[18] Bouts of ten-minute aerobic exercise may be warranted if a client cannot sustain exercise for 30 continuous minutes because of pain. Vigorous cardiorespiratory exercise intensities can be prescribed or progressed to as tolerated by the client and if completed safely. Exercise professionals can consider prescribing non-weight-bearing aerobic exercises if weight-bearing joints are arthritic. Otherwise, exercise modalities can be left to a client's preference to increase exercise adherence. Progression should be slow, increasing exercise time and frequency before intensity.

It is also recommended that clients with arthritis complete resistance exercise two to three days per week, targeting each major muscle group. The resistance applied should be dependent on a client's goals and physical limitations. If a client desires to increase strength and/or muscle mass and is physically capable, a starting intensity between 60 and 80 percent 1RM is acceptable.[19] However, if a client's goal is to increase muscular endurance, is physically limited, or deconditioned, a starting intensity range between 50 and 60 percent 1RM is more appropriate.[20] Otherwise, set and repetition schemes are like those presented in Chapter 2. Like cardiorespiratory exercise, progression should be slow, and modifications to sets and repetitions should be made prior to the applied resistance.

There are several safety considerations that exercise professionals must take into account when serving clients with arthritis. First, all exercise programs should be completed with minimal pain, and every effort must be made to ensure no joint damage occurs. This means exercise professionals should emphasize technique, promote adherence by selecting exercise intensities and ground-impact exercises that limit delayed onset muscle soreness and other inflammatory responses, and chose modalities that can be successfully and enjoyably completed by clients. During acute "flare-ups," exercise professionals should encourage clients to gently move joints through their full range of motion and consider flexibility exercises to limit joint stiffness.[21] Exercise professionals can consider aquatic exercises in warm pool water (83–88 degrees Fahrenheit).[22] Lastly, exercise professionals should make sure clients wear appropriate shoes and clothing to reduce the risk of injury, communicate with physicians concerning worsening conditions, and comply with any physician orders.

Demonstration Case Study 7.2

Exercise Prescription for Clients with Arthritis

Asia is an exercise physiologist specializing in training clients with arthritis. Her most recent client is Paul. Paul is a 47-year-old male, 220 pounds, BMI = 30.1 kg/m², and sedentary with bilateral hip osteoarthritis. Paul reported to Asia's clinic seeking an exercise program to help improve the quality of his life, reduce chronic pain, and improve his overall health. Paul was fully cleared by his physician with orders to exercise with minimal pain—no more than a three on a zero- to ten-point pain scale. Paul told Asia that he would enjoy exercises that are not weight bearing.

After completing a series of exercise tests, the following fitness data were obtained: (1) estimated $\dot{V}O_{2max}$ of 23.5 mL/kg · min using the Astrand-Rhyming cycle protocol, (2) chest press 1RM = 120 pounds, (3) leg press 1RM = 200 pounds, (4) seated shoulder press 1RM = 80 pounds, (5) seated crunch 1RM = 100 pounds, (6) leg extension 1RM = 80 pounds, (7) leg curl 1RM = 60 pounds, (8) body fat percentage = 30 percent, and (9) sit-and-reach score was poor.

After analyzing Paul's medical history, exercise preferences, and exercise test scores, Asia begins to write a comprehensive exercise prescription. First, Asia recommends cardiorespiratory exercises to be completed three days per week consisting of three ten-minute bouts. Further, cardiorespiratory exercises should be completed on non-weight-bearing modalities given the client's preferences. Asia determines that the initial cardiorespiratory exercise intensity should be 40 percent of Paul's $\dot{V}O_2R$ or at or below the pain threshold ordered by Paul's physician. Asia's metabolic calculations for the Monark cycle and arm ergometers is shown next.

$\dot{V}O_2R$ Calculations:

$\dot{V}O_2R = \dot{V}O_{2max} - 3.5$ mL/kg · min

$\dot{V}O_2R = 23.5$ mL/kg · min $- 3.5$ mL/kg · min

$\dot{V}O_2R = 20$ mL/kg · min

40 percent of $\dot{V}O_2R = (20$ mL/kg · min x .4$) + 3.5$ mL/kg · min

40 percent of $\dot{V}O_2R = 11.5$ mL/kg · min

<u>Cycling Calculations:</u>

Asia feels that Paul can comfortably cycle at 50 revolutions per minute and, therefore, uses the cycle equation to calculate the resistance necessary to elicit 40 percent of Paul's $\dot{V}O_2R$.

$$11.5 \text{ mL/kg} \cdot \text{min} = (1.8 \times 50 \times \text{resistance} \times 6/100 \text{ kg}) + 7$$

Resistance = 0.83 kp

<u>Arm Cycling Calculations:</u>

Asia feels that Paul can comfortably arm cycle at 70 revolutions per minute and, therefore, uses the arm cycle equation to calculate the resistance necessary to elicit 40 percent of Paul's $\dot{V}O_2R$.

$$11.5 \text{ mL/kg} \cdot \text{min} = (3 \times 70 \times \text{resistance} \times 2.4/100 \text{ kg}) + 3.5$$

Resistance = 1.59 kp

Asia designs an exercise progression scheme that limits pain and muscle soreness. As such, Asia decides to increase exercise time, per ten-minute interval, by one minute each week. Once Paul can exercise for 60 minutes per exercise session, Asia will add an additional day of training per week every other week. Eventually, Paul will be performing cardiorespiratory exercises five days per week, 60 minutes each exercise session, at an intensity of 40 percent of $\dot{V}O_2R$. At that point, Asia will increase exercise intensity as tolerated. Asia also wants to include aquatic exercises to provide variety and limit joint pain.

After writing a cardiorespiratory exercise prescription, Asia moves to design a resistance training regimen. Asia recommends that Paul perform resistance exercises two days per week, two sets for each exercise, eight repetitions per set, at an intensity of 50 percent 1RM. This means Paul will chest press 60 pounds, leg press 100 pounds, shoulder press 40 pounds, crunch 50 pounds, leg extend 40 pounds, and leg curl 30 pounds. Asia decides to add one set to each exercise every two weeks until four sets per exercise are being completed. After that, Asia wants to increase each set by one repetition every week until four sets of 12 repetitions are being performed. At that point, Asia will increase the resistance as tolerated. Asia reiterates that all resistance exercises are to be performed at or below the pain threshold ordered by Paul's physician.

To limit joint stiffness, Asia provides Paul with flexibility exercise recommendations. She suggests that Paul target the major muscle-tendon groups (two sets) with static stretches. Asia states that each stretch should be held for 30 seconds without pain. Asia will add sets as tolerated and progress to dynamic stretches.

FIBROMYALGIA

Fibromyalgia is a syndrome characterized by widespread pain, limited pain threshold, and secondary symptoms, such as the inability to obtain restorative sleep, fatigue, muscle and joint stiffness, emotional disturbance, memory loss, and headache.[23,24,25]

Fibromyalgia is rooted in both neurological and psychological symptoms, although, unlike arthritis, fibromyalgia clients do not experience inflammation and joint or muscle degradation.[26,27] The exact etiology and pathology of fibromyalgia are largely unknown. However, the symptoms brought on by fibromyalgia contribute to diminished physical activity and exercise, leading to muscle loss, decreased aerobic capacity, and the onset of cardiometabolic diseases.[28,29]

Once diagnosed, the medical management of fibromyalgia is complex and often centers on symptom management. From an exercise professional's standpoint, regular exercise has been shown to be effective at managing many of the symptoms associated with fibromyalgia. Regular exercise has been linked to improvements of the health-related components of physical fitness, cardiometabolic disease risk reduction, reduced joint and muscle pain, improved self-efficacy, reduced anxiety and depressive-like symptoms, improved overall well-being, and improved functional capacity among individuals with fibromyalgia.[30,31,32,33] For all these reasons, regular exercise should be recommended for most clients with fibromyalgia, and exercise professionals need to be prepared for the challenges of designing exercise programs for these clients.

EXERCISE TESTING FOR CLIENTS WITH FIBROMYALGIA

Exercise testing should be considered when serving clients with fibromyalgia. However, exercise test selection is largely dependent on a client's pain level and symptoms.[34] Pain and symptoms are not only uncomfortable and discouraging for clients, but they can also limit the accuracy of exercise test results. Exercise professionals, therefore, must make any modifications necessary to limit pain and symptoms. Such practices include individualized exercise test protocols, equipment modifications (i.e., seat height), consideration of non-weight-bearing and client preferred modalities, adequate rest of stressed and painful muscle groups between tests, and the frequent use of pain scales.[35] Submaximal cardiorespiratory and muscular fitness tests are preferred protocols, although maximal protocols could be selected for asymptomatic and regularly active clients. Further, honest communication with clients regarding the probability of mild pain with exercise should occur, as this can improve exercise adherence. Lastly, constant encouragement may be needed, as many clients with fibromyalgia may become discouraged by the experience of pain or other symptoms.

Demonstration Case Study 7.3

Exercise Test Selection for Clients with Fibromyalgia

Boomer is an exercise professional who specializes in training clients with widespread pain. His newest client is Trinity, a 41-year-old female with chronic widespread pain and a diagnosis of fibromyalgia. Because of Trinity's fibromyalgia, she has been sedentary for the last two years and has gained weight and lost strength over that time. Trinity is limited in her ability to carry out her activities of daily living and as result started experiencing signs of depression. Trinity and her physician decided that exercise could help her manage her condition and prevent the onset of cardiometabolic diseases. Trinity reports to Boomer with full medical clearance to participate in an exercise program so long as pain stays below a three out of ten on a zero- to ten-point pain scale.

Boomer reviews Trinity's medical history, physician orders, and goals. Then, to encourage and promote adherence, Boomer decides to be open and transparent with Trinity about the exercise tests he wishes to perform. Boomer offers the following comments to Trinity:

> *I want to see how you respond to exercise before I write you an exercise plan. To do this, I want to conduct a series of exercise tests that assess your cardiorespiratory and muscular fitness and flexibility. You may experience some discomfort during these tests, which is to be expected and is normal. Slight discomfort does not mean your condition is worsening. If you do experience pain, I want you to indicate how severe that pain is on this zero- to ten-point pain scale. I will be sure to stop the tests if your pain gets too severe.*
>
> *The first test I am going to conduct is an Astrand-Rhyming cycle test. This test will let me estimate your cardiorespiratory fitness. This test is not very intense and lasts six minutes, and the resistance and peddle frequency will be the same throughout. I chose this test because I want to limit the pain you might feel with another test, like a treadmill or step test. Throughout this test, I will record your heart rate and blood pressure. Just be sure to communicate any pain you have, and if you need to stop, let me know.*
>
> *The next set of tests I will have you complete are simple body weight exercises. These tests will give me an idea of what kinds of muscular fitness exercises I can recommend. I am only going to have you complete two of these tests. The first is a sit-to-stand test. Here, I will place a chair behind you, and I want you to sit and stand up as many times as you can. I will ask you about any pain you have throughout the test and stop the test if you start to strain noticeably. The second test I will ask you to complete is a modified push-up test. Here you will use your knees as a pivot and complete as many push-ups as you can. I will coach you through the technique and stop the test when you break form. As with the other tests, let me know if you are experiencing pain. You may request to stop these tests at any time.*
>
> *Lastly, I want to test your lower body flexibility. Over the past couple of years, you have been sedentary. Being sedentary can cause your muscles to tighten, which can limit your range of motion. I am going to ask you to complete a sit-and-reach test so that we can track your improvements throughout the exercise program. To complete the sit-and-reach test, you will sit down on a floor mat, place your feet flat against the sit-and-reach box, place one hand on top of the other, and bend forward at your hips and slowly reach forward. You will do this three times. Make sure you let me know about any pain, and you may request to stop at any time.*

EXERCISE PRESCRIPTION FOR CLIENTS WITH FIBROMYALGIA

Cardiorespiratory, resistance, and flexibility exercises are all beneficial for clients with fibromyalgia. However, because of the variability among symptoms, there are many modifications that should be made to the FITT-VP. It is unrealistic to suspect asymptomatic responses from all clients with fibromyalgia, but exercise professionals must make every effort possible to limit the occurrence of symptoms and pain, as these can negatively influence overall exercise adherence. Exercise adherence is key, and encouragement and limitation of painful responses to exercise go a long way!

Clients with fibromyalgia should be encouraged to complete cardiorespiratory exercise up to three days per week. Not all clients are capable of this and thus deconditioned clients or clients who frequently experience symptoms should start with one or two cardiorespiratory exercise sessions per week.[36] Exercise professionals should make sure that adequate recovery occurs. This means that exercise sessions should be separated by at least 48 hours—especially when the same muscle groups are targeted through training. Exercise professionals should initially prescribe low-intensity cardiorespiratory exercise (i.e., 30-39 percent of HRR/$\dot{V}O_2R$).[37] Clients with fibromyalgia should start with 10-minute exercise sessions and slowly progress to 30- to 60-minute exercise sessions.[38] The modalities selected are largely based on a client's preference and symptoms. Aquatic exercises can be considered to add variety and/or to limit high-impact, weight-bearing exercise. The progression of cardiorespiratory fitness is very slow. It is important for exercise professionals to note that exercise adherence is key and any spike in pain or symptoms felt by the client may result in the termination of exercise as a new lifestyle behavior.

Resistance training can also be included in a client's program. The frequency of resistance exercise remains the same as for healthy adults. However, intensity and time are generally different. First, the resistance applied should be dependent on a client's goals and physical limitations. For deconditioned clients or clients seeking to increase muscular endurance, 40–60 percent 1RM is a recommended starting point. For clients experiencing less pain, who have a history of resistance exercise, or who seek to increase muscular strength, a starting intensity of 60–80 percent 1RM is appropriate. Initially, selected exercises should be completed for one set of four to five repetitions.[39] Slow progression to two to four sets and 8 to 12 repetitions is recommended. For extremely deconditioned clients or clients with more frequent pain, resistance bands can be used. Adequate recovery time is necessary—at least 48 hours between sessions. The flexibility recommendations for clients with fibromyalgia are like those with arthritis. However, starting with one day of flexibility exercise per week may be appropriate given the frequency at which pain occurs.[40]

Demonstration Case Study 7.4

Exercise Prescription for Clients with Fibromyalgia

Lucie is an exercise physiologist specializing in training clients with fibromyalgia. Her most recent client is Heather. Heather is a 44-year-old female, 180 pounds, BMI

= 32.7 kg/m², sedentary, and has fibromyalgia. Heather has not exercised since first experiencing symptoms five years prior. Since then, Heather's pain occurrences have been frequent and intense. Heather and her physician agreed that an exercise program may be beneficial for symptom management. Heather was fully cleared by her physician with orders to exercise with minimal pain—no more than three on a zero- to ten-point pain scale. Heather told Lucie that walking anywhere causes pain to occur. Heather also told Lucie lifting heavy weights triggers pain.

After completing a series of exercise tests, the following fitness data were obtained: (1) estimated $\dot{V}O_{2max}$ of 17.5 mL/kg · min using the Astrand-Rhyming cycle protocol, (2) sit-to-stand test = 3 repetitions, (3) modified push-ups = 4 repetitions, (4) body fat percentage = 38 percent, and (5) sit-and-reach score was poor.

After analyzing Heather's medical history and exercise test scores, Lucie begins to write a comprehensive exercise prescription. First, Lucie recommends cardiorespiratory exercises to be completed one day per week consisting one ten-minute bout. Further, cardiorespiratory exercises should be completed on non-weight-bearing modalities given the client's preferences. Lucie determines that the initial cardiorespiratory exercise intensity should be 30 percent of Heather's $\dot{V}O_2R$ or at or below the pain threshold ordered by Heather's physician. Lucie's metabolic calculations for the Monark cycle and arm ergometers are shown next.

$\dot{V}O_2R$ Calculations:

$\dot{V}O_2R = \dot{V}O_{2max} - 3.5$ mL/kg · min

$\dot{V}O_2R = 17.5$ mL/kg · min $- 3.5$ mL/kg · min

$\dot{V}O_2R = 14$ mL/kg · min

30 percent of $\dot{V}O_2R = (14$ mL/kg · min x .3) $+ 3.5$ mL/kg · min

30 percent of $\dot{V}O_2R = 7.7$ mL/kg · min

Cycling Calculations:

Lucie feels it is best to control the resistance on the flywheel to reduce the likelihood of pain. Lucie believes that 0.25 kp of resistance is sufficient for keeping Heather below the recommended pain threshold and to elicit 30 percent of Heather's $\dot{V}O_2R$. Lucie then solves for peddle frequency on the Monark cycle.

7.7 mL/kg · min = (1.8 x frequency x 0.25 x 6/81.81 kg) + 7

Peddle frequency = 21 revolutions per minute

Arm Cycling Calculations:

Lucie feels it is best to control the resistance on the flywheel to reduce the likelihood of pain. Lucie believes that 1.2 kp of resistance is sufficient for keeping Heather below the recommended pain threshold and to elicit 30 percent of Heather's $\dot{V}O_2R$. Lucie then solves for peddle frequency on the Monark arm cycle.

7.7 mL/kg · min = (3 x frequency x 1.2 x 2.4/81.81 kg) + 3.5

Peddle frequency = 40 revolutions per minute

Lucie then designs an exercise progression scheme that limits pain. Realizing that Heather frequently experiences pain with movement, Lucie plans to increase exercise time by two minutes each week but only as tolerated. Once 30 minutes of continuous exercise occurs per day, then Lucie will add an extra day of training every other week. Lucie will not increase exercise intensity until Heather can complete three days of cardiorespiratory exercise per week, 30 minutes each session, without pain.

After writing a cardiorespiratory exercise prescription, Lucie designs a resistance training program. Given Heather's frequent pain, Lucie decides to write a resistance band program. As a part of this plan, Lucie will initially recommend completing eight resistance band exercises, five repetitions of each exercise, two days per week. A period of at least 48 hours will separate exercise sessions. Lucie will progress repetitions and sets before suggesting machine-based weight training.

Lastly, to improve range of motion and overall functional capability, Lucie wants Heather to complete flexibility exercises. She suggests that Heather target the major muscle-tendon groups with one static stretch. Lucie recommends that each stretch should be held for 10 to 30 seconds without pain. Stretches will be initially completed after each cardiorespiratory exercise session. Lucie will progress Heather as pain permits.

OSTEOPOROSIS

Osteoporosis is a disease characterized by bone mineral loss. This bone mineral loss increases the likelihood of fracture, which can be catastrophic for the short- and long-term health and mortality of older adults.[41] Osteoporosis is highly prevalent in the United States, with approximately 10 million adults suffering from the disease and nearly 45 million adults with abnormally low bone mineral density.[42] Osteoporosis primarily occurs in females, particularly after menopause but can also occur in men.

Exercise is an important lifestyle modification for individuals with osteoporosis, and the benefits of regular exercise can positively influence the disease process and reduce health risks associated with osteoporosis. First, exercise promotes favorable improvements in proprioception, which can limit the risk of suffering fractures from falling.[43] Second, exercise can stimulate increases in bone mineral density. Load-bearing exercises of increasing intensity facilitate the absorption of calcium in bones, thus increasing bone mineral density.[44,45] This benefit is particularly useful in the prevention of low bone mineral levels from progressing to osteoporosis. Third, as with other populations, exercise offers benefits that favorably alter cardiometabolic disease risk in clients with osteoporosis.

EXERCISE TESTING FOR CLIENTS WITH OSTEOPOROSIS

In general, exercise testing is regarded as safe for individuals with osteoporosis. Exercise testing procedures for all health-related components of physical fitness are similar to the healthy adult population.[46] However, like with other special populations, safety considerations must be at the forefront. With clients suffering from osteoporosis, exercise professionals need to consider modalities and protocols that limit the likelihood of accidents leading to fracture. This means exercise tests need to be selected according to not only the client's disease status but exercise history as well. Non-weight-bearing modalities should be used when client's regularly experience pain or have severe vertebral osteoporosis. Maximal effort protocols can be considered for regularly active, asymptomatic, and nonsevere osteoporosis; however, it is possible that ventilation may be compromised because of structural changes to the vertebral column and or thoracic cavity.[47] Lastly, given the susceptibility of fracture, clients with osteoporosis should undergo balance testing or a fall risk assessment.[48]

Demonstration Case Study 7.5

Exercise Testing for Clients with Osteoporosis

Buck is an exercise physiologist at a health-fitness center within a retirement village. Buck serves a lot of clients with osteoporosis, and his most recent client was recently diagnosed with osteoporosis. Gina, a 67-year-old female, has been regularly active in her retirement but has ultimately avoided high-impact exercises. She recently read that exercise can help manage osteoporosis and reduce her risk of falling and fracturing bones. For this reason, she visit's Buck's health-fitness center.

Buck notices that Gina has been regularly active and received physician clearance to participate in exercise. Despite Gina's regular activity, Buck does not wish to conduct maximal effort tests simply since Gina has avoided high-impact exercises. Therefore, Buck conducts a submaximal Bruce protocol test, a series of repetition-based muscular fitness tests, and basic anthropomorphic assessments. Following these tests, Gina thinks she is finished for the day, but Buck alerts her to one more test he would like to perform. Buck told Gina that he would like to get an idea of how well she can balance herself. Buck explained to Gina that he wants to make sure he prescribes safe exercises, and he wants to track her progress, as neuromotor exercises will be included in her exercise prescription to reduce her fall risk.

EXERCISE PRESCRIPTION FOR CLIENTS WITH OSTEOPOROSIS

A key characteristic of exercise program design for clients with osteoporosis is that selected exercises should be weight bearing and progress to higher velocity and vigorous movement and intensities.[49,50] The simple rationale for this is bones will not sufficiently remodel unless they are adequately stressed.[51] Accordingly, both cardiorespiratory and resistance exercises that induce vertical loading and high-velocity muscle contractions should be included in the exercise prescription. Further, neuromotor exercises, such as balance and agility drills should be considered as a means to improve proprioception and thereby reduce fall risk. Although the aforementioned recommendations have scientific merit, exercise professionals must not sacrifice the safety of the client in hopes of better physiological/anatomical adaptations. Exercise professionals will need to limit pain when possible, stay within physician orders, ensure proper exercise technique, and individualize exercise prescriptions to the physical limitations of each client.

The cardiorespiratory exercise recommendations are similar for intensity and time as for healthy adults. One difference is exercise frequency. It is beneficial for clients with osteoporosis to perform cardiorespiratory exercises four or more days per week.[52] For exercise type, whenever possible, exercise modalities should be load bearing. Progression through a cardiorespiratory exercise program is like healthy adults with exercise time being increased before intensity. The goal of cardiorespiratory exercise should be to eventually progress the client to higher-intensity exercises, as these exercises provide greater stress on bones, which elicits more favorable adaptations in bone mineral density.

Resistance exercise is prescribed in a different manner for clients with osteoporosis so as not to cause injury. First, exercise frequency starts out with one day per week and eventually progresses to three days per week.[53] The intensity is selected not by percentage of 1RM but rather by the challenging nature of the final two repetitions per set. Therefore, of the 8 to 12 repetitions per set initially recommended, the final two repetitions per set should be somewhat difficult—without risking injury.[54] The starting point for sets is one that eventually progresses to two. Overall, the accumulation of resistance exercises performed over the course of a week should at least target each major muscle group once. Progression through a resistance training program is like healthy populations with the eventual goal of high-intensity training as tolerated. Lastly, flexibility exercises should be completed on most days in accordance with the recommendations discussed in Chapter 2.

Demonstration Case Study 7.6

Exercise Prescription for Clients with Osteoporosis

Hernando is an exercise physiologist specializing in training clients with osteoporosis. His most recent client is Grace. Grace is a 71-year-old female, 105 pounds, BMI = 19 kg/m², and modestly physically active; she has moderate osteoporosis of the lumbar vertebra. Grace reported to Hernando's clinic seeking an exercise program to help slow her bone mineral loss and to aid in reducing fall and fracture risk. Grace was fully cleared by her physician to participate in an exercise program.

After completing a series of exercise tests, the following fitness data were obtained: (1) estimated $\dot{V}O_{2max}$ of 25 mL/kg · min using the Naughton protocol, (2) chest press 8RM = 50 pounds, (3) leg press 8RM = 75 pounds, (4) seated row 8RM = 60 pounds, (5) seated back extension 8RM = 30 pounds, (6) leg extension 8RM = 50 pounds, (7) leg curl 8RM = 50 pounds, (8) body fat percentage = 18 percent, (9) balance score = normal, and (10) sit-and-reach score was below average.

After analyzing Grace's medical history and exercise test scores, Hernando begins to write a comprehensive exercise prescription. First, Hernando recommends weight-bearing cardiorespiratory exercises to be completed four days per week, 30 minutes per day. Hernando chose this starting point and exercise type because weight-bearing exercises are beneficial for osteoporosis clients, and Grace's balance score indicates she can perform these exercises safely. Further, given Grace's modest physical activity history, Hernando determines that the initial cardiorespiratory exercise intensity should be 55 percent of Grace's $\dot{V}O_2R$. Hernando's metabolic calculations for walking and stepping are shown next.

$\dot{V}O_2R$ Calculations:

$$\dot{V}O_2R = \dot{V}O_{2max} - 3.5 \text{ mL/kg} \cdot \text{min}$$

$$\dot{V}O_2R = 25 \text{ mL/kg} \cdot \text{min} - 3.5 \text{ mL/kg} \cdot \text{min}$$

$$\dot{V}O_2R = 21.5 \text{ mL/kg} \cdot \text{min}$$

$$55 \text{ percent of } \dot{V}O_2R = (21.5 \text{ mL/kg} \cdot \text{min} \times .55) + 3.5 \text{ mL/kg} \cdot \text{min}$$

$$55 \text{ percent of } \dot{V}O_2R = 15.33 \text{ mL/kg} \cdot \text{min}$$

Walking Calculations:

Hernando believes that walking at 3.5 mph will be sufficient to elicit increases in bone mineral density and can be completed safely. Therefore, Hernando uses the walking equation to calculate the incline necessary to elicit 55 percent of Grace's $\dot{V}O_2R$.

$$15.33 \text{ mL/kg} \cdot \text{min} = (0.1 \times 3.5 \times 26.8) + (1.8 \times 3.5 \times 26.8 \times \text{incline}) + 3.5$$

$$\text{Incline} = 1.45 \text{ percent}$$

Stepping Calculations:

Hernando believes that stepping at a rate of 20 steps per minute will be sufficient to elicit increases in bone mineral density and can be completed safely. Therefore, Hernando uses the stepping equation to calculate the step height necessary to elicit 55 percent of Grace's $\dot{V}O_2R$.

$$15.33 \text{ mL/kg} \cdot \text{min} = (0.2 \times 20) + (1.33 \times 1.8 \times \text{step height} \times 20) + 3.5$$

$$\text{Step height} = 0.163 \text{ meters} = 16.3 \text{ cm}$$

Hernando chooses a progression scheme that eventually has Grace performing vigorous-intensity exercise. However, Hernando wants to progress her there slowly. Hernando decides to increase exercise time by 5 percent each week until Grace is able to perform cardiorespiratory exercises four days per week, 45 minutes per day. Then Hernando will add an additional day of training per week before slowly increasing exercise intensity as tolerated.

After writing a cardiorespiratory exercise prescription, Hernando designs a resistance training program. Hernando intends to have Grace complete the chest press, leg press, seated row, seated back extension, seated leg extension, and seated leg curl once per week at her 8RM. Hernando decides to progress her repetitions for each exercise weekly until 12 repetitions are completed. At that point, Hernando will add an extra set, followed by an additional training day. Hernando decides only to increase exercise intensity once Grace can complete her resistance exercises three days per week, 12 repetitions per exercise.

Hernando realizes balance and neuromotor exercises are important for reducing Grace's fall risk. Therefore, Hernando will incorporate stability disc and BOSU ball exercises into Graces exercise routine. Hernando plans to have Grace perform these exercises before she walks on the treadmill or does stepping exercises. As Grace adapts, Hernando will challenge her by having her complete neuromotor exercises after she has finished her cardiorespiratory exercise sessions. Lastly, following each exercise training session, Hernando will have Grace complete two to four stretches for each major muscle group and hold each stretch for 10 to 30 seconds.

Student Case Study 7.1

Exercise Testing and Prescription for Clients with Arthritis: Comprehensive Case Study

An exercise physiologist works for a health-fitness facility serving clients with neuro-musculoskeletal conditions. He thoroughly collected the following data from his most recent client:

Demographics: (1) male and (2) 55 years old

Family History: (1) father died of cancer at 71, (2) mother developed bilateral hip arthritis leading to a left hip replacement

Biometrics: (1) resting heart rate = 80 beats per minute; (2) resting blood pressure = 120/80 mmHg; (3) LDL-c = 120 mg/dL, HDL-c = 41 mg/dL, triglycerides = 144 mg/dL; (4) glycosylated hemoglobin = 6.4 percent and blood glucose = 100 mg/dL; and (5) weight = 250 lbs., BMI = 33 kg/m^2

Medical Diagnoses: (1) bilateral knee osteoarthritis

Medications: (1) nonsteroidal anti-inflammatory agent

Symptoms: (1) moderate knee pain during weight-bearing movements

Exercise History: (1) no recent exercise history, (2) does not tolerate weight-bearing movements

Exercise Goals and Needs: (1) pain reduction, (2) decrease chronic disease risk, and (3) improve quality of life

1. Should the exercise physiologist conduct a maximal or submaximal cardiorespiratory fitness test? In four to five sentences, provide a defense for the decision based on the client's profile.
2. Which cardiorespiratory fitness test should be conducted? In four to five sentences, provide a defense for the decision based on the client's profile.
3. Given limitless resources, which body composition test should the exercise physiologist conduct? In four to five sentences, provide a defense for thc dcci sion based on the client's profile.
4. Given minimal resources with a small budget, which body composition test should be conducted? In four to five sentences, provide a defense for the decision based on the client's profile.

5. Specific to this case, which body composition test would be preferred? In four to five sentences, provide a defense for the decision based on the client's profile.
6. To assess muscular fitness, should muscular endurance assessments or muscular strength assessments be conducted, or both? In four to five sentences, provide a defense for the decision based on the client's profile.
7. Provide a list of four specific muscular fitness tests to be conducted on the client. Then provide a four- to five-sentence defense supporting the selections.
8. Provide a list of four specific muscular fitness tests to be conducted on the client. Then provide a four- to five-sentence defense supporting the selections.
9. List all the ways the exercise physiologist can enhance safety during exercise testing procedures that assess cardiorespiratory fitness, muscular fitness, and flexibility.
10. Based on the answer for questions 1 and 2, calculate the client's $\dot{V}O_{2\,max}$ from the most appropriate of the following cardiorespiratory fitness tests (Figures 7.1–7.5).

Figure 7.1 This table depicts hypothetical data from a YMCA cycle test

YMCA Cycle Test

Stage	Kpm/ min	Heart Rate	Blood Pressure	RPE	ECG	Symptoms/ Comments
Resting	0	80	120/80	NA	Sinus	No symptoms
I	150	111	130/78	12	Sinus	No symptoms
II	300	122	150/78	14	Sinus	Pain, 1 out of 10
Immediate	100	120	148/80	NA	Sinus	Pain, 1 out of 10
Recovery 1 min	50	104	132/80	NA	Sinus	No symptoms
Recovery 5 min	25	86	122/76	NA	Sinus	No symptoms

Figure 7.2 Students may use these gridlines to graph data from the YMCA cycle test

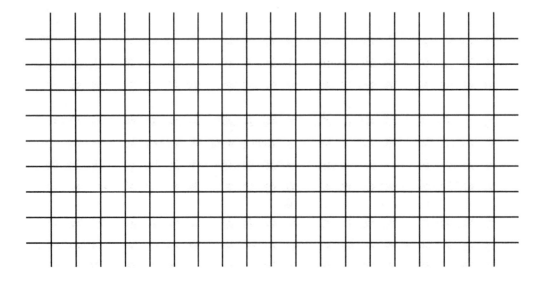

Figure 7.3 This table depicts hypothetical data from a submaximal treadmill test

Submaximal Bruce Protocol

Stage	Speed (mph)	Grade %	Heart Rate	Blood Pressure	RPE	ECG	Symptoms
Resting	0	0	80	120/80	NA	Sinus	No symptoms
I	1.7	10.0	100	132/80	10	Sinus	Pain, 1 out of 10
II	2.5	12.0	120	144/80	13	Sinus	Pain, 2 out of 10
III	3.4	14.0	140	166/80	15	Sinus	Pain, 3 out of 10
Immediate	1.5	0	141	168/80	NA	Sinus	Pain, 3 out of 10
Recovery 1 min	1.5	0	115	140/78	NA	Sinus	No symptoms
Recovery 5 min	1	0	85	122/78	NA	Sinus	No symptoms

Figure 7.4 This table depicts hypothetical data from a maximal treadmill test

Maximal Treadmill Test

Stage	Time	Speed (mph)	Grade %	Blood Pressure	$\dot{V}O_2$ (mL/kg · min)	Blood Lactate (mmol)	RPE	Heart Rate	RER
Resting	NA	0	0	120/80	4.1	NA	NA	80	0.84
I	2:00	3.5	2	150/80	16.7	2.1	13	126	0.99
II	4:00	4.5	4	188/86	22.2	5.7	19	170	1.06
Immediate	NA	1.5	0	190/86	22.8	NA	NA	161	1.08
Recovery 1 min	NA	1.5	0	168/84	19.3	NA	NA	140	1.04
Recovery 5 min	NA	1	0	138/82	8.9	NA	NA	81	1.01

Comments: **Test terminated because of client's desire to stop. Seven out of ten pain recorded**

Figure 7.5 This table depicts hypothetical data from a maximal cycle test

Maximal Cycle Test

Stage	Time	Kpm /min	Heart Rate	Blood Pressure	RPE	$\dot{V}O_2$ (mL/kg · min.)	RER	Blood Lactate (mmol)	ECG
Resting		0	80	120/80	NA	4.1	0.81	NA	Sinus
I	2:00	600	115	140/80	11	8.8	0.9	2.0	Sinus
II	4:00	900	129	160/80	14	16.2	1.0	4.0	Sinus
III	6:00	1200	141	178/82	15	24.9	1.04	6.1	Sinus
IV	8:00	1500	160	190/82	18	26.0	1.17	8.0	Sinus
Immediate	NA	300	159	188/80	NA	25.9	1.12	NA	Sinus
Recovery 1 min	NA	150	130	160/80	NA	16.1	1.00	NA	Sinus
Recovery 5 min	NA	75	88	132/78	NA	10.7	0.95	NA	Sinus

Comments: **Test terminated because of volitional fatigue. Pain, 3 out of 10 recorded**

11. For the cardiorespiratory fitness test chosen to interpret the answer for question 10, should the test have been terminated prior to completion? Explain why or why not.

12. Assuming the skinfold assessment for body composition test was selected, calculate body fat percentage from the following seven-site skinfold data (Figure 7.6).

Figure 7.6 This table depicts hypothetical data from a seven-site skinfold assessment

Site	Trial 1	Trial 2	Trial 3	Average
Triceps	17	19	18	mm
Subscapular	21	22	22.5	mm
Chest	22	23	23	mm
Abdominal	25	27	25.75	mm
Suprailiac	27	23	22.75	mm
Midaxillary	21	19.75	20.75	mm
Thigh	27	29	28.25	mm

13. Assuming muscular strength was selected, interpret and classify the client's leg and chest press strength from the following data (Figure 7.7).

Figure 7.7 This table depicts hypothetical data from a 3–5RM test

Leg Press Strength Test

Trial 1	5	repetitions
	185	weight
Trial 2	4	repetitions
	195	weight
Trial 3	3	repetitions
	205	weight
Best Trial	3	repetitions
	205	weight

Chest Press Strength Test

Trial 1	5	repetitions
	110	weight

(Continued)

Figure 7.7 This table depicts hypothetical data from a 3–5RM test (Continued)

Chest Press Strength Test

Trial 2	_____5_____ repetitions
	_____120_____ weight
Trial 3	_____5_____ repetitions
	_____125_____ weight
Best Trial	_____5_____ repetitions
	_____125_____ weight

14. Calculate a heart rate range based on the heart rate reserve that the client should maintain during aerobic exercise. Is this the most reliable method for quantifying cardiorespiratory endurance exercise? Why or why not?

15. Calculate a $\dot{V}O_2$ range based on the $\dot{V}O_2$ reserve that the client should maintain during aerobic exercise.

16. Provide an exercise type (be specific), frequency, and time at the $\dot{V}O_2$ range found in question 15 for the client to improve his cardiorespiratory fitness and manage symptoms.

17. Suggest four possible aerobic exercises that would be appropriate for this client.

18. Provide a resistance and arm crank frequency for arm cycling to elicit the lower end of the $\dot{V}O_2$ range listed in question 15.

19. Provide a resistance and peddle frequency for leg cycling to elicit the upper end of the $\dot{V}O_2$ range listed in question 15.

20. Suggest a progression scheme for improving cardiorespiratory fitness. Would vigorous-intensity or high-intensity interval training be warranted? Why or why not?

21. Provide a range for weight that the client should chest press.

22. Provide a range for weight that the client should leg press.

23. Provide a resistance exercise prescription for frequency and number of exercises, sets, and repetitions to improve muscular fitness.

24. Suggest at least four specific resistance training exercises that are appropriate for this client.

25. Suggest a progression scheme to help the client improve overall muscular fitness.

26. Provide the frequency, intensity, number of stretches, sets, and amount of time each stretch should be to help improve the client's flexibility.

27. Are there other exercises that may be appropriate for this client (cardiorespiratory, resistance, flexibility, neuromotor, etc.)? Provide a justification for the response.

28. Provide a list consisting of all safety considerations that should be considered when supervising this client's exercise program. Would these considerations be different if the client had rheumatoid arthritis? Explain why or why not.

Exercise Testing and Prescription for Clients with Fibromyalgia: Comprehensive Case Study

An exercise physiologist works for a health-fitness facility serving clients with neuro-musculoskeletal conditions. He thoroughly collected the following data from his most recent client:

<u>Demographics:</u> (1) female and (2) 50 years old

<u>Family History:</u> (1) father developed type II diabetes at age 45, (2) mother was diagnosed with depression at age 60

<u>Biometrics:</u> (1) resting heart rate = 75 beats per minute; (2) resting blood pressure = 132/74 mmHg; (3) LDL-c = 129 mg/dL, HDL-c = 40 mg/dL, triglycerides = 149 mg/dL; (4) glycosylated hemoglobin = 6.4 percent and blood glucose = 125 mg/dL; and (5) weight = 196 lbs., BMI = 34.9 kg/m^2

<u>Medical Diagnoses:</u> (1) fibromyalgia and (2) chronic fatigue

<u>Medications:</u> (1) milnacipran (antidepressant)

<u>Symptoms:</u> (1) widespread pain (2) sleeplessness (3) depressive symptoms (4) headache

<u>Exercise History:</u> (1) no recent exercise history; (2) pain is triggered by fast and vigorous movements, pain with weight-bearing movement; and (3) physician ordered no exercise at pain exceeding three out of ten

<u>Exercise Goals and Needs:</u> (1) pain reduction, (2) decrease chronic disease risk, and (3) improve quality of life

1. Should the exercise physiologist conduct a maximal or submaximal cardio-respiratory fitness test? In four to five sentences, provide a defense for the decision based on the client's profile.
2. Which cardiorespiratory fitness test should be conducted? In four to five sentences, provide a defense for the decision based on the client's profile.
3. Given limitless resources, which body composition test should the exercise physiologist conduct? In four to five sentences, provide a defense for the decision based on the client's profile.
4. Given minimal resources with a small budget, which body composition test should be conducted? In four to five sentences, provide a defense for the decision based on the client's profile.
5. Specific to this case, which body composition test would be preferred? In four to five sentences, provide a defense for the decision based on the client's profile.
6. To assess muscular fitness, should muscular endurance assessments or muscular strength assessments be conducted, or both? In four to five sentences, provide a defense for the decision based on the client's profile.
7. Provide a list of four specific muscular fitness tests to be conducted on the client. Then provide a four- to five-sentence defense supporting the selections.

8. Provide a list of four specific muscular fitness tests to be conducted on the client. Then provide a four- to five-sentence defense supporting the selections.
9. List all the ways the exercise physiologist can enhance safety during exercise testing procedures that assess cardiorespiratory fitness, muscular fitness, and flexibility.
10. Based on the answer for questions 1 and 2, calculate the client's $\dot{V}O_{2max}$ from the most appropriate of the following cardiorespiratory fitness tests (Figures 7.8–7.9).

Figure 7.8 This table depicts hypothetical data from an Astrand-Rhyming cycle test

Astrand-Rhyming Cycle Test

Stage/Minute	Kpm/m	Heart Rate	Blood Pressure	RPE	ECG	Symptoms
Resting		75	132/74	NA	Sinus	No symptoms
I	300	135	166/76	13	Sinus	No symptoms
II	300	141	168/76	13	Sinus	Pain, 1 out of 10
III	300	142	170/78	14	Sinus	Pain, 2 out of 10
IV	300	143	172/78	14	Sinus	Pain, 2 out of 10
V	300	144	174/78	15	Sinus	Pain, 3 out of 10
VI	300	144	176/78	16	Sinus	Pain, 3 out of 10
Immediate	150	130	178/80	NA	Sinus	Pain, 3 out of 10
Recovery 1 min	75	117	150/74	NA	Sinus	No symptoms
Recovery 5 min	50	107	142/72	NA	Sinus	No symptoms

Figure 7.9 This table depicts hypothetical data from a submaximal treadmill test

Submaximal Bruce Protocol

Stage	Speed (mph)	Grade %	Heart Rate	Blood Pressure	RPE	ECG	Symptoms
Resting	0	0	75	132/74	NA	Sinus	No symptoms
I	1.7	10.0	111	170/78	14	Sinus	Pain, 3 out of 10
II	2.5	12.0	129	190/78	15	Sinus	Pain, 6 out of 10
III	3.4	14.0	138	200/80	18	Sinus	Pain, 9 out of 10
Immediate	1.5	0	137	200/80	NA	Sinus	Pain, 9 out of 10
Recovery 1 min	1.5	0	122	180/80	NA	Sinus	Pain, 7 out of 10
Recovery 5 min	1	0	100	148/76	NA	Sinus	Pain, 5 out of 10

11. For the cardiorespiratory fitness test chosen to interpret the answer for question 10, should the test have been terminated prior to completion? Explain why or why not.

12. Assuming the skinfold assessment for body composition test was selected, calculate body fat percentage from the following seven-site skinfold data (Figure 7.10).

Figure 7.10 This table depicts hypothetical data from a seven-site skinfold assessment

Site	Trial 1	Trial 2	Trial 3	Average
Triceps	20	22	20.25	mm
Subscapular	24	25	25.25	mm
Chest	25	26	27	mm
Abdominal	28	30	28.75	mm
Suprailiac	30	26	25.75	mm
Midaxillary	24	27.25	23.5	mm
Thigh	30	32	30.75	mm

13. Assuming muscular strength was selected, interpret and classify the client's leg and chest press strength from the following data (Figure 7.11).

Figure 7.11 This table depicts hypothetical data from a 3–5RM test

Leg Press Strength Test

Trial 1	5 repetitions 70 weight
Trial 2	4 repetitions 75 weight
Trial 3	3 repetitions 80 weight
Best Trial	3 repetitions 80 weight

Chest Press Strength Test

Trial 1	5 repetitions 25 weight
Trial 2	5 repetitions 30 weight

(Continued)

Chest Press Strength Test

Trial 3	_____3_____ repetitions
	_____35_____ weight
Best Trial	_____3_____ repetitions
	_____35_____ weight

14. Calculate a heart rate range based on the heart rate reserve that the client should maintain during aerobic exercise. Is this the most reliable method for quantifying cardiorespiratory endurance exercise? Why or why not?

15. Calculate a $\dot{V}O_2$ range based on the $\dot{V}O_2$ reserve that the client should maintain during aerobic exercise.

16. Provide an exercise type (be specific), frequency, and time at the $\dot{V}O_2$ range found in question 15 for the client to improve her cardiorespiratory fitness and manage symptoms.

17. Suggest four possible aerobic exercises that would be appropriate for this client.

18. Provide a resistance and arm crank frequency for arm cycling to elicit the lower end of the $\dot{V}O_2$ range listed in question 15.

19. Provide a resistance and peddle frequency for leg cycling to elicit the upper end of the $\dot{V}O_2$ range listed in question 15.

20. Suggest a progression scheme for improving cardiorespiratory fitness. Would vigorous-intensity or high-intensity interval training be warranted? Why or why not?

21. Provide a range for weight that the client should chest press.

22. Provide a range for weight that the client should leg press.

23. Provide a resistance exercise prescription for frequency, number of exercises, sets, and repetitions to improve muscular fitness.

24. Suggest at least four specific resistance training exercises that are appropriate for this client.

25. Suggest a progression scheme to help the client improve overall muscular fitness.

26. Provide the frequency, intensity, number of stretches, sets, and amount of time each stretch should be to help improve the client's flexibility.

27. Are there other exercises that may be appropriate for this client (cardiorespiratory, resistance, flexibility, neuromotor, etc.)? Provide a justification for the response.

28. Provide a list consisting of all safety considerations that should be considered when supervising this client's exercise program.

Exercise Testing and Prescription for Clients with Osteoporosis: Comprehensive Case Study

An exercise physiologist works for a health-fitness facility serving clients with neuro-musculoskeletal conditions. He thoroughly collected the following data from his most recent client:

Demographics: (1) female and (2) 65 years old

Family History: (1) father died of natural causes at age 91, (2) mother died of natural causes at the age of 96

Biometrics: (1) resting heart rate = 60 beats per minute; (2) resting blood pressure = 116/70 mmHg; (3) LDL-c = 95 mg/dL, HDL-c = 48 mg/dL, triglycerides = 120 mg/dL; (4) glycosylated hemoglobin = 6.3 percent and blood glucose = 99 mg/dL; and (5) weight = 120 lbs., BMI = 21.1 kg/m^2

Medical Diagnoses: (1) osteoporosis

Medications: (1) ibandronate

Symptoms: (1) none

Exercise History: (1) leg cycling daily for 30 minutes at a moderate intensity

Exercise Goals and Needs: (1) increase/maintain bone mineral density, (2) decrease fall risk

Strength Test Data: (1) chest press 8RM = 55 pounds, (2) leg press 8RM = 65 pounds, (3) seated row 8RM = 45 pounds, (4) seated back extension 8RM = 35 pounds, (5) leg extension 8RM = 30 pounds, (6) leg curl 8RM = 25 pounds

1. Should the exercise physiologist conduct a maximal or submaximal cardio-respiratory fitness test? In four to five sentences, provide a defense for the decision based on the client's profile.
2. Which cardiorespiratory fitness test should be conducted? In four to five sentences, provide a defense for the decision based on the client's profile.
3. Given limitless resources, which body composition test should the exercise physiologist conduct? In four to five sentences, provide a defense for the decision based on the client's profile.
4. Given minimal resources with a small budget, which body composition test should be conducted? In four to five sentences, provide a defense for the decision based on the client's profile.
5. Specific to this case, which body composition test would be preferred? In four to five sentences, provide a defense for the decision based on the client's profile.
6. To assess muscular fitness, should muscular endurance assessments or muscular strength assessments be conducted, or both? In four to five sentences, provide a defense for the decision based on the client's profile.

7. Provide a list of four specific muscular fitness tests to be conducted on the client. Then provide a four- to five-sentence defense supporting the selections.
8. Are there other types of fitness tests that should be considered for this client? If so, broadly explain the fitness tests and why they should be conducted.
9. List all the ways the exercise physiologist can enhance safety during exercise testing procedures that assess cardiorespiratory fitness, muscular fitness, and flexibility.
10. Based on the answer for questions 1 and 2, calculate the client's $\dot{V}O_{2max}$ from the most appropriate of the following cardiorespiratory fitness tests (Figures 7.12–7.14).

Figure 7.12 This table depicts hypothetical data from a submaximal treadmill test

Submaximal Bruce Protocol

Stage	Speed (mph)	Grade %	Heart Rate	Blood Pressure	RPE	ECG	Symptoms
Resting	0	0	60	116/70	NA	Sinus	No symptoms
I	1.7	10.0	85	130/68	10	Sinus	No symptoms
II	2.5	12.0	113	146/68	11	Sinus	No symptoms
III	3.4	14.0	126	160/68	13	Sinus	No symptoms
Immediate	1.5	0	137	160/68	NA	Sinus	No symptoms
Recovery 1 min	1.5	0	122	130/66	NA	Sinus	No symptoms
Recovery 5 min	1	0	100	116/66	NA	Sinus	No symptoms

Figure 7.13 This table depicts hypothetical data from an Astrand-Rhyming cycle test

Astrand-Rhyming Cycle Test

Stage/Minute	Kpm/m	Heart Rate	Blood Pressure	RPE	ECG	Symptoms
Resting		60	116/70	NA	Sinus	No symptoms
I	450	135	130/70	10	Sinus	No symptoms
II	450	141	134/68	11	Sinus	No symptoms
III	450	142	136/68	11	Sinus	No symptoms
IV	450	143	136/68	11	Sinus	No symptoms
V	450	144	136/68	11	Sinus	No symptoms
VI	450	144	136/66	11	Sinus	No symptoms
Immediate	150	130	134/66	NA	Sinus	No symptoms
Recovery 1 min	75	117	124/66	NA	Sinus	No symptoms
Recovery 5 min	50	107	116/66	NA	Sinus	No symptoms

Figure 7.14 This table depicts hypothetical data from a maximal treadmill test

Maximal Treadmill Test

Stage	Time	Speed (mph)	Grade %	Blood Pressure	$\dot{V}O_2$ (mL/kg · min)	Blood Lactate (mmol)	RPE	Heart Rate	RER
Resting	NA	0	0	116/70	3.7	NA	NA	60	0.79
I	2:00	3.5	2	120/70	16.7	1.9	13	80	0.90
II	4:00	4.5	4	160/72	28.2	4.4	15	137	1.07
III	6:00	5.5	6	184/72	31.5	6.9	18	154	1.15
Immediate	NA	1.5	0	180/72	22.8	NA	NA	161	1.13
Recovery 1 min	NA	1.5	0	140/70	19.3	NA	NA	136	1.10
Recovery 5 min	NA	1	0	120/74	8.9	NA	NA	71	0.98

Comments: Test terminated because of volitional fatigue. No pain recorded

11. For the cardiorespiratory fitness test chosen to interpret the answer for question 10, should the test have been terminated prior to completion? Explain why or why not.
12. Calculate a heart rate range based on the heart rate reserve that the client should maintain during aerobic exercise. Is this the most reliable method for quantifying cardiorespiratory endurance exercise? Why or why not?
13. Calculate a $\dot{V}O_2$ range based on the $\dot{V}O_2$ reserve that the client should maintain during aerobic exercise.
14. Provide an exercise type (be specific), frequency, and time at the $\dot{V}O_2$ range found in question 13 for the client to improve her cardiorespiratory fitness and manage symptoms.
15. Should cardiorespiratory exercise be load bearing for this client? Defend the response in two to three sentences.
16. Suggest four possible aerobic exercises that would be appropriate for this client.
17. Provide a step height and stepping frequency to elicit the lower end of the $\dot{V}O_2$ range listed in question 13.
18. Provide a running speed and incline to elicit the upper end of the $\dot{V}O_2$ range listed in question 13.
19. Provide a resistance and peddle frequency for leg cycling to elicit the upper end of the $\dot{V}O_2$ range listed in question 13.
20. Suggest a progression scheme for improving cardiorespiratory fitness. Would vigorous-intensity or high-intensity interval training be warranted? Why or why not?
21. Provide a range for weight that the client should chest press.
22. Provide a range for weight that the client should leg press.
23. Provide a resistance exercise prescription for frequency and number of exercises, sets, and repetitions to improve muscular fitness.

24. Suggest at least four specific resistance training exercises that are appropriate for this client.

25. Suggest a progression scheme to help the client improve overall muscular fitness.

26. Provide the frequency, intensity, number of stretches, sets, and amount of time each stretch should be to help improve the client's flexibility.

27. Are there other exercises that may be appropriate for this client (cardiorespiratory, resistance, flexibility, neuromotor, etc.)? Provide a justification for the response.

28. Provide a list consisting of all safety considerations that should be considered when supervising this client's exercise program. Would these considerations be different if the client had rheumatoid arthritis? Explain why or why not.

REFERENCES

1. K. E. Barbour, C. G. Helmick, M. Boring, and T. J. Brady. "Vital Signs: Prevalence of Doctor-Diagnosed Arthritis and Arthritis-Attributable Activity Limitation—United States, 2013–2015," *Morbidity and Mortality Weekly Report* 66 (2017): 246–53.

2. B. Walitt, R. L. Nahin, R. S. Katz, et al., "The Prevelance of Fibromyalgia in the 2012 National Health Interview Survey," *PLoS One* 10, no. 9 (2015): e0138024.

3. N. C. Wright, A. C. Looker, K. G. Saag, et al., "The Recent Prevalence of Osteoporosis and Low Bone Mass in the United States Based on Bone Mineral Density at the Femoral Neck or Lumbar Spine," *Journal of Bone and Mineral Research* 29 (2014): 2520–26.

4. American College of Sports Medicine, *ACSM's Guidelines for Exercise Testing and Prescription*, 11th ed. (Philadelphia: Wolters Kluwer Health, 2022).

5. American College of Sports Medicine, *ACSM's Exercise Management for Persons with Chronic Diseases and Disabilities*, 4th ed (Champaign, IL: Human Kinetics, 2016).

6. American College of Sports Medicine, *ACSM's Guidelines*.

7. American College of Sports Medicine, *ACSM's Exercise*.

8. M. Shih, J. Hootman, J. Kruger, and C. Hemlick, "Physical Activity in Men and Women with Arthritis," *American Journal of Preventive Medicine* 30, no. 5 (2006): 385–93.

9. A. J. Busch, S. C. Webber, M. Brachaniec, et al., "Exercise Therapy for Fibromyalgia," *Current Pain and Headache Reports* 15, no. 5 (2011): 358.

10. N. J. Bosomworth, "Exercise and Knee Osteoarthritis: Benefit or Hazard?," *Canadian Family Physician* 55, no. 9 (2009): 871–8.

11. American College of Sports Medicine, *ACSM's Guidelines*.

12. Barbour et al., "Vital Signs."

13. I. B. McInnes and G. Schett. "The Pathogenesis of Rheumatoid Arthritis," *New England Journal of Medicine* 365, no. 23 (2011): 2205–19.

14. American College of Sports Medicine, *ACSM's Guidelines*.

15. ibid.

16. P. L. Ritter, V. M. Gonzalez, D. D. Laurent, and K. R. Lorig, "Measurement of Pain Using the Visual Numeric Scale," *Journal Rheumatology* 33, no. 3 (2006): 574–80.

17. American College of Sports Medicine, *ACSM's Guidelines*.

18. ibid.

19. ibid.

20. ibid.

21. ibid.

22. ibid.

23. F. Wolfe, "The Fibromyalgia Syndrome: A Consensus Report on Fibromyalgia and Disability," *Journal of Rheumatology* 23 (1996): 534–39.

24. A. J. Busch, C. L. Schachter, T. J. Overend, et al., "Exercise for Fibromyalgia: A Systematic Review. *Journal of Rheumatology* 35, no. 6 (2008): 1130–44.

25. American College of Sports Medicine, *ACSM's Guidelines.*

26. D. L. Goldenberg, C. Burckhardt, and L. Crofford, "Management of Fibromyalgia Syndrome," *JAMA* 292, no. 19 (2004): 2388–95.

27. American College of Sports Medicine, *ACSM's Guidelines.*

28. F. Wolfe, K. Michaud, T. Li, and R. S. Katz, "Chronic Conditions and Health Problems in Rheumatic Diseases: Comparisons with Rheumatoid Arthritis, Noninflammatory Rheumatic Disorders, Systemic Lupus Erythematosus, and Fibromyalgia," *Journal of Rheumatology* 37, no. 2 (2010): 305–15.

29. American College of Sports Medicine, *ACSM's Guidelines.*

30. Busch et al., "Exercise for Fibromyalgia."

31. D. S. Rooks, C. B. Silverman, and F. G. Kantrowitz, "The Effects of Progressive Strength Training and Aerobic Exercise on Muscle Strength and Cardiovascular Fitness in Women with Fibromyalgia: A Pilot Study," *Arthritis Care Research* 47, no. 1 (2002): 22–8.

32. H. Valkeinen, M. Alen, A. Hakkinen, et al., "Effects of Concurrent Strength and Endurance Training on Physical Fitness and Symptoms in Postmenopausal Women with Fibromyalgia: A Randomized Controlled Trial," *Archives of Physical Medicine and Rehabilitation* 89, no. 9 (2008): 1660–66.

33. S. E. Gowans, A. DeHueck, S. Voss, et al., "Effect of a Randomized, Controlled Trial of Exercise on Mood and Physical Function in Individuals with Fibromyalgia," *Arthritis Care Research* 45, no. 6 (2001): 519–29.

34. American College of Sports Medicine, *ACSM's Guidelines.*

35. Ritter et al., "Measurement of Pain."

36. ibid.

37. ibid.

38. ibid.

39. ibid.

40. ibid.

41. P. Haentjens, J. Magaziner, C. S. Colon-Emeric, et al., "Meta-Analysis: Excess Mortality After Hip Fracture among Older Women and Men," *Annals of Internal Medicine* 152, no. 6 (2010): 380–90.

42. Wright et al., "The Recent Prevalence."

43. D. De Kam, E. Smulders, V. Weerdesteyn, and B. C. Smits-Engelsman, "Exercise Interventions to Reduce Fall-Related Fractures and Their Risk Factors in Individuals with Low Bone Density: A Systematic Review of Randomized Controlled Trials," *Osteoporosis International* 20, no. 12 (2009): 2111–25.

44. J. Iwamoto, T. Takeda, and S. Ichimura, "Effect of Exercise Training and Detraining on Bone Mineral Density in Postmenopausal Women with Osteoporosis," *Journal of Orthopaedic Science* 6, no. 2 (2001): 128–32.

45. B. L. Specker, "Evidence for an Interaction between Calcium Intake and Physical Activity on Changes in Bone Mineral Density," *Journal of Bone and Mineral Research* 11, no. 10 (1996): 1539–44.

46. American College of Sports Medicine, *ACSM's Guidelines.*

47. ibid.

48. ibid

49. ibid.

50. S. L. Watson, B. K. Weeks, L. J. Weis, et al., "High Intensity Resistance and Impact Training Improves Bone Mineral Density and Physical Function in Postmenopausal Women with Osteopenia and Osteoporosis: The LIFTMOR Randomized Controlled Trial," *Journal of Bone and Mineral Research* 33, no. 2 (2018): 211–20.

51. Watson et al., "High Intensity Resistance."

52. American College of Sports Medicine, *ACSM's Guidelines.*

53. ibid.

54. ibid.

Exercise Testing and Prescription for Clients with Multiple Diseases

INTRODUCTION

THE DISEASES, RISK factors, and conditions discussed in this text oftentimes do not occur in isolation. Consider obesity. Obesity is one of the root causes of hypertension, dyslipidemia, and type II diabetes.[1,2,3] Thus it is not uncommon for exercise professionals to encounter clients with all four conditions.

Metabolic syndrome is one example of multiple conditions where a person has high abdominal fat, high blood glucose, dyslipidemia, and high blood pressure. However, there are many other combinations of conditions that do not have a specific name.

With the aging population, high prevalence of sedentary behaviors, and advances in medical technology, exercise professionals will be serving clients with more than one disease more frequently.[4] Unfortunately, exercise guidelines for each possible disease combination do not exist. Accordingly, it is necessary for exercise professionals to be prepared to think critically and creatively to meet the needs of these populations.

To address the challenges of serving clients with multiple diseases, students will have to reflect on previous chapters in this text. Further, recollection of exercise prescriptions for clients with a single disease or health condition is necessary to complete the case studies in this chapter. On completion of the case studies within this chapter, students will be able to achieve the following:

1. Analyze a client's profile and select appropriate exercise tests
2. Analyze a client's profile and select the appropriate disease or medical condition for which exercise prescriptions should be based
3. Articulate the most appropriate cardiorespiratory, muscular fitness, and flexibility FITT-VP recommendations and modifications to clients with multiple diseases
4. Suggest safety considerations for clients with multiple diseases and highlight strategies for promoting exercise adherence

EXERCISE TESTING AND PRESCRIPTION FOR CLIENTS WITH MULTIPLE DISEASES

Currently, exercise guidelines do not exist to address the countless possibilities of multiple disease combinations. To account for the dearth of research in this area, exercise professionals need to be able to critically think about a client's disease status and select exercise tests and prescriptions that will address the conditions safely. To accomplish this, the ACSM[5] recommends that exercise professionals consider the following when serving clients with multiple diseases: (1) thoroughly conduct pre-participation and pre-exercise evaluations; (2) frequently communicate concerns and new findings with prescribing physicians and make sure all present diseases are medically stable; (3) take into account clients' medical histories and physical limitations when choosing exercise tests and writing exercise prescriptions; (4) consider client goals and remember the principle of specificity; (5) follow the exercise recommendations for the disease with the most conservative guidelines, as these diseases likely pose the greatest risk and are usually most detrimental for activities of daily living and exercise adherence (i.e., fibromyalgia has more conservative guidelines than dyslipidemia); (6) use strategies that promote exercise adherence; (7) frequently monitor clients for signs and symptoms and stay below exercise intensities that elicit them; and (8) err on the side of caution and start clients at low intensities and progress them slowly. Demonstration Case Study 8.1 provides a hypothetical scenario of an exercise professional designing an exercise testing and prescription plan for a client with multiple diseases.

Demonstration Case Study 8.1

Exercise Testing and Prescription for Clients with Multiple Diseases

An exercise physiologist works for a health-fitness facility that serves populations with chronic diseases. The data for her most recent client is provided next, along with the exercise physiologist's actions from pre-participation screening to exercise prescription.

Demographics: (1) male, (2) 46 years old, (3) quit smoking one pack per day four months prior

Family History: (1) father had coronary artery bypass graft of the left main and left anterior descending coronary arteries at the age of 54, (2) mother had a percutaneous transluminal coronary angioplasty of the right marginal coronary artery at the age of 66

Biometrics: (1) resting heart rate = 62 beats per minute; (2) resting blood pressure = 140/88 mmHg; (3) LDL-c = 131 mg/dL, HDL-c = 41 mg/dL, triglycerides = 155 mg/dL; (4) glycosylated hemoglobin = 6.6 percent and blood glucose = 120 mg/dL; and (5) weight = 260 lbs., BMI = 38 kg/m^2

Medical Diagnoses: (1) rheumatoid arthritis, (2) type II diabetes, (3) metabolic syndrome (obesity, dyslipidemia, insulin resistance, and hypertension)

<u>Medications:</u> (1) methotrexate, (2) carvedilol, (3) metformin, (4) simvastatin

<u>Symptoms:</u> (1) knee pain, (2) fatigue with exertion

<u>Exercise History:</u> (1) daily stretches to alleviate knee pain, (2) no history of cardiorespiratory exercise, (3) resistance training in college, (4) does not enjoy weight-bearing activities, (5) physician clearance to participate in any exercise program obtained 13 months prior

<u>Exercise Goals and Needs:</u> (1) weight loss, (2) lower lipids and body fat, (3) manage blood pressure and blood glucose, (4) reduce pain

Exercise Professional's Actions:

<u>Pre-participation Health Screening (ACSM's Pre-Participation Screening Algorithm 6):</u> (1) Client does not meet the criteria for being physically active, (2) client has type II diabetes, and (3) client experiences fatigue upon exertion. Because of experiencing fatigue upon exertion (a symptom of cardiovascular disease) and having a metabolic disease, the exercise professional recommends physician clearance prior to completing an exercise test and participating in an exercise program.

<u>Cardiovascular Risk Assessment:</u> The exercise professional wants to track and monitor improvements in as many health-related outcomes as possible. Accordingly, the exercise professional conducts a cardiovascular risk assessment from the client's medical records. The following are the positive risk factors (no negative risk factors present): (1) age, (2) family history, (3) smoking, (4) physical inactivity, (5) obesity, (6) hypertension, (7) dyslipidemia, and (8) diabetes.

<u>Pre-Exercise Physical Examination:</u> Given the clients multiple diseases and many cardiovascular disease risk factors, the exercise professional will conduct an abbreviated physical examination consisting of (1) apical and radial pulses (determines resting heart rate and possible underlying/undetected atrial or ventricular ectopy), (2) blood pressure (assesses resting systolic and diastolic blood pressure and determines if resting blood pressure meets the criteria for postponing exercise testing, which is less than 200/110 mmHg), (3) skin assessment for ankle edema (given the known cardiovascular risk factors, ankle edema can indicate deep vein thrombosis, venous insufficiency, or heart failure), (4) skin assessment for xanthomas (the client has dyslipidemia and may have developed new cholesterol deposits unknown to the client or his physician), (5) open foot sores or blisters (the client has type II diabetes and wounds heal slowly, especially if peripheral neuropathy is present; sores and open wounds, if present, need to be monitored and prevented from worsening), and (6) pulmonary function testing (smoker 45 years of age or older).

<u>Exercise Test Selection:</u> Because of the client's physical inactivity and multiple disease status, submaximal tests are selected. For cardiorespiratory fitness testing, an individualized arm cycle protocol was chosen because of knee pain, physical

inactivity, and class II obesity, which could make sitting on a cycle seat uncomfortable. For muscular fitness testing, body weight muscular endurance tests were chosen because of regular knee pain and extensive physical inactivity. For body composition, waist circumference was chosen because of obesity and the limitations that poses on the accuracy of skinfolds and other body composition assessments. Lastly, for flexibility, the simple sit-and-reach test was chosen.

Exercise Test Safety Considerations: Because of the client's type II diabetes, precautions need to be made to detect silent ischemia; therefore, ECG monitoring is chosen. In addition, checking for open foot sores and a blood glucose concentration between 100 and 250 mg/dL will be carried out. During the test, the exercise professional will monitor for chronotropic incompetence (failure of heart rate to rise with submaximal intensities or decrease 12 bpm in the first minute of recovery and 22 bpm by the second minute), signs of hypoglycemia, normal pressor responses (increase of 10 mmHg for systolic blood pressure per one MET increase in intensity and no more than a 10 mmHg in diastolic blood pressure), and avoid spikes in blood pressure by having the client avoid the Valsalva maneuver. Because of the client's rheumatoid arthritis, the exercise professional will ensure that the client is not experiencing acute systematic inflammation and will provide encouragement during the test should minor pain occur. Lastly, the exercise professional will follow the ACSM's[7] exercise test termination criteria to determine if a test should be stopped prior to completion.

Exercise Prescription: Although the pressing health issues for the client center on his cardiometabolic conditions and risk factors, the best exercise prescription recommendation to follow is the most conservative. Therefore, the exercise professional selects the exercise prescription recommendations for rheumatoid arthritis from which to base her prescription. The exercise professional suggests that the client initially perform non-weight-bearing cardiorespiratory exercises three times per week, three ten-minute bouts per session, at an intensity of 40 percent $\dot{V}O_2R$. The exercise professional then recommends two days per week of resistance exercise targeting each major muscle group twice for 12 repetitions. Since muscular endurance exercises were chosen, no 1RM was established, and the intensity for resistance training will be the resistance that can successfully be overcome 12 times per set. Lastly, the exercise professional recommends daily static stretching, targeting each major muscular-tendon group twice per day, holding each stretch for 10–30 seconds below the threshold of pain. All progressions will center on increasing time and frequency before intensity and the overall progression will be slow.

Exercise Safety Considerations: The exercise professional plans to monitor signs of silent ischemia, chronotropic incompetence, pressor responses, glycemic responses, developing sores and wounds, joint pain, systematic inflammation, and myalgia throughout the exercise program. Should minor abnormalities occur, the exercise professional will modify the FITT-VP to a "lower level" to accommodate the client. Should unusual or alarming issues occur, such as persistent myalgia, chronotropic incompetence, exercise-induced hypo/hyperglycemia, or hypertension/hypotension, the exercise professional will contact the client's supervising physician and refer the client to medical care as warranted.

Student Case Study 8.1

Exercise Testing and Prescription for Clients with Multiple Diseases

An exercise physiologist works for a health-fitness facility that serves populations with chronic diseases. The data of his most recent client is provided next.

Demographics: (1) female, (2) 54 years old, (3) quit smoking one pack per day seven months prior

Family History: (1) father had coronary artery bypass graft of the left main and left anterior descending coronary arteries at the age of 56, (2) mother had a percutaneous transluminal coronary angioplasty of the right marginal coronary artery at the age of 64

Biometrics: (1) resting heart rate = 70 beats per minute; (2) resting blood pressure = 120/90 mmHg; (3) LDL-c = 123 mg/dL, HDL-c = 39 mg/dL, triglycerides = 145 mg/dL; (4) glycosylated hemoglobin = 6.4 percent and blood glucose = 126 mg/dL; and (5) weight = 190 lbs., BMI = 32 kg/m^2

Medical Diagnoses: (1) obesity (2) dyslipidemia (3) hypertension

Medications: (1) losartan, (2) atenolol, (3) atorvastatin

Symptoms: (1) ankle swelling, (2) sleeplessness, (3) anxiety, (4) occasional rapid heartbeat

Exercise History: (1) daily light paced walking for 20 minutes, (2) no history of resistance exercise, (3) does not enjoy cycling or walking stairs, (4) no official physician clearance to exercise

Exercise Goals and Needs: (1) weight loss, (2) lower lipids and body fat, (3) manage blood pressure, (4) reduce chronic disease risk

1. Using the PAR-Q+ and ePARmed-X+, if necessary, make a recommendation for the client regarding the need for medical clearance prior to exercise testing and participation. Why was this recommendation made?
2. Using the Exercise Pre-participation Health Screening Questionnaire for Exercise Professionals, make a recommendation for the client regarding the need for medical clearance prior to exercise testing and participation. Why was this recommendation made?
3. Using the ACSM's Pre-participation Health Screening Algorithm, make a recommendation for the client regarding the need for medical clearance prior to exercise testing and participation. Why was this recommendation made?

4. Was the recommendation regarding medical clearance different among any of the prescreening tools in questions 1 through 3? If differences are noted, what would be the professional implication for prescreening clients with chronic diseases?

5. What are the positive risk factors that the client has for cardiovascular disease? Why is each considered a risk factor?

6. What, if any, physical examination findings would be concerning to the client's exercise trainer? Why?

7. Taking in all of the presented information, can the client proceed to exercise testing, prescription, and participation without having sought medical clearance? Why or why not?

8. Should the exercise physiologist conduct a maximal or submaximal cardiorespiratory fitness test? In four to five sentences, provide a defense for the decision based on the client's profile.

9. Which cardiorespiratory fitness test should be conducted? In four to five sentences, provide a defense for the decision based on the client's profile.

10. Is the client taking any medications or have any health conditions that may limit the accuracy of a heart rate–dependent submaximal cardiorespiratory fitness test? If so, in two to three sentences, explain how.

11. Given limitless resources, which body composition test should the exercise physiologist conduct? In four to five sentences, provide a defense for the decision based on the client's profile.

12. Given minimal resources with a small budget, which body composition test should be conducted? In four to five sentences, provide a defense for the decision based on the client's profile.

13. Specific to this case, which body composition test would be preferred? In four to five sentences, provide a defense for the decision based on the client's profile.

14. To assess muscular fitness, should muscular endurance assessments or muscular strength assessments be conducted, or both? In four to five sentences, provide a defense for the decision based on the client's profile.

15. Provide a list of four specific muscular fitness tests to be conducted on the client. Then provide a four- to five-sentence defense supporting the selections.

16. Provide a list of all safety considerations the exercise physiologist should take into account when conducting exercise tests on this client. In two to three sentences, explain why each consideration needed to be taken into account.

17. For which of the client's diseases or health conditions should the exercise physiologist's exercise prescription be based? In four to five sentences, provide a defense in support of the selection.

18. Provide an initial cardiorespiratory exercise prescription (FITT-VP) for this client. Be sure to list specific exercise modalities. In four to five sentences, provide a defense in support of the overall prescription.

19. Provide an initial muscular fitness exercise prescription (FITT-VP) for this client. Be sure to list at least six specific resistance training exercises. In four to five sentences, provide a defense in support of the overall prescription.

20. Provide an initial flexibility exercise prescription (FITT-VP) for this client. Be sure to list at least six specific stretches. In two to three sentences, provide a defense in support of the overall prescription.
21. Provide a list of all safety considerations the exercise physiologist should take into account when prescribing and/or monitoring an exercise program for this client. In two to three sentences, explain why each consideration needed to be taken into account.

Student Case Study 8.2

Exercise Testing and Prescription for Clients with Multiple Diseases

An exercise physiologist works for a health-fitness facility that serves populations with chronic diseases. The data of his most recent client is provided next.

Demographics: (1) male, (2) 50 years old, (3) smokes one cigar daily

Family History: (1) father had a hemorrhagic stroke at the age of 70, (2) mother had a myocardial infarction at the age of 75

Biometrics: (1) resting heart rate = 80 beats per minute; (2) resting blood pressure = 128/82 mmHg; (3) LDL-c = 100 mg/dL, HDL-c = 55 mg/dL, triglycerides = 120 mg/dL; (4) glycosylated hemoglobin = 6.3 percent and blood glucose = 121 mg/dL; and (5) weight = 185 lbs., BMI = 27.2 kg/m²

Medical Diagnoses: (1) type I diabetes (2) bilateral hip osteoarthritis

Medications: (1) NovoLog (rapid-acting insulin), (2) Lantus (long-acting insulin), (3) ibuprofen

Symptoms: (1) pain during weight-bearing movements, (2) hypoglycemia with vigorous exertion

Exercise History: (1) moderate-intensity jogging four times per week, 30 minutes per day, for the last ten years, (2) no resistance training in the last ten years, (3) open to any exercise so long as it doesn't amplify hip pain, (4) physician clearance to exercise 24 months prior

Exercise Goals and Needs: (1) pain reduction, (2) better control of type I diabetes

1. Using the PAR-Q+ and ePARmed-X+, if necessary, make a recommendation for the client regarding the need for medical clearance prior to exercise testing and participation. Why was this recommendation made?
2. Using the Exercise Pre-participation Health Screening Questionnaire for Exercise Professionals, make a recommendation for the client regarding the need for medical clearance prior to exercise testing and participation. Why was this recommendation made?
3. Using the ACSM's Pre-participation Health Screening Algorithm, make a recommendation for the client regarding the need for medical clearance prior to exercise testing and participation. Why was this recommendation made?

4. Was the recommendation regarding medical clearance different among any of the prescreening tools in questions 1 through 3? If differences are noted, what would be the professional implication for prescreening clients with chronic diseases?

5. What are the positive risk factors that the client has for cardiovascular disease? Why is each considered a risk factor?

6. What, if any, physical examination findings would be concerning to the client's exercise trainer? Why?

7. Taking in all of the presented information, can the client proceed to exercise testing, prescription, and participation without having sought medical clearance? Why or why not?

8. Should the exercise physiologist conduct a maximal or submaximal cardiorespiratory fitness test? In four to five sentences, provide a defense for the decision based on the client's profile.

9. Which cardiorespiratory fitness test should be conducted? In four to five sentences, provide a defense for the decision based on the client's profile.

10. Is the client taking any medications or have any health conditions that may limit the accuracy of a heart rate–dependent submaximal cardiorespiratory fitness test? If so, in two to three sentences, explain how.

11. Given limitless resources, which body composition test should the exercise physiologist conduct? In four to five sentences, provide a defense for the decision based on the client's profile.

12. Given minimal resources with a small budget, which body composition test should be conducted? In four to five sentences, provide a defense for the decision based on the client's profile.

13. Specific to this case, which body composition test would be preferred? In four to five sentences, provide a defense for the decision based on the client's profile.

14. To assess muscular fitness, should muscular endurance assessments or muscular strength assessments be conducted, or both? In four to five sentences, provide a defense for the decision based on the client's profile.

15. Provide a list of four specific muscular fitness tests to be conducted on the client. Then provide a four- to five-sentence defense supporting the selections.

16. Provide a list of all safety considerations the exercise physiologist should take into account when conducting exercise tests on this client. In two to three sentences, explain why each consideration needed to be taken into account.

17. For which of the client's diseases or health conditions should the exercise physiologist's exercise prescription be based? In four to five sentences, provide a defense in support of the selection.

18. Provide an initial cardiorespiratory exercise prescription (FITT-VP) for this client. Be sure to list specific exercise modalities. In four to five sentences, provide a defense in support of the overall prescription.

19. Provide an initial muscular fitness exercise prescription (FITT-VP) for this client. Be sure to list at least six specific resistance training exercises. In four to five sentences, provide a defense in support of the overall prescription.

20. Provide an initial flexibility exercise prescription (FITT-VP) for this client. Be sure to list at least six specific stretches. In two to three sentences, provide a defense in support of the overall prescription.

21. Provide a list of all safety considerations the exercise physiologist should take into account when prescribing and/or monitoring an exercise program for this client. In two to three sentences, explain why each consideration needed to be taken into account.

Student Case Study 8.3

Exercise Testing and Prescription for Clients with Multiple Diseases

An exercise physiologist works for a health-fitness facility that serves populations with chronic diseases. The data of her most recent client is provided next.

Demographics: (1) female, (2) 53 years old, (3) no tobacco use

Family History: (1) father had renal failure at age 64, (2) mother developed chronic obstructive pulmonary disease at age 66

Biometrics: (1) resting heart rate = 91 beats per minute; (2) resting blood pressure = 138/88 mmHg; (3) LDL-c = 127 mg/dL, HDL-c = 42 mg/dL, triglycerides = 149 mg/dL; (4) glycosylated hemoglobin = 6.4 percent and blood glucose = 123.6 mg/dL; and (5) weight = 222 lbs., BMI = 37 kg/m²

Medical Diagnoses: (1) moderate lumbar osteoporosis, (2) fibromyalgia, (3) obesity

Medications: (1) risedronate, (2) pregabalin, (3) orlistat

Symptoms: (1) widespread pain, (2) depressive symptoms, (3) anxiety, (4) chronic fatigue, (5) weakness, (6) headache

Exercise History: (1) no exercise in the previous five years; (2) jogging daily, until five years prior; and (3) physician clearance to exercise five months prior

Exercise Goals and Needs: (1) pain reduction, (2) reduction of depressive symptoms, (3) improved bone mineral density, (4) improved quality of life and activities of daily living, (5) does not tolerate pain well and wishes to experience minimal pain during exercise training

1. Using the PAR-Q+ and ePARmed-X+, if necessary, make a recommendation for the client regarding the need for medical clearance prior to exercise testing and participation. Why was this recommendation made?

2. Using the Exercise Pre-participation Health Screening Questionnaire for Exercise Professionals, make a recommendation for the client regarding the need for medical clearance prior to exercise testing and participation. Why was this recommendation made?

3. Using the ACSM's Pre-participation Health Screening Algorithm, make a recommendation for the client regarding the need for medical clearance prior to exercise testing and participation. Why was this recommendation made?

4. Was the recommendation regarding medical clearance different among any of the prescreening tools in questions 1 through 3? If differences are noted, what would be the professional implication for prescreening clients with chronic diseases?

5. What are the positive risk factors that the client has for cardiovascular disease? Why is each considered a risk factor?

6. What, if any, physical examination findings would be concerning to the client's exercise trainer? Why?

7. Taking in all of the presented information, can the client proceed to exercise testing, prescription, and participation without having sought medical clearance? Why or why not?

8. Should the EP conduct a maximal or submaximal cardiorespiratory fitness test? In four to five sentences, provide a defense for the decision based on the client's profile.

9. Which cardiorespiratory fitness test should be conducted? In four to five sentences, provide a defense for the decision based on the client's profile.

10. Is the client taking any medications or have any health conditions that may limit the accuracy of a heart rate-dependent submaximal cardiorespiratory fitness test? If so, in two to three sentences explain how.

11. Given limitless resources, which body composition test should the exercise physiologist conduct? In four to five sentences, provide a defense for the decision based on the client's profile.

12. Given minimal resources with a small budget, which body composition test should be conducted? In four to five sentences, provide a defense for the decision based on the client's profile.

13. Specific to this case, which body composition test would be preferred? In four to five sentences, provide a defense for the decision based on the client's profile.

14. To assess muscular fitness, should muscular endurance assessments or muscular strength assessments be conducted, or both? In four to five sentences, provide a defense for the decision based on the client's profile.

15. Provide a list of four specific muscular fitness tests to be conducted on the client. Then provide a four- to five-sentence defense supporting the selections.

16. Provide a list of all safety considerations the exercise physiologist should take into account when conducting exercise tests on this client. In two to three sentences, explain why each consideration needed to be taken into account.

17. For which of the client's diseases or health conditions should the exercise physiologist's exercise prescription be based? In four to five sentences, provide a defense in support of the selection.

18. Provide an initial cardiorespiratory exercise prescription (FITT-VP) for this client. Be sure to list specific exercise modalities. In four to five sentences, provide a defense in support of the overall prescription.

19. Provide an initial muscular fitness exercise prescription (FITT-VP) for this client. Be sure to list at least six specific resistance training exercises. In four to five sentences, provide a defense in support of the overall prescription.

20. Provide an initial flexibility exercise prescription (FITT-VP) for this client. Be sure to list at least six specific stretches. In two to three sentences, provide a defense in support of the overall prescription.

21. Provide a list of all safety considerations the exercise physiologist should take into account when prescribing and/or monitoring an exercise program for this client. In two to three sentences, explain why each consideration needed to be taken into account.

REFERENCES

1. D. Leroith, "Pathophysiology of the Metabolic Syndrome: Implications for the Cardiometabolic Risks Associated with Type 2 Diabetes. *American Journal of the Medical Sciences* 343, no. 1 (2012): 13–16.

2. Y. E. Bogaert and S. Linas, "The Role of Obesity in the Pathogenesis of Hypertension," *Nature Reviews Nephrology* 5, no. 2 (2009): 101–11.

3. D. C. J. Goff, A. G. Bertoni, H. Kramer, et al., "Dyslipidemia Prevelance, Treatment, and Control in the Multi-Ethnic Study of Atherosclerosis: Gender, Ethnicity, and Coronary Artery Calcium," *Circulation* 113, no. 5 (2006): 647–56.

4. American College of Sports Medicine. *ACSM's Guidelines for Exercise Testing and Prescription, 10th ed* (Philadelphia: Wolters Kluwer Health, 2018).

5. ibid.

6. ibid.

7. ibid.